AF323277

WITHDRAWN

WITHDRAWN

RESEARCH IN
IMMUNOCHEMISTRY AND IMMUNOBIOLOGY

VOLUME 3

Although the articles for RESEARCH IN IMMUNO-CHEMISTRY AND IMMUNOBIOLOGY are usually written by invitation, the Editorial Board will be pleased to receive suggestions and proposals for topics and articles on theoretical, methodological, and applicable aspects of immunochemistry and immunobiology. An honorarium is paid for accepted articles.

VOLUME 3

Research in Immunochemistry and Immunobiology

Scientific Editor-in-Chief

J. B. G. KWAPINSKI, M.D., Ph.D., F.A.A.M.
University of Manitoba
Winnipeg, Manitoba, Canada

Associate Editor

E. D. DAY, Ph.D.
Duke University Medical Center
Durham, North Carolina, U.S.A.

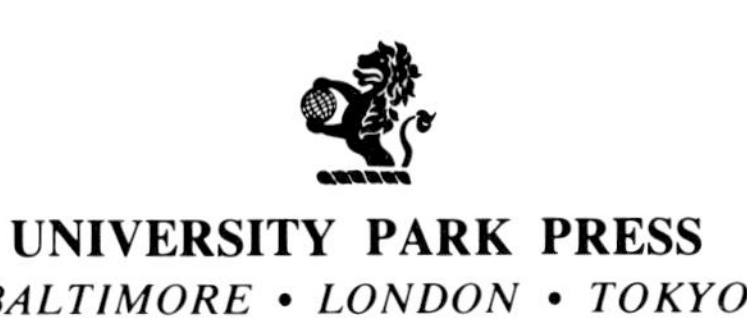

UNIVERSITY PARK PRESS
BALTIMORE • LONDON • TOKYO

CONTENTS

Preface: A Concept of Modern Immunochemistry
and Immunobiology   *vii*
J. B. G. Kwapinski and E. D. Day

Immunochemistry of Bacterial Polysaccharides   *1*
Michael Heidelberger

Immunological Distribution Analysis   *41*
Eugene D. Day

Comparative Immunochemistry of IgA   *91*
J. P. Vaerman

Methods of Labeling Antibodies for Electron
Microscopic Localization of Antigens   *185*
Manfred Wagner

Immunochemistry of Fusobacteria   *253*
Tore Kristoffersen and Tor Hofsted

Index   *285*

PREFACE

A Concept of Modern Immunochemistry and Immunobiology

J. B. G. KWAPINSKI AND E. D. DAY

Modern immunochemistry and immunobiology may be defined as a branch of science that is concerned with the states of specific excitation of dynamic molecules in a subject responding to the introduction of structural units possessing alien conformations.

The quantum principle has reduced all chemistry and all chemical compounds to the dynamics of a system of moving point charges recognizable by quantum mechanics. By applying the quantum principle to immunochemistry, all immunobiologically active bodies may be regarded as quantum states of excitation of a dynamic geometry. Immunological interactions as different in strength as ionic forces, homopolar forces, and van der Waals forces, originate from elemental electrostatics.

At the outset of an immune response, electrons of atoms in an immunocompetent cell absorb energy from an antigen molecule, and are then excited to a higher energy quantum. The energy absorbed is quantitized, and the quantum is then passed to the progeny cells. In response, electrons of the nascent immunoglobulins are excited to a specific energy quantum that is compatible with the dynamic energy state of the original antigen. Essentially, the above phenomena rely on the absorption and emission of specific frequencies of electromagnetic radiation. Only the antigen and antibody molecules formed by the absorption and transmission of energy quanta, and differing in respect to outer-orbital energy of their electrons, may interact to yield products of an immunoreaction. In contrast, antigen and antibody molecules having exactly the same outer-orbital energy cannot react with each other because their outer orbits are degenerate.

In the light of quantum immunochemistry, immunochemical specificity depends on a quantum of energy existing in a particular space and time in the conformational area of a nascent molecule site. This definable quantum of energy is transmitted by electrical contact to the conformationally complementary sites of certain host-molecules, charging them in accordance with the conformation of the inducer-molecule, so that in time sufficient numbers of such immunologically conformant molecules are present to be detected by immunological tests, in which the charge is lost. The original quantum of energy is usually exhausted after a time, although it may persist in some cells to be "reactivated" by a secondary stimulus of an identical conformational unit, thus giving impetus to a second, chain-like energy reaction, which results in the accumulation of immunobiologically active and detectable immunoglobulins.

Because immunochemistry and immunobiology are closely linked to biochemistry, physical chemistry, biophysics, microbiology, pathology, molecular biology, genetics, and quantum chemistry, their rapid development in recent years has been reflected by an ever-increasing number of publications dealing entirely or in part with various aspects of this group of disciplines. The significance of these publications usually remains concealed until they are evaluated and interpreted in terms of our current knowledge of immunochemistry, immunobiology, and quantum chemistry. With these objectives in mind, RESEARCH IN IMMUNOCHEMISTRY AND IMMUNOBIOLOGY presents significant ideas and data on various subjects of immunochemistry and immunobiology, obtained from the research work and experience of leading scientists, and supplemented by a comprehensive yet concise and critical discussion of the pertinent literature. Although both specialized and broad knowledge of different aspects of immunochemistry and immunobiology will be balanced against each other in these books, it is our sincere desire to lead this scientific endeavor through Molecular Immunobiology into its future, Quantum Immunobiology.

Literature Cited

Alford, W. P. 1962. Atomic structure. *In* M. Florkin and E. H. Stotz (eds.), Comprehensive biochemistry, Vol. 1, pp. 1–33. Elsevier, New York.

Pullman, B. 1968. (ed.). Molecular associations in biology. Academic Press, New York.

Wheeler, J. A. 1971. From Mendeléev's atom to the collapsing star. Trans. New York Acad. Sci. 33: 745–779.

Immunochemistry of Bacterial Polysaccharides

MICHAEL HEIDELBERGER

Emeritus Professor of Immunochemistry, Dept. of Medicine, Columbia University, and Adjunct Professor, Dept. of Pathology, New York University, New York, U.S.A.

Contents

I. Introduction 1
II. Polysaccharides of Pneumococci 2
III. Streptococcal Polysaccharides 11
IV. Polysaccharides of Meningococci 16
V. Polysaccharides of *Salmonella* and Other Enterobacteriaceae 17
VI. Polysaccharides of *Klebsiella* (*Aerobacter aerogenes*) 22
VII. Polysaccharides of Other Bacteria 24
VIII. Conclusion 28
    Literature Cited 29

I. Introduction

The bacterial polysaccharides have come into prominence not only because they are often determinants of group-specificity and type-specificity of many microorganisms but also because of their crucial use as reagents in the development of modern immunology. Not surprisingly, a number of relatively recent comprehensive reviews have been written [Heidelberger, 1960; Krause, 1963; How, Brimacombe, and Stacey, 1964; Staub and Westphal, 1964; Lüderitz, Staub, and Westphal, 1966; Ørskov et al., 1967; Jeanes, 1968; Lüderitz, Jann, and Wheat, 1968; Nikaido, 1968; Baddiley, 1970; Halliday, 1971 (immunological paralysis)].

The present review attempts to supplement previous surveys and to deal more extensively with the chemical relationships of polysaccharides responsible for numerous instances of cross-reactivity, often between widely divergent species of living organisms.* Use is made mainly of immune precipitation in disclosing these relationships.

Agglutination is one of the most widely used of the visible immune reactions of microorganisms. It is, however, actually a precipitin reaction at the surfaces of the cells (Heidelberger and Kabat, 1937). Although immune precipitation is somewhat less sensitive than agglutination, it lends itself more readily to exact microquantitation, permitting the measurement of antibodies in micrograms (Heidelberger, 1939a,b). If only minimal quantities of polysaccharides or antisera are available, one may often profitably resort to the micromethod for the quantitative fixation of complement (Wassermann and Levine, 1961).

A word of caution is perhaps useful at this point. Precipitin reactions with periodate-oxidized polysaccharides may yield illusory results, particularly in sera of high antibody content. The aldehydes formed by the action of IO_4^- are capable of combining covalently with proteins (Rebers, Estrada-Parra, and Heidelberger, 1963). Complexes of this nature may include nonspecific protein and are often soluble in alkali only with difficulty (Heidelberger and Rao, 1966; Heidelberger and Slodki, 1968). It is therefore advisable to reduce periodate-oxidized polysaccharides with borohydride before use in quantitative analyses of antisera.

II. Polysaccharides of Pneumococci

In 1917 Dochez and Avery described a specific soluble substance, which was elaborated by virulent pneumococci and which precipitated antipneumococcal (anti-Pn) sera of the same serological type. Its constitution was polysaccharidic (Heidelberger and Avery, 1923, 1924), and this established for the first time an immunological function for polysaccharides (Avery and Heidelberger, 1925). The soluble specific substances of pneumococcal types I, II, and III were shown to differ from each other chemically and physically.† Now some 80 serological types of pneumococcus have been recognized, and in each

---

*The present review appeared in its original French version as Chapter 4 of Immunologie, Paul Bordet, ed., Flammarion, Paris, 1972.

†In this review pneumococcal type-specific polysaccharides are abbreviated S I, S II, S III, etc. Antipneumococcal sera are designated anti-Pn I, etc.

instance in which the structure of the type-specific (capsular) substance has been studied, the polysaccharide has been shown to differ from others. A group-specific, or C-polysaccharide, has also been recognized as a component of even nonencapsulated pneumococci (Tillett and Francis, 1930; Tillett, Goebel, and Avery, 1930; Heidelberger and Kendall, 1931) and its constitution studied (Goebel et al., 1943; Liu and Gotschlich, 1963; Gotschlich and Liu, 1967; Tomasz, 1967; Brundish and Baddiley, 1967, 1968; Mosser and Tomasz, 1970).

Although the total number of sugars which occur in polysaccharides is close to that of the amino acids which form the building blocks of proteins, and although the molecular weights of polysaccharides can be of the same order as those of proteins, the chemistry of the polysaccharides is simpler. This is partly because many are characterized by the repetition of units which rarely contain more than three, four, or five different sugars. Moreover, the methods for the study of fine structure, for determination of the order and linkages of the sugars, are more precise and more easily available and interpretable than those applicable to proteins. The structures of the polysaccharides are also usually more open than those, for example, of the globular proteins. Table 1 shows the probable structures of a number of pneumococcal capsular polysaccharides. Table 2 lists the component sugars of the polysaccharides of pneumococcal types for which the structure has not been elucidated, together with the principal antigenic determinant, if known, as well as any di- or oligo-saccharides isolated on partial hydrolysis. In these and the following tables the sugars are considered to be in the pyranose form unless furanose (f) is added. Abbreviations used are: gal, galactose; galA, galacturonic acid; glc, glucose; glcA, glucuronic acid; man, mannose; rham, rhamnose; fuc, fucose; galN, galactosamine; galNAc, N-acetylgalactosamine; glcN, glucosamine; glcNAc, N-acetylglucosamine; manN, mannosamine; manNAc, N-acetylmannosamine; fucN, fucosamine; fucNAc, N-acetylfucosamine.

Comments on Tables 1 and 2

"C-substance" (Table 2): If this is a single substance it appears to be both a polysaccharide and a teichoic acid. Phosphorylcholine is an

Table 1. Structures proposed for pneumococcal capsular polysaccharides

Serological type	Proposed structure

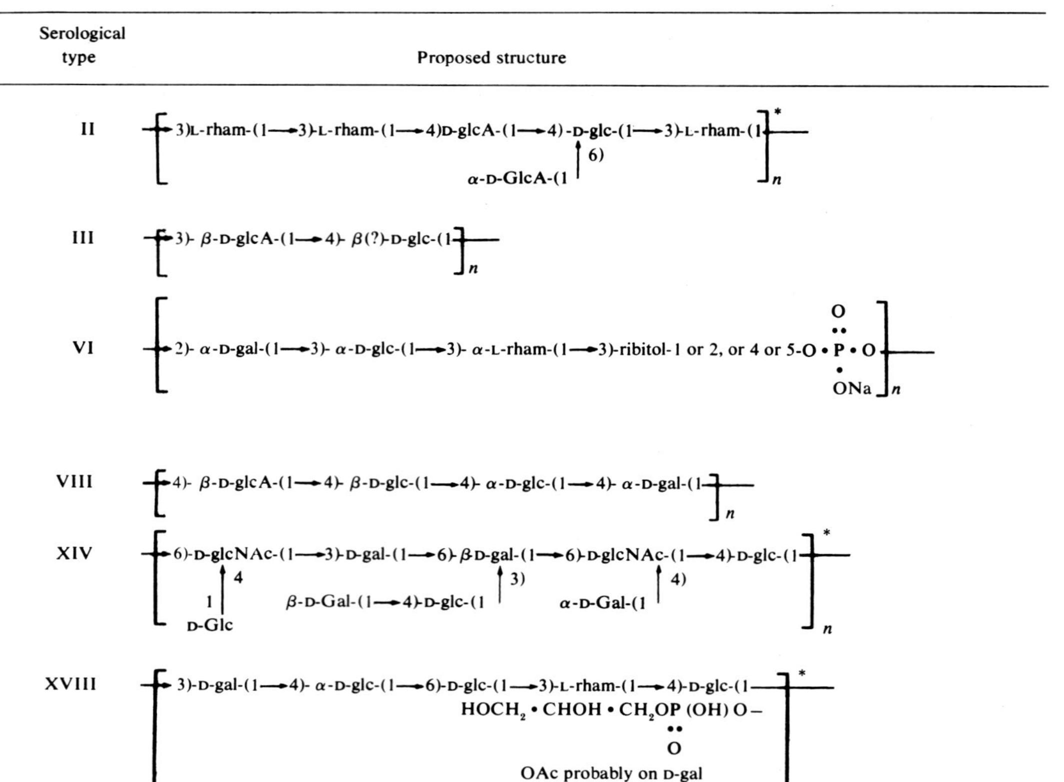

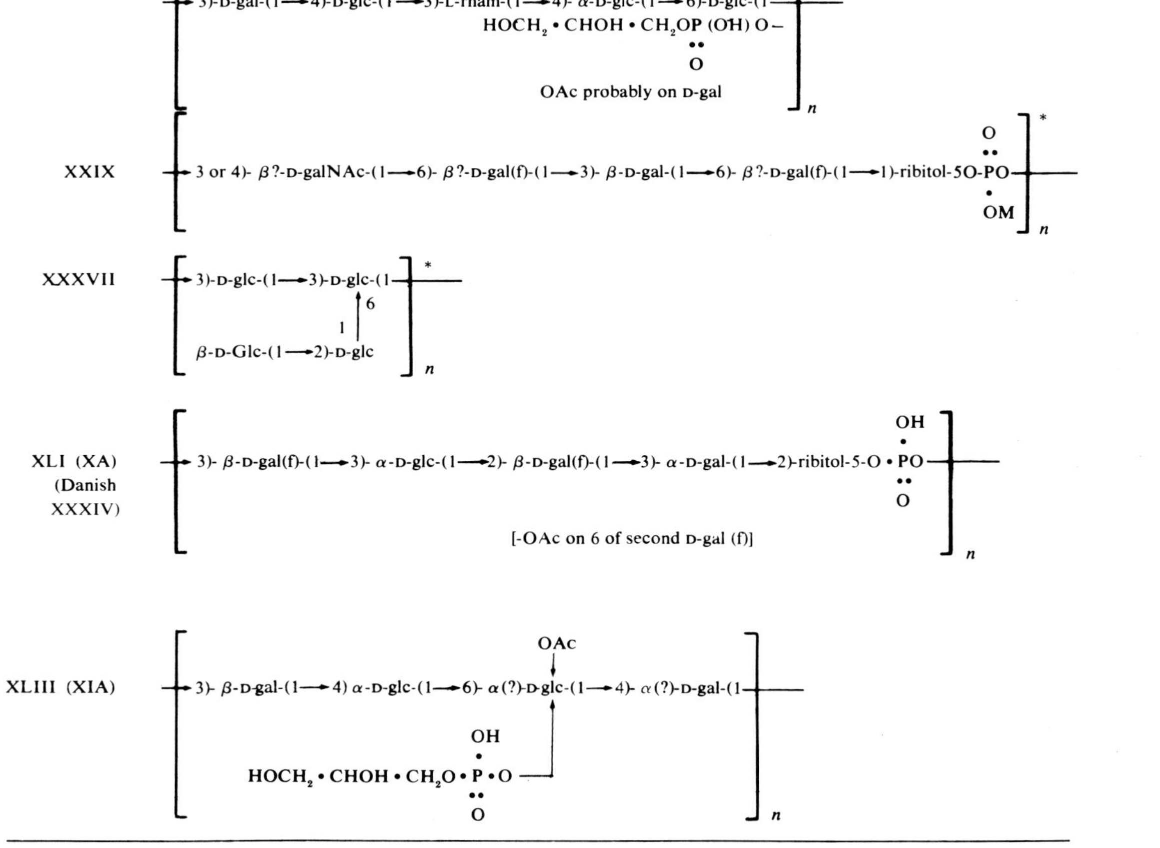

or

3)-D-gal-(1→4)-D-glc-(1→3)-L-rham-(1→4)-α-D-glc-(1→6)-D-glc-(1 *
HOCH₂ · CHOH · CH₂OP (OH) O—
O
OAc probably on D-gal
n

XXIX   3 or 4)- β?-D-galNAc-(1→6)- β?-D-gal(f)-(1→3)- β-D-gal-(1→6)- β?-D-gal(f)-(1→1)-ribitol-5O-PO *
O
OM
n

XXXVII   3)-D-glc-(1→3)-D-glc-(1 *
6
1
β-D-Glc-(1→2)-D-glc
n

XLI (XA)   3)- β-D-gal(f)-(1→3)- α-D-glc-(1→2)- β-D-gal(f)-(1→3)- α-D-gal-(1→2)-ribitol-5-O · PO
(Danish   OH
XXXIV)   O
[-OAc on 6 of second D-gal (f)]
n

XLIII (XIA)   3)- β-D-gal-(1→4) α-D-glc-(1→6)- α(?)-D-glc-(1→4)- α(?)-D-gal-(1
OAc
OH
HOCH₂ · CHOH · CH₂O · P · O
O
n

*Not uniquely determined

Table 2. Constituents of other pneumococcal polysaccharides

"C," group-specific polysaccharide, of all types and rough strains: mucopeptide + poly-galNAc.PO_4 (Gotschlich and Liu, 1967); galNAc, PO_4, 2AcNH-4NH_2-2,4,6-trideoxyhexose, ribitol PO_4, glc, phosphorylcholine (Tomasz, 1967; Mosser and Tomasz, 1970; Brundish and Baddiley, 1968).

Capsular polysaccharides, type	Constituents
I	D-GalA,glc,galN,glcN. Oligosaccharides indicated: galA-(1→3)-glcN-(1→3)galA, galA→galN, galA→glcN
IV	D-Gal, D-galNAc, manNAc, fucNAc, pyruvic acid apparently on D-gal.
V	D-Gal, D-glc, D-glcA, "Pneumosamine" 2-AcNH-2,6-dideoxy-L-talose, 2AcNH-2,6-dideoxy-L-galactose(L-fucosamine). Oligosaccharides indicated: →2)- β-D-glcA-(1→3)-L-fucN, D-glcA-(1→3)-L-fucN-(1→4)-D-glc
VII	D-Gal, D-glc, L-rham, galNAc, D-glcNAc. Nonreducing end groups: mainly β-D-gal, also D-glcNAc
IX	D-Glc, D-glcA, D-glcNAc, manNAc. Oligosaccharides indicated: - α-D-glcA-(1→3)-D-glc, -glcA-(1→3)-glcNAc, -manNAc-(1→3)-glc-(1→3)-manNAc
X	Gal(f), galN, glcN, ribitol, PO_4
XI	Gal, glc, glcN, ribitol, PO_4
XII	D-Gal, D-glc, D-galN, L-fucN. Oligosaccharide: possibly-D-glc-(1→2)-D-glc-
XIII	Gal, glc, glcN, ribitol, PO_4
XV	Gal, glc, galN, glcN, glycerol, PO_4
XVI	Gal, glc, rham, galN, glcN, glycerophosphate
XVII	Gal, glc, rham, polyol, unidentified sugar
XIX	Glc, rham, D-manNAc, PO_4, 1 : 2 : 1 : 1; or gal, glc, rham, galN, glcN, PO_4. Strain 39458: glc, rham, ribose, manN
XX	Gal, glc, glcN, PO_4
XXI	Gal, glc, glcN, PO_4
XXII	D-Glc, uronic acid
XXIII	D-Gal, D-glc, L-rham, 5 : 2 : 2. [L-Rham-(1] ; →2(-L-rham-(1 − ; →4)-D-glc-(1 −]$_n$
XXIV	Glc, rham, ribose, glcN, ribitol, PO_4
XXVII	Gal, glc, rham, glcN, PO_4, pyruvic acid
XXVIII	Glc, rham, glycerol, PO_4
XXX	Gal, glc, galN, ribitol, PO_4
XXXI	D-Gal, L-rham, glcA, 2 : 2 : 1, also OAc. GlcA →gal
XXXIII	Gal, glc, D-galA
XXXIV	Gal, glc, ribitol, PO_4

immunological determinant (Heidelberger, Gotschlich, and Higgin-botham, 1972) and seems to be the portion of the molecule responsible for precipitation of C-reactive protein and certain myeloma proteins (Kaplan and Volanakis, 1971; Leon and Young, 1971). Of the amino acids of C-substance, glutamic was all D, lysine all L, and alanine D to the extent of 25–33% in three different preparations (Manning, 1971). A capsular polysaccharide, thus far indistinguishable from C-substance, has been isolated (Bornstein et al., 1968).

Type I (Table 2): The data are from Guy et al., 1967.

Type II (Table 1): Several structures are possible, but one recently proposed (Barker, Somers, and Stacey, 1967), which postulates end groups of cellobiouronic acid, is incompatible with tests of the inhibition of the type II system by neutralized solutions of the glcA-(1——►4)-glc and glcA-(1——►6)-glc aldobiouronic acids (Heidelberger, Roy, and Glaudemans, 1969).* Actually, cellobiouronic acid inhibits less than glcA, and the best inhibitor is α-D-glcA-(1——►6)-D-glc, in accord with one of the possible structures indicated by the work of Butler and Stacey (1955).

Oxidation of S II by periodate involves not only the nonreducing end groups of D-glcA (Barker et al., 1967) but also glcA linked 1,4 and the 1,4,6-linked glc. These changes greatly reduce precipitation in anti-Pn II, but even slightly increase the cross-reaction in anti-Pn VI, this being caused by the oxidation-resistant 1,3-linked L-rham (Rebers et al., 1962).

Type III (Reeves and Goebel, 1941) and type VIII (Jones and Perry, 1957) (Table 1): Recent experiments on their enzymatic degradation have shown that anti-Pn III and anti-Pn VIII are directed against more than one repeating unit (Mage and Kabat, 1963; Campbell and Pappenheimer, 1966), as had already been indicated with S III by direct analysis of the specific precipitates (Heidelberger and Kendall, 1937). The type III system is strongly inhibited by cellobiouronic acid (Heidelberger, Roy, and Glaudemans, 1969).

Type IV (Table 2): S IV contains about 9% of pyruvic acid (Heidelberger, Dudman, and Nimmich, 1970), bound as a ketal, probably to D-galactose, another constituent. D-GalN, manN, and fucN are

---

*Note added to proof. — New structural studies have confirmed the presence of end groups of α-D-glcA-(1——►6)-D-glc and not that of 1,4-linked glcA [see next paragraph (Larm et al., 1972)].

also present, probably as their N-acetyl derivatives (Higginbotham and Heidelberger, 1972). Removal of pyruvic acid results in reduction of type-specificity and emergence of group-specificity. Depyruvylated S IV not only reacts with antibodies to pneumococcal C-substance but even precipitates C-reactive protein quantitatively in the presence of Ca^{++} (Higginbotham, Heidelberger, and Gotschlich, 1970).

Type V (Table 2): Barker et al. (1966) described the first natural occurrence of two amino sugars in this substance. It is related to type II because its 1,2-linked D-glcA mimics end groups (Heidelberger, 1962).

Type VI (Table 1): The only remaining uncertainty is the linkage of PO_4 to ribitol (Rebers and Heidelberger, 1959, 1961). S VI provides one of the few instances in carbohydrate chemistry in which the phosphate-free repeating unit may be obtained almost quantitatively in crystalline form. Although a polysaccharide, S VI is related to the teichoic acids (Baddiley, 1970), as the units are bound together by ribitol phosphate. 1,2-linked D-gal and 1,3-linked L-rham are principal antigenic determinants (Heidelberger and Rebers, 1960).

Type VII (Table 2): Nonreducing end groups of D-gal were first indicated by the cross-reaction of S VII in anti-Pn XIV (Heidelberger and Tyler, 1964). These were identified as in the β-form by the cross-reactions of polysaccharides with known β-D-gal end groups and by inhibition experiments, both in anti-Pn VII sera (Tyler and Heidelberger, 1968). A mixture of D-gal and L-rham inhibited the homologous reaction moderately. End groups of D-glcNAc, as well as those of D-gal, have also been found by methylation (Chaudhari, Bishop, and Fielder, 1972. Carbohydr. Res. 25: 161–172).

Type IX (Table 2): S IX (Rao and Heidelberger, 1966) is more complex than originally believed. The principal antigenic determinant appears to be α-D-glcA-(1⟶3)-D-glc. This apparently occurs in the main chain, with few or no end groups of glcA, since there is no cross-reaction in anti-Pn II (Higginbotham, Das, and Heidelberger; Das, Higginbotham and Heidelberger, 1972).

Types X, XI, XIII, XV, XVI, XX, XXI, XXIV, XXVIII, XXX and XXXIV (Table 2): The sugars and components listed for each of these types are those given by Shabarova, Buchanan, and Baddiley (1962) for preparations isolated by Brown (1939) and Brown and Robinson (1943).

Type XII (Table 2): Constituent sugars were identified by Cifonelli et al. (1966). The amino sugars are probably present as their N-acetyl derivatives and the hexoses may be linked 1,2 (*cf.* also Goodman and Kabat, 1960; Suzuki and Hehre, 1964).

Type XIV (Table 1): The structure given is one of several alternatives and is adapted from the review of How et al. (1964). The principal antigenic determinants are the multiple (Heidelberger and Kendall, 1935) nonreducing end groups of D-gal (Heidelberger, 1955).

Type XVII (Table 2): Constituent sugars were listed by J. K. N. Jones (personal communication). There is a massive two-way cross-reaction between group F type IV streptococcus (*cf.* also Table 3) and Pn XVII (Heidelberger, Willers, and Michel, 1969).

Type XVIII (Table 1): The alternative structures differ only in the position of the maltosyl residues (Estrada-Parra and Heidelberger, 1963). The location of the glycerophosphate side chain is unknown. The O-acetylated sugar, the principal antigenic determinant, is probably D-gal. Isomaltosyl is also a determinant.

Type XIX (Table 2): Miyazaki and Yadomae (1971) have found S XIX to contain glc, rham, D-manNAc, and PO_4 in the ratio 1 : 2 : 1 : 1, while Shabarova et al. (1962) report gal, glc, rham, galN, glcN, PO_4, and in strain 39453, glc, rham, ribose, manN, PO_4.

Cross-reactions, often reciprocal, between the pneumococcal types II–XIX, II–XX, VII–XIV, VII–XVIII, VII–XIX, VIII–XVIII, VIII–XIX, X–XIV, and X–XX have been instructive (Heidelberger and Tyler, 1964) but would have yielded far more information if the structures of more of the type-specific polysaccharides had been known. Only after a study of the cross-reactions of the type II polysaccharide of streptococcal group F (Heidelberger, Willers, and Michel, 1969), the structure of which was known (Michel, van Vonno, and Krause, 1969) (Table 3), was it possible to ascribe the pneumococcal VIII-XIX cross-reaction to residues of β-1,4-linked D-glc which occur in S VIII, strep. FII, and presumably in S XIX.

Type XXII (Table 2): Cross-reactions in anti-Pn XXII with polysaccharides and carbohydrates containing D-glc or D-glcA indicate that S XXII contains D-glc and that its uronic acid (Brown, 1939) is probably D-glcA (Heidelberger, 1960).

Type XXIII (Table 2): The presence of end groups of L-rhamnose in S XXIII is indicated not only by the rapid appearance of this sugar on mild hydrolysis (Jones and Perry, personal communication) but also by the marked cross-reactivity of S XXIII in antistreptococcal group B and G sera (Heidelberger, Davie, and Krause, 1967). The principal antigenic determinant of the group B and G polysaccharides has been shown to be rhamnose (Curtis and Krause, 1964). Perry (personal communication) has found D-gal, D-glc, and L-rham, 2 : 2 : 5, in S XXIII, confirming multiple end groups of L-rham by methylation as well as finding this sugar linked 1,2. D-Gal apparently forms branch points.

Type XXV (Table 2): The uronic acid of S XXV has been identified as galA (Das, Heidelberger, and Brown, unpublished observations), at least in part the D-isomer.

Type XXVII (Table 2): The marked cross-reactivity of pyruvate-containing capsular polysaccharides of *Rhizobium trifolii* in anti-Pn XXVII led to the recognition of pyruvic acid in S XXVII (Dudman and Heidelberger, 1969). Similarly, precipitation of both anti-Pn XXVII and anti-Pn IV by *Klebsiella* polysaccharide K32 led to the finding of pyruvic acid in S IV and K 32 and the surmise that a cross-reaction must exist between Pn IV and Pn XXVII (Heidelberger, Dudman, and Nimmich, 1970). Although a reciprocal cross-reaction was found, it is actually larger with depyruvylated S IV and S XXVII than with the intact substances.

Type XXIX (Table 1): The structure given was assigned by Rao et al. (1969). Precipitation of 40% of the antipolysaccharide in anti-Pn XXIX by streptococcal group F type I substance was ascribed to the probable presence of D-galNAc and D-gal(f) in similar linkages in both S XXIX and strep. F1 (Heidelberger, Willers, and Michel, 1969).

Type XXXI (Table 2; Roy, Carroll, and Glaudemans, 1970): Deacetylation reduces the homologous reaction.

Type XXXIII (Table 2; Mills et al., 1960): The substance gives a small cross-reaction in certain antisera to Pn I.

Type XXXVII (Knecht, Schiffman, and Austrian, 1970): The capsular substance of this avirulent pneumococcal type is a polyglucose which is not degraded by enzymes of serum or saliva. A possible repeating unit is given in Table 1.

Type XLI (Danish XXXIV) (XA) (Table 1): The structure was proposed by Chittenden et al. (1968). Assignation of an immunologically important O-acetyl (OAc) group to position 6 of the second D-gal(f) in alternate repeating units is indicated by the work of Dixon et al. (1968) and Roy and Glaudemans (1968).

Type XLIII (XIA) (Table 1): A structure for the repeating unit has been proposed by Kennedy, Buchanan, and Baddiley (1969), who also ascribed the cross-reaction with type XVIII (Eddy, 1944) to occurrence of the monoacetylated sequence α-3-D-gal-(1$\longrightarrow$4)-D-glc-(1$\longrightarrow$6)-D-glc in S XLIII and one of the structures assigned to S XVIII (Table 1).

III. Streptococcal Polysaccharides

Lancefield's classical studies (reviewed by McCarty, 1954) began contemporaneously with those of Avery's group on pneumococci. Her work showed clearly that the immunochemical organization of streptococcal group A, responsible for so many human infections, was quite different from that of the pneumococci. Lancefield was able to separate the streptococci into a number of large groups, each characterized by a group-specific polysaccharide, but the type-specific components of group A, designated M and T, proved to be proteins (Lancefield, 1962). On the other hand, the type-specific substances thus far characterized in streptococcal groups B, C, D, etc., are polysaccharides. The composition and immunological determinants of the group-specific and type-specific polysaccharides, insofar as they are known, are given below and are summarized in Table 3.

Group A and A-variant (V) strains (McCarty and Lancefield, 1955; McCarty, 1956, 1958): In the polysaccharides of the intermediate and V strains, end groups or side chains of β-D-glcNAc have been stripped off to varying extents, with resulting changes in specificity. The greater reactivity of V than A in anti-Pn II and anti-Pn VI helped to show that Pn II and Pn VI were related through the occurrence in each capsular polysaccharide of multiple residues of 1,3-linked L-rham (Heidelberger and Rebers, 1960). This also showed for the first time that at least part of the rham in A was linked 1,3 (Estrada-Parra, Heidelberger, and Rebers, 1963). Confirmation followed through methylation studies conducted simultaneously by Hey-

Table 3. Polysaccharides of streptococci

Group	Type	Sugars (%)	Immunodominant groups
A		L-Rham, 60; glcNAc, 30	β-D-GlcNAc
A-intermediate		L-Rham, 70; glcNAc, 17	L-Rham, glcNAc
A-variant		L-Rham, 85; glcNAc, 3	-L-rham-(1⟶3)-L-rham-(1—
B		D-Gal, 10; L-rham, 50; glcNAc, 12	$\left[\text{L-Rham-(1}\right]_n$
	II	D-Gal, D-glc, glcNAc, sialic acid	$\left[\beta\text{-D-Gal-(1}\right]_n$
C		L-Rham, 42; D-galNAc, 40; glcNAc, 5	$\left[\text{GalNAc-(1}\longrightarrow\text{?)-L-rham-(1}\right]_n$
C-intermediate		L-Rham, 59; D-galNAc, 22; glcNAc, 4	
C-variant		L-Rham, 88; D-galNAc, 2; glcNAc, 3	$\left[\text{L-Rham-(1}\right]_n$
D		Intracellular teichoic acid, with attached residues of kojibiose, kojitriose	
	I	D-Glc, rham, D-glcNAc, galN, ribitol teichoic acid	α-D-Glc, D-glcNAc
	XXVI	Glc, rham, galN, glcN	
E		D-Glc, 22, L-rham, 44, glcNAc, 2	$\left[\beta\text{-D-Glc-(1}\longrightarrow\text{?)-L-rham}\right]_n$

F	D-Glc, 14.5; rham, 35; galNAc, 18.5	β-D-Glc-(1⟶3)-galNAc-rham—
I	Gal, 46.5; glc, 21.5; rham, 23; galNAc, 16.5	
II	Gal, 12, glc, 26, rham, 24.5, galNAc, 19.5	
	β-D-GalNAc-(1⟶2)- α-D-gal-(1⟶2)- α-rham-(1⟶4)- β-D-glc-(1⟶4)-D-glc-	
III	Gal, 31; glc, 44; rham, 9	β-D-Glc, α-D-gal?
IV	Gal, 31; glc, 35; rham, 26; glcN, 8	β-D-Gal-
V	Gal, 19; glc, 9; rham, 50; galN, 14.5	β-D-Glc?
G	D-Gal, 23.5; L-rham, 40.5; galNAc, 25.5	$\left[\text{L-Rham-(1}\right]_n$
H–S	Usually gal, glc, rham; occasionally galN, glcN. Man in group K.	
z1	Glc, 31; rham, 47; glcN, 6	L-Rham-(1——
z2	Gal, 11; rham, 30; glcN, 30.5	
z3	Rham, 50; glcNAc, 17.5; galNAc, 16.5	3-O- α-glcNAc-galNAc-
z4	Gal, 12; rham, 48; glcN, 38.5	$\left[\text{D-Gal-(1}\right]_n$
z6	Gal, 11.5; glc, 15.5; rham, 47; glcN, 23.	

mann et al. (1963), and these workers also showed (Heymann et al., 1964) that several residues of L-rham were linked together in A.

Groups B and G: The reciprocal cross-reactions of these groups were first elucidated by Curtis and Krause (1964) and were further clarified in connection with the cross-precipitation of both substances in anti-Pn XXIII (Heidelberger, Davie, and Krause, 1967). The latter study made it probable that the B and G substances and S XXIII owed their cross-reactivity to multiple nonreducing end groups of L-rham.

By methylation and inhibition Chionglo and Hayashi (1969) found that the end groups of L-rhamnose are linked α-1$\longrightarrow$2 to the next sugar in group B and α-1$\longrightarrow$4 in group G.

The type II substance of group B (Lancefield and Freimer, 1966; Freimer, 1967) is partially degraded by treatment with hot dilute acid. Sialic acid is split off (Lancefield, personal communication), and the remainder of the molecule no longer precipitates B II antibodies completely. Additional evidence for the nonreducing end groups of D-gal believed to occur in B II was found in the strong cross-reaction in anti-Pn XIV and a weaker precipitation of anti-Pn VII.

Group C (Krause and McCarty, 1962): The group substances show behavior similar to those of group A, with which there is a cross-reaction, presumably caused by multiples of 1,3-linked L-rham in the polysaccharides of both groups. However, the immunodominant sugar of group C is D-galNAc. Optical rotatory dispersion shows its linkage to be α (Beychok, Hammarström, and Kabat, 1971).

Group D: The group-specific substance is an intracellular teichoic acid with attached residues of kojibiose and kojitriose (Wicken, Elliott, and Baddiley, 1963). In this group the type I polysaccharide has been studied more thoroughly than that of type XXVI (Bleiweis and Krause, 1965, 1967).

Nonreducing end groups of β-D-glcNAc have been found in the cell-wall polysaccharide of *Streptococcus bovis* S 19, a strain of group D (Kane and Karakawa, 1969). These account for the reciprocal cross-reaction with streptococcal group A. In the walls of another strain, N, of group D, two polysaccharides were found, one consisting of gal, glc, rham, and galNAc, the other containing D-gal and D-glc (Pazur, Anderson, and Karakawa, 1971). Both precipitated antistrain N, and the reaction was inhibited by lactose > allolactose > D-gal. Chromatographic evidence of lactosyl and gentiobiosyl residues was obtained, and the former are probably present as side chains.

Group E (Slade, Lüderitz, and Westphal, 1965).

Group F: Separation of group and type (T) antigens was described by Michel and Krause (1967) following earlier studies (Willers et al., 1964; Michel and Willers, 1964). More recently a third class of polysaccharides, termed "zero" or z antigens, has been isolated. These occur, with a type antigen of one of several groups, including F, in strains which cannot be classified in any of the recognizable streptococcal groups (Michel and Krause, 1967; Willers and Alderkamp, 1967). Their cross-reactions were extensively studied (Heidelberger, Willers and Michel, 1969) in connection with those of group F, and are therefore mentioned at this point.

Group F polysaccharide is the only one thus far to which the sequence β-D-glc-(1——➤3)-D-galNAc ——➤rham has been attributed (Michel and Willers, 1964). Substance z1 precipitates a portion of the same antibody from anti-Pn XXIII as do the streptococcal B and G antigens. This identifies at least part of its rham as L-rham in the form of nonreducing end groups or 2-substituted L-rham. Cross-reactivity of z2 in anti-Pn VII was with a portion of the antibodies precipitated by T IV. Substance z4 reacted heavily in anti-Pn VII, and with much of the fraction precipitated by T IV. The cross-reactions of z6 were similar to those of z1.

T 1 precipitates anti-Pn XXIX massively, indicating that it contains D-gal(f) and possibly D-galNAc in linkages similar to those in Pn S XXIX (Table 1).

T II is the only antigen of group F for which a complete structure has been proposed, and this knowledge has been useful in two respects. From the cross-reactions of z1, z2, and T II in anti-Pn VII and their overlapping on cross-absorption, it was concluded that z1, z2, and S VII, like T II, contained 1,2-linked L-rham or a few nonreducing end groups of this sugar. The latter would be expected to react much like the former, in analogy with the experience with multiples of similarly linked D-gal in the Pn VI system (Heidelberger and Rebers, 1960). It now appears that the rham in S VII is linked as end groups (C. Bishop, personal communication). Knowledge of the structure of T II also showed the well-known cross-reaction of Pn VIII and Pn XIX (and that of T II in anti-Pn VIII and XIX) to be caused partly by the presence of β-1,4-linked D-glc in the antigenic determinants of all three types.

Cross-reactivities of T III were attributed to the sequence gal-glc,

while those of T IV overlapped to some extent with cross-precipi-
tations of T II and z4. T IV precipitated a portion of the same antibody
as did T II from anti-Pn VIII and XIX, identifying at least part of its
glc as D-glc. T IV was distinctive in giving massive reciprocal crossing
with Pn XVII. This reaction, and a strong precipitation in anti-Pn
XVI, are probably caused by the presence in T IV of multiple nonreducing end groups of D-gal.

Groups H–S: The chemistry of these substances was studied by
Slade and Slamp (1962). Montague and Knox (1969) found 72 of 91
strains of *Streptococcus salivarius* classifiable as types I or II, but only
the former reacted with group K antisera. The principal determinant of
type I specificity appeared to be β-D-gal-(1⟶6)-D-gal. Other disaccharides isolated were β-D-glc-(1⟶6)-D-gal and β-D-glc-
(1⟶3)-D-gal.

Cross reactions between streptococcal groups other than A and
C, and B and G have been recorded. Jelinkova, Bicova, and Rotta
(1967) found such a relation between groups A and L, and Elliott,
Hayward, and Liu (1971) noted an antigen like that of the A variant in
group N, as well as in groups D, E, G, and M. Other serologically
active polysaccharides were also found.

Teichoic acid extracted from freeze-dried whole cells of groups A,
D, E, O, and T (Matsumo and Slade, 1970) reacted with antisera to
groups B, C, F, G, H, K–N, P, Q, and R, but not S. Material from
group A had glcN⟶glycerol linkages, ester-bound alanine, and PO_4,
and reacted with anti-E. Material from T reacted with anti-O, but the
reverse reactions did not occur. Precipitation was inhibited by glcNAc.

IV. Polysaccharides of Meningococci

The group-specific carbohydrate of group A is mainly a 1⟶6-
linked polymer of manN phosphate, partly O- and N-acetylated (Liu et
al., 1971); those of groups B and C are immunologically different
polysialic acids (Gotschlich, Liu, and Artenstein, 1969). Robinson and
Apicella (1970) also identified the group C-substance as a
poly-N-acetylneuraminic acid and noted that those of groups X and Y
failed to give tests for sialic acids.

V. Polysaccharides of Salmonella *and Other Enterobacteriaceae*

A comprehensive review by many of the workers in the field has appeared in *Ann. N.Y. Acad. Sci.* 133:277–786 (1966) and another has been written on O antigens of *Shigella flexneri* (Simmons, 1971).

Studies on the biosynthesis of the lipopolysaccharides have been facilitated by the use of mutants defective in one or another step of the pathway between the "core polysaccharide" and the attachment of the various lateral chains to form the completed "O" antigen. Other approaches have also been useful (Nikaido, 1968; Osborn and Tze-Yuen, 1968; Osborn and Weiner, 1968; Kent and Osborn, 1968; Droege et al., 1968). Sarvas and Nikaido (1971) have traced the steps leading to gal(f) and ribose(f) in T1 antigens.

Chermann, Digeon, and Raynaud (1967; Digeon, Chermann, and Raynaud, 1967) found that precipitation of lipopolysaccharides by polyethyleneglycol avoided the contamination by nucleic acids occurring with the phenol method, and that there was less degradation when the extraction from the cells was made with NaCl-citrate solution. EDTA has also been recommended for the latter reason (Leive, Shovlin, and Mergenhagen, 1968).

Hellerqvist et al. (1968, 1969) have proposed a structure for the O-specific side chains of group B on the basis of studies with *Salmonella bredeney* and *S. typhimurium* (Table 4). In this group, α-D-glc attached to D-gal at position 6 results in antigen 1, whereas if it is linked to position 4, antigen 12_2 is produced. Of two strains of *S. typhimurium,* 395MS and LT2, the latter has OAc at position 2 of only about one-half of the gal. An "M" or mucoid antigen from *S. typhimurium* 395 MRO-M2 has pyruvic acid linked as a ketal to positions 3 and 4 of terminal β-D-gal (Lindberg, personal communication). However, the M1 antigen of *S. typhimurium* 395 MRO-M1 has acetaldehyde as a substituent on the gal, with the structure

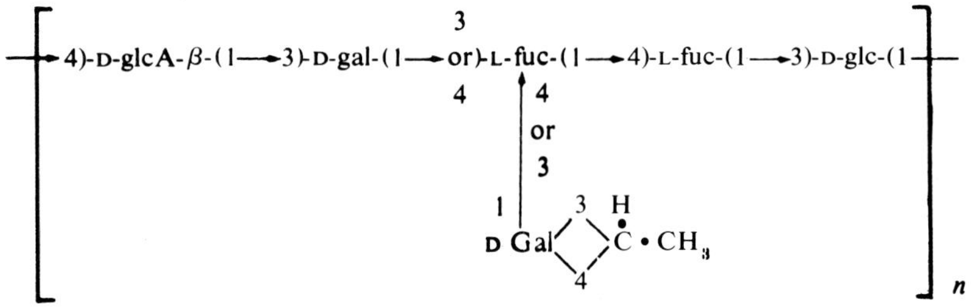

$$
\left[\begin{array}{c}
\overset{\textstyle 3}{} \\
\text{—4)-D-glcA-}\beta\text{-(1}\longrightarrow\text{3)-D-gal-(1}\longrightarrow\text{or)-L-fuc-(1}\longrightarrow\text{4)-L-fuc-(1}\longrightarrow\text{3)-D-glc-(1—} \\
\underset{\textstyle 4}{} \qquad \overset{\displaystyle 4}{\underset{\displaystyle\ \,3}{\big\uparrow\text{or}}} \\[4pt]
\underset{\text{D Gal}}{\overset{\textstyle 1}{\big|}}\ \ {}^{3}\diagup\diagdown{}^{H}\hspace{-2pt}\overset{\bullet}{C}\cdot CH_3
\end{array} \right]_{n}
$$

(Garegg et al., 1969).

The O-chains of *S. münster* and *S. senftenberg* were also studied (Hellerqvist et al., 1971). No OAc was found in the former; otherwise the results resembled those of Robbins et al. (1965) with *S. anatum.* The conclusions of earlier workers on *S. senftenberg* were confirmed and extended to the determination of the anomeric forms of the sugars.

A modified structure for the repeating unit of the O-specific side chains of *S. typhi* and *S. enteritidis,* group D, is given by Hellerqvist et al. (1969) (Table 4). The most definite difference between them is the dearth of OAc groups in the latter.

Oligosaccharides isolated after partial hydrolysis of the polysaccharide of *S. strasbourg,* group D_2, were α-gal-(1——→6)-α-man(1——→4)-rham and the two constituent disaccharides (Nghiem, Bagdian, and Staub, 1967). Oxidation showed tyvelose (tyv), the immunodominant sugar of antigens 9 and 46, to be linked 1——→3 to man.

O antigens of *Salmonella* strains of group A (chemotype XV) are characterized by the Kauffmann factors 1, 2, 12, in which paratose, D-glc, and L-rham have been shown to be the immunodominant sugars (Lüderitz, Staub, and Westphal, 1966). However, the acetylphosphogalactan of *Sporobolomyces* yeast, containing about 15% of D-glc, precipitated more than 60% of the antibodies in two different antiparatyphoid A sera even after the removal of OAc, the terminal D-gal, and phosphate, and still reacted heavily (30%) after oxidation by periodate*, which would remove terminal D-glc (Heidelberger and Slodki, 1968, 1970). It was concluded that possibly two residues of D-gal (the cross-precipitation being so massive) occurred linked 1,3 and/or 1,6 in the side chains of the O antigen of *S. paratyphi* A, constituting an essential portion of one or more of antigens 1, 2, and 12. Dagorn and Staub (personal communication) have now shown that the galactan reacts with antibodies to factor 1 (α-D-glc-(1——→6)-D-gal . . .), that glc is a good inhibitor of the cross-reaction, and that gal is also an inhibitor, but weaker, as would be anticipated from the chemistry of factor 1. It is apparent from both the old and the new results that not more than one gal per repeating unit can be involved, but that gal is, as originally stated (Heidelberger and Slodki, 1968, 1970), an immunologically important component of the specificity of *S. paratyphi* A.

---

*Note added to proof.—Dagorn and Staub (see below) have found that deacetylation followed by oxidation abolishes the cross-reaction.

Table 4. Structures of O-specific side chains of lipopolysaccharides of *Salmonella* groups D_1 and B

Group

D₁

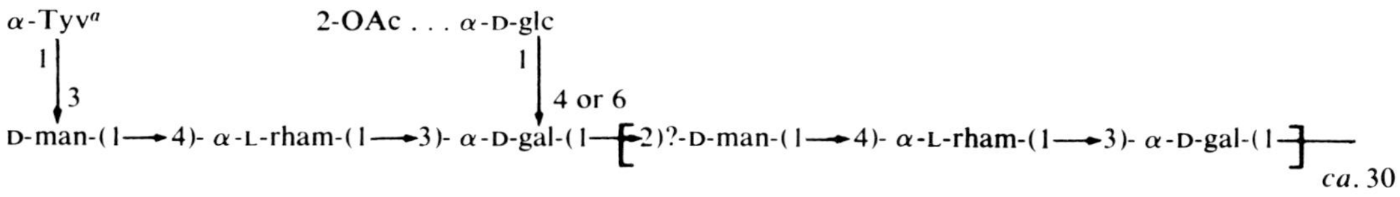

α-Tyv[a]　　　　　　　　2-OAc . . . α-D-glc
　1│　　　　　　　　　　　　　1│
　　↓3　　　　　　　　　　　　　↓4 or 6
D-man-(1→4)- α-L-rham-(1→3)- α-D-gal-(1→[2)?-D-man-(1→4)- α-L-rham-(1→3)- α-D-gal-(1]

ca. 30

B

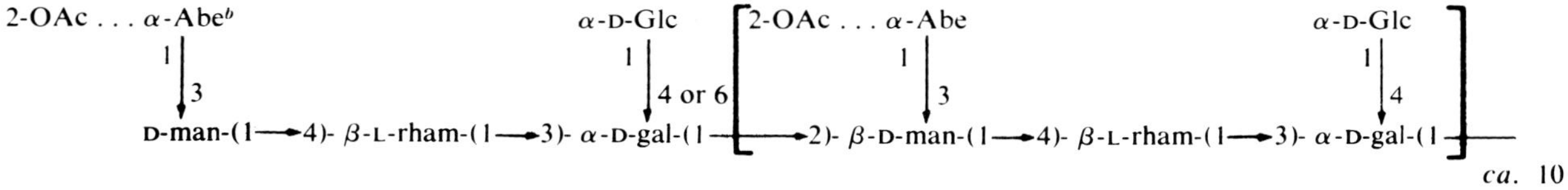

2-OAc . . . α-Abe[b]　　　　　　α-D-Glc　[2-OAc . . . α-Abe　　　　　　α-D-Glc]
　1│　　　　　　　　　　　　　1│　　　　　1│　　　　　　　　　　　1│
　　↓3　　　　　　　　　　　　　↓4 or 6　　　↓3　　　　　　　　　　　↓4
D-man-(1→4)- β-L-rham-(1→3)- α-D-gal-(1→[2)- β-D-man-(1→4)- β-L-rham-(1→3)- α-D-gal-(1]

ca. 10

[a] Tyv, tyvelose (3,6-dideoxy-D-arabinohexose).
[b] Abe, abequose (3,6-dideoxy-D-xylohexose).

The "common core polysaccharide" to which the O-antigenic side chains of *Salmonella* are attached was found to be different in different mutants of *S. typhimurium* and to have alkali-labile groups which were not OAc (Hellerqvist and Lindberg, 1971).

Among the changes caused in *Salmonella* by their phages is the displacement by phage 14 of glc in the lipopolysaccharide of *S. cholerae suis* from one mannose to another:

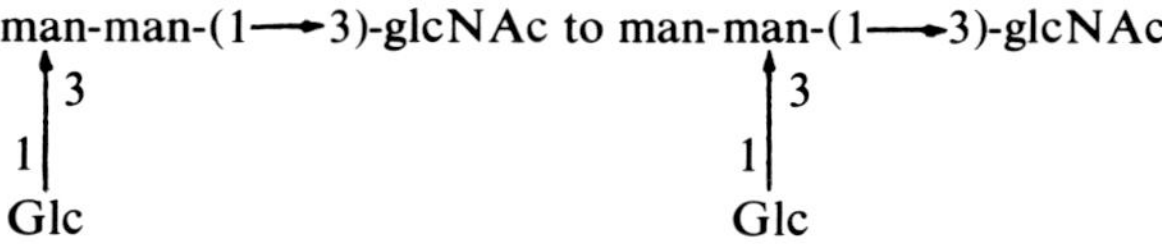

(Fuller and Staub. 1968: Fuller. Etievant, and Staub. 1968).

Attention has also been given to the amino sugars. ManN has been found in groups J and T and also in *S. arizona* 15; quinovose has been found in the O antigens of group S (O48 and O58) and of *S. arizona* 1.33 (Lüderitz, Gmeiner et al., 1968). The reaction between O48 and homologous antiserum is inhibited by N-acetylneuraminic acid showing this to be one of the antigenic determinants of group S (Kedzierska, Mikulaszek, and Pogonowska-Goldhar, 1968). For the first time L-rhamN (2-amino-2, 6-dideoxy-L-mannose) has been found in a natural substance, the lipopolysaccharide of *E. coli* U41/14 (O3 : K2ab (L) : H2) (Jann and Jann, 1968).

Capsular polysaccharides of *E. coli* have been studied in a number of instances. The K7 substance of strains with antigens O7 and O14 was found to contain D-mannosamineuronic acid (Mayer, 1969), while structures have been given for the repeating units of K27 (Jann et al., 1968), K29 (Nhan, Jann, and Jann, 1971), K30 (Hungerer et al., 1967), K42 (Jann et al., 1965), and K85 (Jann et al., 1966) (Table 5). Analysis of the cross-reactions of the last three has added to the knowledge of these substances (Heidelberger, Jann et al., 1968). K30 and K85 both precipitate anti-Pn II and anti-Pn V, the former more strongly in anti-II, the latter in anti-V, a result opposite to that expected from the structures assigned to these substances (Table 5) and to Pn S II and V (Tables 1 and 2). Oxidation of K85 by periodate predictably diminishes its reactivity in anti-Pn II but more than doubles that in anti-Pn X, indicating that this cross-reaction is caused by glcNAc, linked 1,3 in

Table 5. Structures of capsular polysaccharides of *Escherichia coli*

Poly-saccharide	Structure
K27	$\left[\begin{array}{l}\text{Gal}\\1\downarrow\\3\end{array}\;?\text{)glc-}(1\rightarrow3)\text{-glcA-}(1\rightarrow3)\text{-fuc}\right]_n$
K29	$\left[6)\text{-man-}(1\rightarrow3)\text{-glc-}(1\rightarrow6)\text{-man-}(1\rightarrow3)\text{-glc-}(1\rightarrow3)\text{-}\beta\text{-D-glcA-}(1\rightarrow3)\text{-}\alpha\text{-gal-}(1\right]_n$
K30	$\left[3)\text{-man-}(1\rightarrow2)\text{-}\beta\text{-D-glcA-}(1\rightarrow3)\text{-D-gal-}(1\right]_n$
K42	$\left[3)\text{-D-gal-}(1\rightarrow3)\text{-D-galA-}(1\rightarrow2)\text{-fuc(f)-}(1\right]_n$
K85	$\left[\overset{2\text{ or}}{\underset{4}{}})\text{glcA-}(1\overset{2\text{ or}}{\underset{6}{\longrightarrow}}\text{-man-}(1\rightarrow3)\text{-man-}(1\rightarrow3)\text{-glcNAc-}(1\rightarrow?)\text{-man-}(1\rightarrow3)\text{-man-}(1\rightarrow3)\text{glcNAc-}(1\right]_n$

For K85: the branch above the first man position is Rham; the branch above the second internal man is Rham with D-GlcA below.

S X also and in the same enantiomorphic form in both K85 and S X. Since all of the rham in K85 exists as nonreducing end groups, this accounts for the cross-reactivity in anti-Pn XXIII. Disappearance of the reaction when K85 is oxidized by periodate and reduced with borohydride is in accord with this interpretation, which also identifies at least a portion of the rham in K85 as the L-isomer. Strangely enough, K42 is one of several polysaccharides which precipitate more "antibody" from the equine anti-Pn XXV available than do several preparations of the homologous polysaccharide S XXV.

Polysaccharides of *E. coli* K235, K12W, M6 mutant of K12, and of a strain isolated from a patient with cystic fibrosis all contained the same proportions of gal, glc, fructose, and glcA and also had OAc (Linker and Evans, 1968). In *E. coli* O100:K? (B):H2 a lipopolysaccharide and an acidic polysaccharide were found, both with O-specificity and both containing gal, rham, glcN and glycerophosphate attached to rham as a phosphodiester (Jann et al., 1970). At least part of the O-specificity was caused by the glycerophosphate.

R strains of *E. coli* have been divided into groups R_1 and R_2 according to their phage-sensitivities. Lipopolysaccharides of R_1 have gal, glc, heptose 2 : 3 : 3; those of R2 have gal, glc, glcN, heptose, 2 : 4 : 1 : 4. Both have similar amounts of ketooctanoic acid, R mutants with incomplete core polysaccharides were also noted (Schmidt, Jann, and Jann, 1969, 1970). Core lipopolysaccharides of different genera of Enterobacteriaceae, except *E. coli* R_1, cross-reacted and contained gal, glc, glcNAc, L-glyceromannoheptose and 3-deoxy-D-mannooctulosonic acid in different proportions (Schmidt, Fromme, and Mayer, 1970). *E. coli* O111 core, with a very low content of gal, was considered to be in a new class R_3.

VI. *Polysaccharides of* Klebsiella (Aerobacter aerogenes)

Klebsiella strains are characterized by group-specific or O antigens and capsular or extracellular type-specific antigens. The relatively few group-specific antigens are lipopolysaccharides (Nimmich and Münter, 1967; Nimmich and Korten, 1970). The type-specific, or K polysaccharides, have been more extensively studied, and those for which at least partial structures have been given are listed in Table 6

Table 6. Capsular or extracellular polysaccharides of *Klebsiella* K serotypes

K type	Structure	
1	D-Glc, D-glcA, L-fuc, mostly linked 1, 3; pyruvic acid	$[\alpha]_D - 105°$
2	—[—3)- β-D-glc-(1 → 4)- β-D-man-(1 → 4)- α-D-glc-(1—]$_n$— 3 ↑ 1 | α-D-GlcA	$[\alpha]_D + 95°$
3	D-Gal, D-man, galA; galA → D-man	$[\alpha]_D + 115°$
8	—[—3- β-D-gal-(1 → 3)- α-D-gal-(1 → 3)- β-D-glc—]$_n$— 4 ↑ 1 | α-D-GlcA	$[\alpha]_D + 95°$
9	[D-GlcA-(1—]$_n$—, D-gal, L-rham; -L-rham-(1 → 3)-L-rham	
47	[L-Rham-(1—]$_n$—, → 3)-D-gal-(1—, → 4)-D-glcA-(1——	
54(A3S1)	[—6)- β-D-glc-(1 → 4)- α-D-glcA-(1 → 3)-L-fuc-(1—]$_n$— 4 ↑ 1 | β-D-Glc	
64	D-Glc, L-rham, D-man, glcA → man	$[\alpha]_D + 29°$

(K type 1: Barker et al., 1963; Gormus, Wheat, and Porter, 1971; 2: Gahan, Sandford, and Conrad, 1967; 3: Eriksen, 1965; 8: Dudman and Wilkinson, 1956; Sutherland, 1970; 54:Sandford and Conrad, 1966; Conrad et al., 1966; 64: Barker et al., 1958a). The sugars of which the K substances of types 1–72 are composed were recorded by Nimmich (1968). Most of the Ks contain glcA, but types 3, 29, 34, 48, 49, 57, and 63 have galA, and the nature of the acid in types 22, 37, 38, and 56 was not determined. The other sugars usually present are gal, glc, man, rham, and sometimes fuc. K types 1–6 and 68 contain pyruvic acid bound as a ketal (Wheat, Dorsch, and Godoy, 1965; Gormus, Wheat, and Porter, 1971); this also occurs in 32 but not in 9, 47, or 52 (Heidelberger, Dudman, and Nimmich, 1970). There is incomplete agreement as to the structure of K type 2 (Barker et al., 1958b; Gahan, Sandford, and Conrad, 1967; Park, Eriksen, and Henriksen, 1967), possibly because different strains and methods were used. Intermediate types (AE) between 1 and 5 (Henriksen and Eriksen, 1959, 1961) and cross-reactions between strains with and without fuc (Henriksen and Eriksen, 1962) have been observed. Other cross-reactions have been indicators of structural characteristics of K9, K32, and K47 (Heidelberger, Dudman, and Nimmich, 1970; B. Lindberg, personal communication) (Table 6).

Like the O antigens of Enterobacteriaceae, those of *Klebsiella* contained 2-keto-3-deoxyoctanoic acid, heptose, glcN, and glc. Of O groups 1–12, O1, 2, 6, 8, 9 held much gal, while man was the main component of O3 and 5, with some 3-OMe-man in O5. Groups O4 and 11 had about 20% each of gal and ribose, O7 and 10 had glc, rham, and ribose, while O12 had gal instead of ribose. Group O10 also contained 3-OMe-rham (Björndal, Lindberg, and Nimmich, 1970). Moreover, O4 has almost the same composition as *Salmonella* T1, but the two do not cross-react and show differences on oxidation with periodate (Nimmich, 1970).

VII. Polysaccharides of Other Bacteria

Teichoic acids of staphylococci with immunodominant α-D-glc or α-D-glcNAc were shown to precipitate with concanavalin A by Reeder and Eckstedt (1971), while those with these sugars in the β-form were shown not to. *Staphylococcus aureus,* phage type 187, was found to contain ribitol, P, galN, and D-ala. GalNAc was the principal antigenic determinant, and ester-bound alanine was a second one (Karakawa and Kane, 1971). The teichuronic acid of cell walls of *Bacillus licheniformis* (Hughes and Thurman, 1970) gave, on partial hydrolysis, glcA-(1——→3)-galNAc. GlcA was substituted in position 4 and there were reducing end groups of galNAc.

The cell walls of *Micrococcus* sp. A_1 contained a polymer of glc and galNAc-1-PO_4 (Partridge, Davison, and Baddiley, 1971). Partial hydrolysis gave 6-phosphoryl--α-D-glc-(1——→3)-galNAc. GalNAc was linked 1——→6 through PO_4 to glc.

The polysaccharide of the cell wall of *Lactobacillus plantarum,* with gal, glc, rham, glcN, P 1 : 1 : 6 : 1 : 1, was essential for lysis by one of two phages which were virulent for the bacillus (Douglas and Wolin, 1971). A neutral polysaccharide of the cell walls of *Lactobacillus acidophilus* contained gal, glc, rham 1 : 1 : 1, apparently linked to muramic acid by phosphodiester bonds (Coyette and Ghuysen, 1970). There was also a 1,6-linked polyglucose with side chains of α-glycerophosphate at C_2 or C_4. Cell wall composition of a number of strains of *Corynebacteria* was described by Cummins (1971). A *Corynebacterium equi* and *Brevibacterium oleocaptus* grew on *n*-paraffins and formed acidic polysaccharides with $[\alpha]_D + 35°$ and $+ 143.5°$, and containing, respectively, 9% ether soluble, 10% OAc, glc, man 3 : 2, succinic acid, lactic acid 5.7 : 1, and gal, glc, man 2 : 2.5 : 3, pyruvic acid, lactic acid (Kanamaru and Yamatodani, 1969).

Polysaccharides of the cell walls of *Listeria monocytogenes* types I and II (Ullmann and Cameron, 1969) contained mainly rham and glcN; that of type III, gal rham, and glcN; and those of IVa and IVb, gal, glc, and rham. Rham was immunodominant in I and II, gal in IVa, glc in IVb. Type II cross-reacted in anti–IVa.

Autolysis of cell walls of *Bacillus cereus* yielded a neutral polysaccharide (Hughes, 1971) comprising about 40% of the walls and containing glc, galNAc, glcNAc and P, as well as another (12%) with the same amino sugar and unidentified acidic components.

Major constituents of a cell wall antigen of *Rothia dentocariosa* were D-gal, D-glc, fructose, and ribose (Hammond, 1970). Fructose was immunodominant, and there were no cross-reactions with polysaccharides or surface polymers of other oral Actinomycetes or filamentous microorganisms.

Wheat and Ghuysen (1971) found that the muramic acid of cell walls of all Gram-positive bacteria examined contained muramic acid of the gluco-, not galacto-, configuration.

Type-specific polysaccharides of *Pasteurella multocida* contained gal, glc, man, xylose, glcA, OAc, and P in different proportions and linkages (Nashkov et al., 1968). Capsular material from type A was definitely characterized as hyaluronic acid (Cifonelli, Rebers, and Heddleston, 1970).

A soil bacterium originally designated *Neisseria winogradsky,* then *Bacterium anitratum,* and finally *Acinetobacter calco-aceticus* (Baumann, Doudoroff, and Stanier, 1968; Baumann, 1968), possesses a large capsule composed of L-rham and D-glc 4 : 1 (Taylor and Juni, 1961; Juni and Heym, 1964). The substance precipitates heavily in anti-Pn XXIII and streptococcal groups B and G antisera (Heidelberger, Das, and Juni, 1969), showing that it contains nonreducing end groups of L-rham, such as are characteristic of the principal antigenic determinants of Pn XXIII and the group polysaccharides of streptococcal B and G. It also precipitates the same fraction of anti-Pn VI as does Pn S II, showing that the acinetobacter polysaccharide also contains L-rham in 1,3-linkage. This was confirmed by the resistance of a portion of its L-rham to oxidation. Since the acinetobacter substance did not precipitate the antibody from anti-Pn VI reactive with glucans containing 1,3-linked D-glc, this portion of the glc must have formed branch points, possibly linked 1,2,3, 1,2,4, or 1,3,6.

Lipopolysaccharides have been found in rhizobia and agrobacteria, and were separated from extracellular polysaccharides and nucleic acid (Graham and O'Brien, 1968). All contained glc and rham. Other sugars commonly present were glcN, 4-OMeglcA, gal, and fuc. A lipopolysaccharide of *Proteus vulgaris* OX19 containing D-gal, glc, galNAc, glcNAc, fuc, heptose, and 2-keto-3-deoxyoctonic acid cross-reacted with human A_1 and B blood groups (Pardoe, Bird, and Uhlenbruck, 1968). Two fractions of the polysaccharides of the S form of *P. vulgaris* OX19, strain 1959, were studied by Kotelko et al. (1969). Fraction I, the somatic antigen, yielded three disaccharides with galA, galN 1 : 1, one with glcA, galN 1 : 1, another with glcA, galN 1 : 1.5, and oligosaccharides with glc, heptose, galA, glcA, galN, glcN, and glc, glcA, galN. Those containing galA and galN were inhibitors of the homologous system.

Lipopolysaccharides of *Neisseria perflava* and *N. catarrhalis* walls were studied by Adams et al. (1968, 1969). The lipid components of only the former resembled those of the Enterobacteriaceae. D-Glc in the former was partly in a chain linked 1⟶3 and, as was L-rham, partly in side chains. *N. catarrhalis* contained D-gal instead of rham, and also OAc.

Endotoxic lipopolysaccharides of three strains of *Pseudomonas aeruginosa* were studied (Fensom and Gray, 1969) under difficulties caused by the firm binding of lipid. This also complicated the isolation of polysaccharides from *Pseudomonas alkaligenes* (Key, Gray, and Wilkinson, 1970).

The fine structure of an O-methylglucose–containing lipopolysaccharide of *Mycobacterium phlei* has been worked out by Saier and Ballou (1968) as

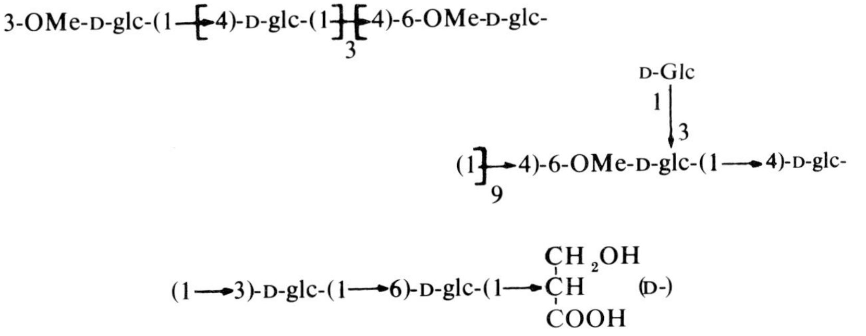

3-OMe-D-glc-(1⟶4)-D-glc-(1⟶4)-6-OMe-D-glc-
(with a branch labeled 3)

D-Glc
1 ↓ 3
(1⟶4)-6-OMe-D-glc-(1⟶4)-D-glc-
(with a branch labeled 9)

$$\text{(1⟶3)-D-glc-(1⟶6)-D-glc-(1⟶}\begin{array}{c}CH_2OH\\|\\CH\\|\\COOH\end{array}\text{ (D-)}$$

with 3 OAc groups, 1 propionate, 1 isobutyrate, 0.3 succinate, and 1 octanoate. Polysaccharides I, II, III, and IV had 0, 1, 2, and 3 succinate in addition. Polysaccharides of *M. phlei* have also been shown to participate in regulation of the activity of a constituent enzyme, fatty acid synthetase (Ilton et al., 1971). In combination with flavin mononucleotide, each of three polysaccharides, I, II, and III, lowered the K_m for acetyl-CoA about 50-fold. I contained about 95% 3-O-Me-man and 5% man, while II and III resembled the above methylglucan.

Cross-reactions between *Brucella* and *M. tuberculosis* have been recorded (Fuks and Serpa, 1962), apparently caused by the presence of glc and glcN in the polysaccharides of both. Wax D of the Aoyama B strain of *M. tuberculosis* has been shown to contain an arabinogalactan as the main serologically active polysaccharide, and also an arabino-mannan (Azuma, Kimura, and Yamamura, 1968).

VIII. Conclusion

In this review we have given a list of microbial polysaccharides of known constitution, omitting a number covered in other reviews. We have also listed cross-reactions of the polysaccharides. These often occur between microbial and other species which are far apart phyloge-netically but which elaborate polysaccharides containing multiples (Heidelberger and Kendall, 1935) of identical or closely similar sugar residues in identical or similar linkages. The cross-reactions are there-fore necessary consequences of the chemical relationships of the cross-reacting structures and are often predictable from the above theory. Some of the consequences of the study of cross-reactions illustrated in the preceding pages are:

1. An immune serum directed against a polysaccharide of known or partially known structure may be used to indicate one or more sugars and even elements of the structure of cross-reacting polysaccha-rides of unknown constitution.

2. Linkages of the sugars, as well as their position, their order, their anomeric form, and sometimes their classification as L or D, may be determined.

3. A cross-reacting polysaccharide of known structure may be used to define the structure of an unknown antigenic determinant for which a precipitating antibody is available.

4. In these ways many rigorous relations between chemical con-stitution and immunological specificity have come to light. Quantitative microanalyses are often essential for this purpose, because cross-reactions are generally only partial and frequently involve too small a fraction of the total antibodies to reduce the residual titer sufficiently for an accurate qualitative test. Quantitative analyses of the

residual antibodies also frequently permit a decision as to which sugar or sugars were involved in a prior cross-reaction.

5. Only positive reactions are of significance. If an antiserum does not react, one raised in another animal, even of the same species, might be positive.

Literature Cited

Adams, G. A., M. Kates, D. H. Shaw, and M. Yaguchi. 1968. Studies on the chemical constitution of cell wall lipopolysaccharides from *Neisseria perflava*. Can. J. Biochem. 46:1175–1184.

Adams, G. A., T. G. Tornabene, and M. Yaguchi. 1969. Cell wall lipopolysaccharides from *Neisseria catarrhalis*. Can. J. Microbiol. 15:365–374.

Annals of the New York Academy of Sciences. 1966. Many of the authors active in the field: Molecular biology of gram-negative lipopolysaccharides. Vol. 133: 277–786.

Avery, O. T., and M. Heidelberger. 1925. Immunological relationships of cell constituents of pneumococcus. II. J. Exp. Med. 42:367–376.

Azuma, I., H. Kimura, and Y. Yamamura. 1968. Chemical and immunological properties of wax D extracted from *Mycobacterium tuberculosis* strain Aoyama B. J. Bacteriol. 96:567–568.

Baddiley, J. 1970. Structure, biosynthesis, and function of teichoic acids. Accts. Chem. Res. 3:98–105.

Barker, S. A., S. M. Bick, J. S. Brimacombe, M. J. How, and M. Stacey. 1966. Structural studies on the capsular polysaccharide of pneumococcus type V. Carbohydr. Res. 2:224–233.

Barker, S. A., J. S. Brimacombe, J. L. Eriksen, and M. Stacey. 1963. Capsular polysaccharide of Klebsiella pneumoniae type A (strain 1265). Nature 197:899–900.

Barker, S. A., A. B. Foster, I. R. Siddiqui, and M. Stacey. 1958a. Structure of an acidic polysaccharide elaborated by Aerobacter aerogenes. Nature 181:999.

Barker, S. A., A. B. Foster, I. R. Siddiqui, and M. Stacey. 1958b. Structure of the capsular polysaccharide of Aerobacter aerogenes, N.C.T.C. 418. J. Chem. Soc. (London), 2358–2367.

Barker, S.A., P. J. Somers, and M. Stacey. 1967. Sequence studies on Diplococcus pneumoniae type II polysaccharide. Carbohydr. Res. 3:261–270.

Baumann, P. 1968. Isolation of Acinetobacter from soil and water. J. Bacteriol. 96:39–42.

Baumann, P., M. Doudoroff, and R. Y. Stanier. 1968. Study of the Moraxella group. II. Oxidative-negative species. J. Bacteriol. 95:1520–1541.

Beychok, S., S. Hammarström, and E. A. Kabat. 1971. Analysis of optical rotatory dispersion and circular dichroism spectra of groups A, A variant, and C streptococcal polysaccharides. Biochemistry 10:1690–1692.

Björndal, H., B. Lindberg, and W. Nimmich. 1970. Structural studies on the lipopoly-saccharide from *Klebsiella* K73:010, I. Methylation analysis, identification and location of 3-O-methyl-L-rhamnose. Acta Chem. Scand. 24:3414–3415.

Bleiweis, A. S., and R. M. Krause. 1965. Cell walls of group D streptococci. I. Immunochemistry of the type I carbohydrate. J Exp. Med. 122:237–249.

Bleiweis, A. S., and R. M. Krause. 1967. II. Chemical studies on the type I antigen, purified from the autolytic digest of cell walls. J. Bacteriol. 94:1381–1387.

Bornstein, D. L., G. Schiffman, H. P. Bernheimer, and R. Austrian. 1968. Capsulation of pneumococcus with soluble C-like (Cs) polysaccharide. I. Biological and genetic properties of Cs pneumococcal strains. J. Exp. Med. 128:1385–1400.

Brown, R. 1939. Chemical and immunological studies of the pneumococcus. V. The soluble specific substances of types I–XXXII. J. Immunol. 37:445–455.

Brown, R., and L. K. Robinson. 1943. VI. The soluble specific substances of new types and subtypes. J. Immunol. 47:7–13.

Brundish, D. E., and J. Baddiley. 1967. Characterization of pneumococcal C-polysaccharide as a ribitol teichoic acid. Biochem. J. 105:30–31c.

Brundish, D. E., and J. Baddiley. 1968. Pneumococcal C-substance, a ribitol teichoic acid containing choline phosphate. Biochem. J. 110:573–582.

Butler, K., and M. Stacey. 1955. Immunopolysaccharides. IV. Structural studies on the type II pneumococcus specific polysaccharide. J. Chem. Soc. (London), 1537–1541.

Campbell, J. H., and A. M. Pappenheimer, Jr. 1966. Quantitative studies of the specificity of antipneumococcal polysaccharide antibodies, types III and VIII. I. Immunochemistry 3:195–212. II. Immunochemistry 213–222.

Chermann, J. C., M. Digeon, and M. Raynaud. 1967. Une nouvelle méthode de purification des endotoxines: la précipitation par le polyéthylène-glycol. Compt. Rend. Acad. Sci., Ser. D., 265:1251–1252.

Chionglo, D. T., and J. A. Hayashi. 1969. Structural basis of group G streptococcal antigenicity. Arch. Biochem. Biophys. 130:39–47.

Chittenden, G. J. F., W. K. Roberts, J. G. Buchanan, and J. Baddiley. 1968. Specific substance from pneumococcus type 34 (41). Biochem. J. 109:597–602.

Cifonelli, J. A., P. A. Rebers, M. B. Perry, and J. K. N. Jones. 1966. The capsular polysaccharide of pneumococcus type XII, S XII. Biochemistry 5:3066–3072.

Cifonelli, J. A., P. A. Rebers, and K. H. Heddleston. 1970. Isolation and character-ization of hyaluronic acid from *Pasteurella multocida*. Carbohydr. Res. 14:272–276.

Conrad, H. E., J. R. Bamburg, J. D. Epley, and T. J. Kindt. 1966. Structure of the Aerobacter aerogenes A3 (S1) polysaccharide. II. Sequence analysis and hydrolysis studies. Biochemistry 5:2808–2817.

Coyette, J., and J. M. Ghuysen. 1970. Structure of the walls of *Lactobacillus acidophilus* strain 63AM Gasser. Biochemistry 9:2935–2943.

Cummins, C. S. 1971. Cell wall composition in *Corynebacteria*. J. Bacteriol. 105:1227–1228.

Curtis, S. N., and R. M. Krause. 1964a. Immunological studies on the specific carbohydrate of group G streptococci. J. Exp. Med. 119:997–1004.

Curtis, S. N., and R. M. Krause. 1964b. Antigenic relationships between groups B and G streptococci. J. Exp. Med. 120:629–637.

Das, A., J. D. Higginbotham, and M. Heidelberger. 1972. Oxidation of the capsular polysaccharide of pneumococcal type IX by periodate. Biochem. J. 126:233–236.

Digeon, M., J. C. Chermann, and M. Raynaud. 1967. Multiplicité des déterminants présents sur la molecule de l'antigène rough lourd des Salmonelles. Ann. Inst. Pasteur 113:843–856.

Dixon, J. R., W. K. Roberts, G. T. Mills, J. G. Buchanan, and J. Baddiley. 1968. O-Acetyl groups of the specific substance from pneumococcus type 34 (U.S. type 41). Carbohydr. Res. 8:262–265.

Dochez, A. R., and O. T. Avery. 1917. The elaboration of specific soluble substance by pneumococcus during growth. J. Exp. Med. 26:477–493.

Douglas, L. J., and M. J. Wolin. 1971. Cell wall polymers and phage lysis of *Lactobacillus plantarum*. Biochemistry 10:1551–1555.

Droege, W., O. Lüderitz, and O. Westphal. 1968. Biochemical studies on lipopolysaccharides of *Salmonella* R mutants. III. Linkage of heptose units. Eur. J. Biochem. 4:126–133.

Droege, W., O. Lüderitz, O. Westphal and E. Ruschmann. 1968. IV. Phosphate groups linked to heptose units and their absence in some R lipopolysaccharides. Eur. J. Biochem. 4:134–138.

Dudman, W. F., and M. Heidelberger. 1969. Immunochemistry of newly found substituents of polysaccharides of *Rhizobium* species. Science 164:954–955.

Dudman, W. F., and J. F. Wilkinson. 1956. Composition of extracellular polysaccharides of *Aerobacter-Klebsiella* strains. Biochem. J. 62:289–295.

Eddy, B. F. 1944. Study of cross-reactions among pneumococci types and their application to identification of types. Publ. Health Repts. (Wash.) 59:451–468.

Elliott, S. D., J. Hayward, and T. Y. Liu. 1971. Presence of a group A variant-like antigen in streptococci of other groups, with special reference to group N. J. Exp. Med. 133:479–493.

Eriksen, J. 1965. Immunochemical studies on some serological cross-reactions in the Klebsiella group. 10. Structure of the capsular polysaccharide of type 3 (C). Acta Pathol. Microbiol. Scand. 64:347–361.

Estrada-Parra, S., and M. Heidelberger. 1963. The specific polysaccharide of type XVIII pneumococcus. III. Biochemistry 2:1288–1294.

Estrada-Parra, S., M. Heidelberger, and P. A. Rebers. 1963. Immunochemical properties of the periodate-oxidized polysaccharide of group A hemolytic streptococcus. J. Biol. Chem. 238:510–512.

Fensom, A. H., and G. W. Gray. 1969. Chemical composition of the lipopolysaccharide of *Pseudomonas aeruginosa*. Biochem. J. 114:185–196.

Freimer, E. H. 1967. Type-specific polysaccharide antigens of group B streptococci. J. Exp. Med. 125:381–392.

Fuks, M. A., and C. E. Serpa. 1962. Utilization of gel-precipitation and passive cutaneous anaphylaxis in the study of cross-reactions between antigenic polysaccharides of Brucella and the tubercle bacillus. Anais Microbiol. Univ. Brasil, A, 10:91–98; through Chem. Abstrs. 1964, 61:16597.

Fuller, N. A., and A. M. Staub. 1968. Immunochemical studies on *Salmonella*. 13, Eur. J. Biochem. 4:286–300.

Fuller, N. A., M. Etievant, and A. M. Staub. 1968. Immunochemical studies on *Salmonella*. 14. Oligosaccharides which determine the specificities 6_2, 7, and 14 in *S. cholerae suis* after conversion by bacteriophage 14(6,7). Eur. J. Biochem. 6:525–533.

Gahan, L. C., P. A. Sandford, and H. E. Conrad. 1967. Structure of the serotype 2 capsular polysaccharide of *Aerobacter aerogenes*. Biochemistry 6:2755–2767.

Garegg, P. J., B. Lindberg, T. Onn, and T. Holme. 1969. M antigen of *Salmonella typhimurium* 395-MRO-M. Acta Chem. Scand. 23:2194–2196.

Goebel, W. F., T. Shedlovsky, G. I. Lavin, and M. H. Adams. 1943. The heterophile antigen of pneumococcus. J. Biol. Chem. 148:1–15.

Goodman, J. W., and E. A. Kabat. 1960. Immunochemical studies on cross-reactions of antipneumococcal sera. I. Cross-reactions of type II and XX antipneumococcal sera with dextrans and of type II anti- pneumococcal sera with glycogen and Friedländer type B polysaccharide. II. Cross-reactions of type IX and XII anti-pneumococcal sera with dextrans. J. Immunol. 84:333–357.

Gormus, B. J., R. W. Wheat, and J. F. Porter. 1971. Occurrence of pyruvic acid in capsular polysaccharides from various *Klebsiella* species. J. Bacteriol. 107:150–154.

Gotschlich, E. C., and T.-Y. Liu. 1967. Structure and immunological studies on the pneumococcal C polysaccharide. J. Biol. Chem. 242:463–470.

Gotschlich, E. C., T.-Y. Liu, and M. S. Artenstein. 1969. Human immunity to the meningococcus. III. Preparation and immunochemical properties of the group A, group B, and group C meningococcal polysaccharides. J. Exp. Med. 129:1349–1365.

Graham, P. H., and M. A. O'Brien. 1968. Composition of lipopolysaccharides from *Rhizobium* and *Agrobacterium*. A. van Leeuwenhoek, J. Microbiol. Serol. 34:326–330, through Chem. Abstrs. 1968, 69:6087.

Guy, R. C. E., M. J. How, M. Stacey, and M. Heidelberger. 1967. The capsular polysaccharide of type I pneumococcus. I. Purification and chemical modification. J. Biol. Chem. 242:5106–5111.

Halliday, W. J. 1971. Immunological paralysis of mice with pneumococcal polysaccharide antigens. Bacteriol. Revs. 35:267–289.

Hammond, B. F. 1970. Isolation and characterization of a cell wall antigen of *Rothia dentocariosa*. J. Bacteriol. 103:634–640.

Heidelberger, M. 1939a. Chemical aspects of the precipitin and agglutinin reactions. Chem. Rev. 24:323–343.

Heidelberger, M. 1939b. Quantitative absolute methods in the study of antigen-antibody reactions. Bacteriol. Rev. 3:49–95.

Heidelberger, M. 1955. Immunological specificities involving multiple units of galactose. II. J. Amer. Chem. Soc. 77:4308–4311.

Heidelberger, M. 1960. Structure and immunological specificity of polysaccharides. Progr. Chem. Org. Natur. Prod. 18:503–536.

Heidelberger, M. 1962. Immunochemistry of pneumococcal types II, V and VI. IV. Cross-reactions of type V antipneumococcal sera and their bearing on the relation between types II and V. Arch. Biochem. Biophys., Suppl. 1:169–173.

Heidelberger, M., and O. T. Avery. 1923. Soluble specific substance of pneumococcus. J. Exp. Med. 38:73–79.

Heidelberger, M., and O. T. Avery. 1924. Soluble specific substance of pneumococcus. J. Exp. Med. 40:301–316.

Heidelberger, M., A. Das, and E. Juni. 1969. Immunochemistry of the capsular polysaccharide of an acinetobacter. Proc. Nat. Acad. Sci. U.S.A. 63:47–50.

Heidelberger, M., J. M. Davie, and R. M. Krause. 1967. Cross-reactions of the group-specific polysaccharides of streptococcal groups B and G in antipneumococcal sera with special reference to type XXIII and its determinants. J. Immunol. 99:794–796.

Heidelberger, M., W. F. Dudman, and W. Nimmich. 1970. Immunochemical relationships of certain capsular polysaccharides of Klebsiella, pneumococci, and Rhizobia. J. Immunol. 104:1321–1328.

Heidelberger, M., W. F. Goebel, and O. T. Avery. 1925. Soluble specific substance of pneumococcus. J. Exp. Med. 42:727–745.

Heidelberger, M., E. C. Gotschlich, and J. D. Higginbotham. 1972. Inhibition experiments with pneumococcal C and depyruvylated type IV polysaccharides. Carbohydr. Res. 22:1–4.

Heidelberger, M., K. Jann, B. Jann, F. Ørskov, I. Ørskov, and O. Westphal. 1968. Relations between structures of three K polysaccharides of *Escherichia coli* and cross-reactivity in antipneumococcal sera. J. Bacteriol. 95:2415–2417.

Heidelberger, M., and E. A. Kabat. 1937. Chemical studies on bacterial agglutination: reaction mechanism and quantitative theory. J. Exp. Med. 65:885–902.

Heidelberger, M., and F. E. Kendall. 1931. Specific and non-specific polysaccharides of type IV pneumococcus. J. Exp. Med. 53:625–638.

Heidelberger, M., and F. E. Kendall. 1935. Precipitin reaction between type III polysaccharide and homologous antibody. III. Quantitative study and a theory of the reaction mechanism. J. Exp. Med. 61:563–591.

Heidelberger, M., and F. E. Kendall. 1937. Quantitative theory of the precipitin reaction. VI. Reaction of pneumococcus specific polysaccharides with homologous rabbit antisera. J. Exp. Med. 65:647–660.

Heidelberger, M., and M. McCarty. 1959. Cross-reactions of streptococcal A and V carbohydrates in type II antipneumococcal horse serum. Proc. Nat. Acad. Sci. U.S.A. 45:235–238.

Heidelberger, M., and C. V. N. Rao. 1966. Immunochemical properties of hualtaco gum. Immunology, 10:543–548.

Heidelberger, M., and P. A. Rebers. 1960. Immunochemistry of the pneumococcal types II, V, and VI. Relation of type VI to type II and other correlations between chemical constitution and precipitation in antisera to type VI. J. Bacteriol. 80:145–153.

Heidelberger, M., N. Roy, and C. P. J. Glaudemans. 1969. Inhibition by aldobiouronates in the pneumococcal type II and type III systems. Biochemistry 8:4822–4824.

Heidelberger, M., and M. E. Slodki. 1968. Predicted and unpredicted cross-reactions of an acetylphosphogalactan of Sporobolomyces yeast. J. Exp. Med. 128:189–196.

Heidelberger, M., and M. E. Slodki. 1970. II. J. Exp. Med. 132:1105–1106.

Heidelberger, M., and J. M. Tyler. 1964. Cross-reactions of pneumococcal types. Quantitative studies with the capsular polysaccharides. J. Exp. Med. 120:711–719.

Heidelberger, M., J. M. N. Willers, and M. F. Michel. 1969. Immunochemical relationships of certain streptococcal group and type polysaccharides to pneumococcal capsular antigens. J. Immunol. 102:1119–1127.

Hellerqvist, C. G., B. Lindberg, S. Svensson, T. Holme, and A. A. Lindberg. 1968. Structural studies on the O-specific side-chains of the cell-wall lipopolysaccharide from *Salmonella typhimurium* 395 MS. Carbohydr. Res. 8:43–55. S. typhimurium LT2. Carbohydr. Res. 9:237–241.

Hellerqvist, C. G., B. Lindberg, S. Svensson, T. Holme, and A. A. Lindberg. 1969. O-specific side-chains of the lipopolysaccharides of *S. typhi* and *S. enteritidis*. Acta Chem. Scand. 23:1588–1596.

Hellerqvist, C. G., O. Larm, B. Lindberg, T. Holme, and A. A. Lindberg. 1969. O-specific side-chains of *S. bredeney*. Acta Chem. Scand. 23:2217–2222.

Hellerqvist, C. G., B. Lindberg, J. Lönngren, and A. A. Lindberg. 1971. Structural studies of the O-specific side-chains of the cell-wall lipopolysaccharide from *S. münster* (3, 10). Carbohydr. Res. 16:289–296.

Hellerqvist, C. G., B. Lindberg, A. Pilotti, and A. A. Lindberg. 1971. O-chains of *S. senftenberg*. Carbohydr. Res. 16:297–302.

Hellerqvist, C. G., and A. A. Lindberg. 1971. Common core polysaccharide of the cell-wall lipopolysaccharide from *Salmonella*. Carbohydr. Res. 16:39–48.

Henriksen, S. D., and J. Eriksen. 1959, 1961. Immunochemical studies on serological cross-reactions in the *Klebsiella* group. 1. Quantitative study of the cross-reactions between type A(1), and E(5) and AE. Acta Pathol. Microbiol. Scand 45:381–386; 3. 51:259–274.

Henriksen, S. D., and J. Eriksen. 1962. V. Reappearance of a fucose-less strain of K. ozaenae type AE. Acta Pathol. Microbiol. Scand. 54:382–386.

Heymann, H., J. M. Manniello, L. D. Zeleznick, and S. S. Barkulis. 1963. Structure of streptococcal cell walls. I. Methylation study of C-polysaccharide. J. Biol. Chem. 238:502–509.

Heymann, H., J. M. Manniello, L. D. Zeleznick, and S. S. Barkulis. 1964. Structure of streptococcal cell walls. II. Group A biose and Group A triose from C-polysaccharide. J. Biol. Chem. 239:1656–1663.

Higginbotham, J. D., A. Das, and M. Heidelberger. 1972. Immunochemical studies on the capsular polysaccharide of pneumococcal type IX. Biochem. J. 126:225–231.

Higginbotham, J. D., and M. Heidelberger. 1972. Specific capsular polysaccharide of pneumococcal type IV. Carbohydr. Res. 23:165–173.

Higginbotham, J. D., M. Heidelberger, and E. C. Gotschlich. 1970. Degradation of a pneumococcal type-specific polysaccharide with exposure of group-specificity. Proc. Nat. Acad. Sci. U.S.A. 67:138–142.

How, M. J., J. S. Brimacombe, and M. Stacey. 1964. Pneumococcal polysaccharides. Adv. Carbohydr. Chem. 19:303–358.

Hughes, R. C. 1971. Autolysis of *Bacillus cereus* cell walls and isolation of structural components. Biochem. J. 121:791–802.

Hughes, R. C., and P. F. Thurman. 1970. Structural features of the teichuronic acid of *Bacillus licheniformis* N.C.T.C. 6346 cell walls. Biochem. J. 117:441–449.

Hungerer, D., K. Jann, B. Jann, and I. Ørskov. 1967. Immunochemistry of K antigens of *Escherichia coli*. 4. K antigen of *E. coli* 09:K30:H12. Eur. J. Biochem. 2:115–126.

Ilton, M., A. W. Jevans, E. D. McCarty, D. Vance, H. B. White, III, and K. Bloch. 1971. Fatty acid synthetase activity in *Mycobacterium phlei:* regulation by polysaccharides. Proc. Nat. Acad. Sci. U.S.A. 68:87–91.

Jann, B., and K. Jann. 1968. 2-Amino-2,6-dideoxy-L-mannose (L-rhamnosamine) isolated from the lipopolysaccharide of *Escherichia coli* O3:K2ab (L):H2. Eur. J. Biochem. 5:173–177.

Jann, B., K. Jann, G. Schmidt, I. Ørskov, and F. Ørskov. 1970. Immunochemical studies of polysaccharide surface antigens of *Escherichia coli* O100:K? (B):H2. Eur. J. Biochem. 15:29–39.

Jann, B., K. Jann, K. F. Schneider, I. Ørskov, and F. Ørskov. 1968. V. The K antigen of *E. coli* O8:K27(A): H⁻. Eur. J. Biochem. 5:456–465.

Jann, K., B. Jann, F. and I. Ørskov, and O. Westphal. 1965. Immunchemische Unter suchungen an K-Antigenen von *Escherichia coli*. II. K-Antigen von *E. coli* O8: 42(A). Biochem. Z. 342:1–22.

Jann, K., B. Jann, F. and I. Ørskov. 1966. Immunchemische Untersuchungen an K-Antigenen von *Escherichia coli*. III. Isolierung und Untersuchung der chemischen Struktur des sauren Polysacchrides aus *E. coli* O141: K85(B):H4 (K85 Antigen). Biochem. Z. 346:368–385.

Jeanes, A. 1968. Microbial polysaccharides. Encycl. Polymer Sci. Technol. 8:693–711.

Jelinkova, J., R. Bicova, and J. Rotta. 1967. Relation between group A and L streptococci. J. Hyg. Epidemiol. Microbiol. Immunol. 11:353–358, through Chem. Abstrs. 1970, 72:75844.

Jones, J. K. N., and M. B. Perry. 1957. Structure of the type VIII pneumococcus specific polysaccharide. J. Amer. Chem. Soc. 79:2787–2793.

Juni, E., and G. A. Heym. 1964. Pathways for biosynthesis of a bacterial capsular polysaccharide. IV. Capsule resynthesis by decapsulated resting-cell suspensions. J. Bacteriol. 87:461–467.

Kanamaru, T., and S. Yamatodori. 1969. Production of heteropolysaccharides from *n*-paraffins. Agr. Biol. Chem. 33:1521–1522.

Kane, J. A., and W. W. Karakawa. 1969. Immunochemical studies on the cross-reactivity between *Streptococcus bovis,* strain S19, and group A streptococcal carbohydrates. J. Immunol. 102:870–876.

Kaplan, M. H., and J. E. Volanakis. 1971. Specificity of C-reactive protein (CRP) for phosphoryl choline and related phosphatides. Interaction of CRP and complement systems. Fed. Proc. 30:471.

Karakawa, W. W., and J. A. Kane. 1971. Immunochemical analysis of a galactosamine-rich teichoic acid of *Staphylococcus aureus,* phage type 187. J. Immunol. 106:900–906.

Kedzierska, B., E. Mikulaszek, and J. Pogonowska-Goldhar. 1968. Immunochemical studies on *Salmonella* serogroup 48. III. N-Acetyl-neuraminic acid as immuno-dominant sugar. Bull. Acad. Polon. Ser. Sci. Biol. 16:673–676; through Chem. Abstrs. 1969, 70:75993.

Kennedy, D. A., J. G. Buchanan, and J. Baddiley. 1969. Type-specific substance from pneumococcus type 11A(43). Biochem. J. 115:37–45.

Kent, J. L., and M. J. Osborn. 1968. Haptenic O-antigen as a polymeric intermediate of *in vivo* synthesis of lipopolysaccharide of *Salmonella typhimurium*. Biochemistry 7:4419–4922.

Key, B. A., G. W. Gray, and S. G. Wilkinson. 1970. Purification and chemical composition of the lipopolysaccharide of *Pseudomonas alkaligenes*. Biochem. J. 120:559–566.

Knecht, J. C., G. Schiffman, and R. Austrian. 1970. Biological properties of pneumococcus type 37 and the chemistry of its capsular polysaccharide. J. Exp. Med. 132:475–487.

Kotelko, K., J. Radziejewska, Z. Sidorczyk, K. Izdebska-Szymona, and J. Zwolinski. 1968. Antigenic structure of *Proteus mirabilis*. II. Oligosaccharides derived from polysaccharides of the S form. Bull. Acad. Polon. Sci., Ser. Sci. Biol. 16:745–750, through Chem. Abstrs. 1969, 70:94951.

Krause, R. M. 1963. Antigenic and biochemical composition of hemolytic streptococcal cell walls. Bacteriol. Revs. 27:369–380.

Krause, R. M., and M. McCarty. 1962a. Studies on the chemical structure of the streptococcal cell wall. II. Composition of group C cell walls and chemical basis for serologic specificity of the carbohydrate moiety. J. Exp. Med. 115:49–62.

Krause, R. M., and M. McCarty. 1962b. Variation in the group-specific carbohydrate of group C hemolytic streptococci. J. Exp. Med. 116:131–140.

Lancefield, R. C. 1962. Current knowledge of the type-specific M antigens of group A streptococci. J. Immunol. 89:307–313.

Lancefield, R. C., and E. H. Freimer. 1966. Type-specific polysaccharide antigens of group B streptococci. J. Hyg. 64:191–203.

Larm, O., B. Lindberg, S. Svensson, and E. A. Kabat. 1972. Structural studies on pneumococcus type II capsular polysaccharide. Carbohydr. Res. 22:391–397.

Leive, L., V. K. Shovlin, and S. E. Mergenhagen. 1968. Physical, chemical, and immunological properties of lipopolysaccharide released from *Escherichia coli* by ethylenediaminetetraacetate. J. Biol. Chem. 243:6384–6391.

Leon, M. A., and N. M. Young. 1971. Specificity for phosphorylcholine of six myeloma proteins with specificity for pneumococcal C-substance and β-lipoproteins. Biochemistry 10:1424–1429.

Linker, A., and L. R. Evans. 1968. Polysaccharide of a mucoid *E. coli* isolated from a patient with cystic fibrosis. Nature 218:774–775.

Liu, T.-Y., and E. C. Gotschlich. 1963. Chemical composition of pneumococcal C-polysaccharide. J. Biol. Chem. 238:1928–1934.

Liu, T.-Y., E. C. Gotschlich, E. K. Jonssen, and J. R. Wysocki. 1971. Studies on meningococcal polysacchrides. I. Composition and chemical properties of the group A polysaccharide. J. Biol. Chem. 246:2849–2858.

Lüderitz, O., J. Gmeiner, B. Kickhofen, H. Mayer, O. Westphal, and R. W. Wheat, 1968. Identification of D-mannosamine and quinovosamine in *Salmonella* and related bacteria. J. Bacteriol. 95:490–494.

Lüderitz, O., K. Jann, and R. Wheat. 1968. Somatic and capsular antigens of gram-negative bacteria. *In* Florkin, M. and E. H. Stotz (eds.), Comprehensive Biochemistry, Vol. 26A, Chapter 3, pp. 105–227, Elsevier, Amsterdam.

Lüderitz, O., A. M. Staub, and O. Westphal. 1966. Immunochemistry of O and R antigens of *Salmonella* and related Enterobacteriaceae. Bacteriol. Rev. 30:192–225.

Mage, R. G., and E. A. Kabat. 1963. Combining regions of type III pneumococcal polysaccharide and homologous antibody. Biochemistry 2:1278–1288.

Manning, J. L. 1971. Chromatographic determination of the D- and L-amino acid residues in pneumococcal C-polysaccharide. J. Biol. Chem. 246:2926–2929.

Matsumo, T., and H. D. Slade. 1970. Composition and properties of a group A streptococcal teichoic acid. J. Bacteriol. 102:747–752.

Mayer, H. 1969. D-Mannosaminuronsäure Baustein des K7-Antigens von *Escherichia coli*. Eur. J. Biochem. 8:139–145.

McCarty, M. 1954. Streptococcal infections, Chapter 1. Columbia University Press, New York.

McCarty, M. 1956. Variation in the group-specific carbohydrate of group A streptococci. II. Studies on the chemical basis for serological specificity of the carbohydrates. J. Exp. Med. 104:629–643.

McCarty, M. 1958. Further studies on the chemical basis for serological specificity of group A streptococcal carbohydrate. J. Exp. Med. 108:311–323.

McCarty, M., and R. C. Lancefield. 1955. Variation in the group-specific carbohydrate of group A streptococci: immunochemical studies on carbohydrates of variant strains. J. Exp. Med. 102:11–28.

Michel, M. F., and R. M. Krause. 1967. Immunochemical studies on the group and type antigens of group F streptococci and the identification of a group-like carbohydrate in a type II strain with an undesignated group antigen. J. Exp. Med. 125:1075–1089.

Michel, M. F., J. van Vonno, and R. M. Krause. 1969. Studies on the chemical structure and the antigenic determinant of type II antigen of group F streptococci. J. Immunol. 102:215–221.

Michel, M. F., and J. M. N. Willers. 1964. Immunochemistry of group F streptococci: isolation of group-specific oligosaccharides. J. Gen. Microbiol. 37:381–389.

Mills, G. T., E. E. B. Smith, H. P. Bernheimer, R. Austrian, and B. Galloway. 1960. Pathway of UDPgalacturonic acid in type 33 pneumococci and its importance in the formation of binary capsulated type 3-33 pneumococci during transformation. Biochem. J. 76:31P.

Miyazaki, T., and T. Yadomae. 1971. Polysaccharides of the type XIX pneumococcus. II. Type-specific polysaccharide and its chemical behavior. Carbohydr. Res. 16:153–159.

Montague, E. A., and K. W. Knox. 1969. Antigenic components of the cell wall of *Streptococcus salivarius*. J. Gen. Microbiol. 54:237–246.

Mosser, J. L., and A. Tomasz. 1970. Choline-containing teichoic acid as a structural component of the pneumococcal cell wall and its role in sensitivity to lysis by an autolytic enzyme. J. Biol. Chem. 245:287–298.

Nashkov, D. K., K. Tsankova, I. Andreev, and I. Khristov. 1968. Polysaccharides of *Pasteurella multocida*. Vet. Med. Nauki (Sofia) 5:11–21, through Chem. Abstrs. 1969, 69:2342.

Nghiem, H. O., G. Bagdian, and A. M. Staub. 1967. Études immunochimiques sur les *Salmonella*. XIII, Détermination de la structure du polyoside spécifique d'une *Salmonella* du group 2 (S. Strasbourg). Eur. J. Biochem. 2:392–398.

Nhan, L.-B., B. Jann, and K. Jann. 1971. Immunochemistry of K antigens of *Escherichia coli*. K29 antigen of *E. coli* O9:K29 (A):H⁻. Eur. J. Biochem. 21:226–234.

Nikaido, H. 1968. Biosynthesis of cell wall lipopolysaccharide in gram-negative enteric bacteria. Adv. Enzymol. 31:77–124.

Nimmich, W. 1968. Zur Isolierung und qualitativen Bausteinanalyse der K-Antigene von Klebsiellen. Z. Med. Mikrobiol. Immunol. 154:117–131.

Nimmich, W. 1970. Vergleichende chemische Untersuchungen an *Klebsiella* O4 und *Salmonella* T1 Antigen. Z. Immunitätsf. 139:347–358.

Nimmich, W., and W. Münter. 1967. Zur Immunchemie der Klebsiella-Antigene. Experimentia 23:907–908.

Nimmich, W., and G. Korten. 1970. Die chemische Zusammensetzung der Klebsiella Lipopolysacchariden (O-Antigene). Pathol. Microbiol. 36:179–190.

Ørskov, F., L. Ørskov, B. Jann, K. Jann, E. Müller-Seitz, and O. Westphal. 1967. Immunochemistry of *Escherichia coli* O antigens. Acta Pathol. Microbiol. Scand. 71:339–358.

Osborn, M. J., and R. Y. Tze-Yuen. 1968. Biosynthesis of a bacterial lipopolysaccharide. J. Biol. Chem. 243:5145–5152.

Osborn, M. J., and I. M. Weiner. 1968. Mechanism of biosynthesis of the lipopolysaccharide of Salmonella. Fed. Proc. 26:70–76.

Pardoe, G. I., G. W. G. Bird, and G. Uhlenbruck. 1968. Structural and serological studies of the lipopolysaccharide of *Proteus vulgaris* OX19. Z. Immunitätsf. 136:488–496.

Park, S. H., J. Eriksen, and S. D. Henriksen. 1967. Structure of the capsular polysaccharide of *Klebsiella pneumoniae* type 2(B). Acta Pathol. Microbiol. Scand. 69:431–436.

Partridge, M. D., A. L. Davison, and J. Baddiley. 1971. Polymer of glucose and N-acetylgalactosamine-1-phosphate in the wall of *Micrococcus* sp. A₁. Biochem. J. 121:695–700.

Pazur, J. H., J. S. Anderson, and W. W. Karakawa. 1971. Glycans from streptococcal cell walls. Immunological and chemical properties of a new diheteroglycan from *Streptococcus faecalis*. J. Biol. Chem. 246:1793–1798.

Rao, C. V. N. and M. Heidelberger. 1966. The capsular polysaccharide of pneumococcus type IX. J. Exp. Med. 123:913–920.

Rao, E. V., M. J. Watson, J. G. Buchanan, and J. Baddiley. 1969. The type-specific substance from pneumococcus type 29. Biochem. J. 111:547–556.

Rebers, P. A., and M. Heidelberger. 1959. The specific polysaccharide of type VI pneumococcus. I. Preparation, properties, and reactions. J. Amer. Chem. Soc. 81:2415–2419. II. The repeating unit. J. Amer. Chem. Soc. 83:3056–3059.

Rebers, P. A., S. Estrada-Parra, and M. Heidelberger. 1963. Immunization of rabbits with periodate-oxidized pneumococcal type III specific capsular polysaccharide coupled to horse antibody. J. Bacteriol. 86:882–883.

Rebers, P. A., E. Hurwitz, M. Heidelberger, and S. Estrada-Parra. 1962. Immunochemistry of pneumococcal types II, V and VI. III. Tests with derivatives of the specific polysaccharides of types II and VI. J. Bacteriol. 83:335–342.

Reeder, W. J., and R. D. Eckstedt. 1971. Study of the interaction of concanavalin A with staphylococcal teichoic acids. J. Immunol. 106:334–340.

Reeves, R. E., and W. F. Goebel. 1941. Chemo-immunological studies on the soluble specific substance of pneumococcus: structure of the type III polysaccharide. J. Biol. Chem. 139:511–519.

Robbins, P. W., J. M. Keller, A. Wright, and R. L. Bernstein. 1965. Enzymatic and kinetic studies on the mechanism of O-antigen conversion by bacteriophage ϵ^{15}. J. Biol. Chem. 240:384–390.

Robinson, J. A., and M. A. Apicella. 1970. Isolation and characterization of *Neisseria meningitides* groups A, C, X, and Y polysaccharide antigens. Infect. Immunol. 1:8–14.

Roy, N., and C. P. J. Glaudemans. 1968. Specific substance from *Diplococcus pneumoniae* type 34 (U.S. type 41): location of the O-acetyl groups. Carbohydr. Res. 8:214–218.

Roy, N., W. R. Carroll, and C. P. J. Glaudemans. 1970. The specific substance from *Diplococcus pneumoniae* type 31. Carbohydr. Res. 12:89–96.

Saier, M. H., Jr. and C. E. Ballou. 1968. 6-O-Methylglucose–containing lipopolysaccharides of *Mycobacterium phlei*. Complete structure of the polysaccharide. J. Biol. Chem. 243:4322–4341.

Sandford, P. A., and H. E. Conrad. 1966. Structure of the *Aerobacter aerogenes* A3(S1) polysaccharide. I. Reexamination using improved procedures for methylation analysis. Biochemistry 5:1508–1517.

Sarvas, M., and H. Nikaido. 1971. Biosynthesis of T1 antigen in *Salmonella*: Origin of D-galactofuranose and D-ribofuranose residues. J. Bacteriol. 105:1063–1072.

Schmidt, G., B. Jann, and K. Jann. 1969, 1970. Immunochemistry of the R lipopolysaccharide of *Escherichia coli*. Different core regions in the lipopolysaccharides of O group 8. Eur. J. Biochem. 10:501–510; 16:382–392.

Schmidt, G., I. Fromme, and H. Mayer. 1970. Immunochemical studies on core lipopolysaccharides of Enterobacteriaceae of different genera. Eur. J. Biochem. 14:357–366.

Shabarova, Z. A., J. G. Buchanan, and J. Baddiley. 1962. Composition of pneumococcus type-specific substances containing phosphorus. Biochim. Biophys. Acta 57:146–148.

Simmons, D.A.R. 1971. Immunochemistry of *Shigella flexneri* O antigens: study of structural and genetic aspects of the biosynthesis of cell-surface antigens. Bacteriol. Rev. 35:117–148.

Slade, H. D., O. Lüderitz, and O. Westphal. 1965. Chemical structure and serological specificity of streptococcal group E cell wall antigens. Bacteriol. Proc., p. 46.

Slade, H. D., and W. S. Slamp. 1962. Cell-wall composition and the grouping antigens of streptococci. J. Bacteriol. 84:345–351.

Staub, A. M., and Westphal, O. 1964. Étude chimique et biochimique de la spécificité immunologique des polyosides bacteriens. Bull. Soc. Chim. Biol. 46:1647–1684.

Sutherland, I. W. 1970. Structure of the *Klebsiella aerogenes* type 8 polysaccharide. Biochemistry 9:2180–2185.

Suzuki, H., and E. L. Hehre. 1964. Differentiation of serotype A and B dextrans by means of partial acetolysis. Arch. Biochem. Biophys. 104:305–313.

Taylor, W. H., and E. Juni. 1961. Pathways for biosynthesis of a bacterial capsular polysaccharide. I. Characterization of the organism and polysaccharide. J. Bacteriol. 81:688–693.

Tillett, W. S., and T. Francis, Jr. 1930. Serological reactions in pneumonia with a non-protein somatic fraction of pneumococcus. J. Exp. Med. 52:561–571.

Tillett, W. S., W. F. Goebel, and O. T. Avery. 1930. Chemical and immunological properties of a species-specific carbohydrate of pneumococci. J. Exp. Med. 52:895–900.

Tomasz, A. 1967. Choline in the cell wall of a bacterium: novel type of polymer-linked choline in pneumococcus. Science 157:694–697.

Tyler, J. M., and M. Heidelberger. 1968. The specific capsular polysaccharide of type VII pneumococcus. Biochemistry 7:1384–1392.

Ullmann, W. W., and J. A. Cameron. 1969. Immunochemistry of the cell walls of *Listeria monocytogenes*. J. Bacteriol. 98:486–493.

Wassermann, E., and L. Levine. 1961. Quantitative micro-complement fixation and its use in the study of antigen-antibody inhibition. J. Immunol. 87:290–295.

Wheat, R. W., C. Dorsch, and G. Godoy. 1965. Occurrence of pyruvic acid in the capsular polysaccharides of *Klebsiella rhinoscleromatis*. J. Bacteriol. 89:539.

Wheat, R. W., and J. M. Ghuysen. 1971. Occurrence of glucomuramic acid in gram-positive bacteria. J. Bacteriol. 105:1219–1221.

Wicken, A. J., S. D. Elliott, and J. Baddiley. 1963. The identity of streptococcal group D antigen with teichoic acid. J. Gen. Microbiol. 31:231–239.

Willers, J. M. N., and G. H. J. Alderkamp. 1967. Loss of type antigen in a type III streptococcus and identification of the determinant disaccharide of the remaining antigen. J. Gen. Microbiol. 49:41–51.

Willers, J. M. N., M. F. Michel, M. J. Sysma, and K. C. Winkler. 1964. Chemical analysis and inhibition reactions of the group and type antigens of group F streptococci. J. Gen. Microbiol. 36:95–105.

Author's address: Prof. M. Heidelberger, Dept. of Pathology, New York University School of Medicine, New York, N.Y. 10016 (U.S.A.).

Immunological Distribution Analysis

Eugene D. Day

Department of Microbiology and Immunology, Duke University Medical Center, Durham, North Carolina, U.S.A.

Contents

I. The Three Parameters of Immunological Specificity and Cross-Reactivity 42
II. Distribution Analysis with Radioantibodies *In Vitro* and *In Vivo* 46
  A. Simple Distribution Analysis *In Vivo* with Radioantibodies 46
    1. Introduction 46
    2. Distribution Analysis within a Tissue Compartment 49
  B. Multicompartment Distribution Analysis *In Vitro* and *In Vivo* with Radioantibodies 55
    1. Introduction 55
    2. The Partitioning Effect 56
    3. Immunozoning 61
    4. Immunozoning by Low-Speed Centrifugation after Adsorption *In Vitro* 65
    5. Immunozoning by Ultracentrifugation after Adsorption *In Vivo* 69
  C. Sequential Adsorption Analysis 72
    1. Introduction 72
    2. The Method 74
    3. Nonselective Adsorption 75
    4. Sequential Adsorption Analysis of Antisynaptosome and Antimyelin Radioantibodies 77
  D. The Kinetics of Radioantibody Localization *In Vivo* 82
    1. Introduction 82
    2. Rate of Localization 82
    3. Stability of Radioantibodies Once Localized 85
    4. Negative Localization 86
Literature Cited 88

This work was supported by contract AT-(40-1)-3195 with the U.S. Atomic Energy Commission.

1. The Three Parameters of Immunological Specificity and Cross-Reactivity

The architecture of antigens is one aspect of tissue immunology; the extent of their reaction with antibodies and/or immune cells is another. There is a third: their distribution. It is held that the full meaning of any particular tissue antigen or set of antigens cannot be obtained without an appreciation of these three parameters of immunological expression.

There are essentially three kinds of immunological specificity, and, to complete the dichotomy, there are essentially three kinds of immunological cross-reactivity. The first kind, which is familiarly known as "chemical" or "true" (Kabat, 1961, p. 405) emphasizes the chemistry of a given antigen and the appropriate spectrum of chemical analogues. In the present context this type of specificity/cross-reactivity will be referred to as *structural* to emphasize its physical as well as chemical make-up.

The second type of immunological specificity and attendant cross-reactivity (as occasioned by the diversity of antibodies raised to a given ligand and as most readily measured by the range of affinity constants that constitute heterogeneity) is referred to here as *affinitive*. It may be argued that this type is nothing more than a variant of the structural kind—and, indeed, variations in the structures of antibody binding sites do account for it—but a moment's reflection will reveal that it does constitute an independent parameter of total specificity/cross-reactivity. Affinitive specificity would be another term for homogeneous binding—antibodies that all display the same affinity constant for a given antigen and an overall Sipsian constant of 1.0. Yet the affinities for analogous antigens would vary, thus accounting for structural cross-reactivity in the face of affinitive specificity. In contrast, affinitive cross-reactivities, which would characterize most reagent antisera, would not interfere with the establishment of structural specificities.

Specificities and cross-reactivities of the third kind—which are sometimes disparagingly termed "pseudo," to contrast them with Kabat's "true,"—emphasize the distribution profile of a given antigenic structure and/or its analogues among the compartments of a given field. If we define a general antigenic system as a field, classical fields would include pneumococci, streptococci, human red cells, human leukocytes, the tissues of various strains of mice, influenza viruses, and genetically polymorphic Bence-Jones proteins, to name a few well-known ones. The compartments of each of these classical fields would be defined by reagent-typing antisera and would consist of the various phenotypes. Other examples of compartmentalized fields *in vivo,* however, may range from plasma with its many protein components, to cells with their many subcellular particles, membranes, and enclosed fluids, to whole animals with their various organs all interconnected by the circulatory system. Examples of fields and their compartments *in vitro* in the laboratory may include density gradients within which tissue homogenates have been distributed, various phases of other fractionating systems (soluble, insoluble, macromolecular, dialyzable, precipitable, filterable, etc.), the regions and subunit components of isolated cell-surface membranes, and purified multichain macromolecules with their range of immunochemically active sequential and conformational determinants. In the present context the type of specificity and accompanying cross-reactivity that characterizes field distribution will be referred to as *compartmental.*

In terms of the example used by Kabat (1961, p. 405), pneumococci types III and VIII would be said to exhibit compartmental cross-reactivity on the basis of their sharing of two antigens: one, a structurally specific "identical" antigen, C substance; the other, a structurally cross-reactive but not identical antigen, the capsular polysaccharide with its aldobiuronic acid residues held in common. Kabat has cautioned that failure to observe this distinction has led to much confusion — the "unfortunate tendency loosely to ascribe relationships of specificity [i.e., structural analogues] to 'common antigens' with the implication that these are identical," or indiscriminately to ascribe "relationships actually due to a common, identical antigen" only to analogous but not structurally identical antigens. Thus, it is absolutely forbidden, in accordance with Kabat's rule, to make decisions concerning structural cross-reactivities and specificities on the basis of compartmental typing analysis.

Today it is essential not only to distinguish among the three immunological parameters — structural, affinitive, and compartmental — but also to recognize that any one parameter should be subordinate to the total concept of specificity.

With the matter of immunological specificity settled in a general, conceptual way, the meaning of nonspecific immunological reactions can also be clarified. Landsteiner (1962, pp. 5–6), in the introduction to his *Specificity of Serological Reactions,* found it "adequate to define serological specificity as the disproportional action of a number of similar agents on a variety of substrata." Reference was made to the relatively nonselective manner in which some plant lectins agglutinated red cells from a number of different species and to the relatively selective manner in which other plant lectins reacted. Landsteiner pointed out that the nonselective agglutinations were "occasionally referred to in the literature as non-specific." We now know that nearly all lectins have a high affinity and structural specificity for one sugar or another, a fact lucidly presented by Boyd (1962), and that the question of selectivity or nonselectivity rests with the distribution of these sugars among the various types of red cells. A lectin whose binding sites happen to complement those of a common ubiquitous substance such as glucose is no less structurally or affinitively specific than one whose reactivity is restricted to a few compartments of the total field, such as lima bean lectin, which is restricted to A-type red cells. Thus, a lectin with a very broad compartmental cross-reactivity for a wide range of red cell species would be nonselective but hardly nonreactive. Clearly, the term "nonspecific" should not be used in view of the high degree of structural (and possible affinitive) specificity that is in evidence. Moreover, Landsteiner's introductory definition for deciding matters of specificity obviously cannot at the same time embrace structural and compartmental types. Kabat's rule forbids it.

The problem of deciding between nonselectivity and nonreactivity to describe the notorious, low-level, broad-spectrum, compartmental cross-reactivity of "normal" immunoglobulins for tissues, cells, and cell components is not so easily settled. It is now well understood that there is no such entity as a "normal" immunoglobulin devoid of reactivity for something. All "normal" immunoglobulins contain combining sites and are in essence antibodies in search of complementary ligands. Since much less than a nanogram of uninstructed antibody per milliliter of serum (less than one part per ten million) may be expected to react with any particular ligand, as one might safely project from the data presented by Haimovich et al. (1970), it is clear that at the usual levels of detection normal globulins would be considered nonreactive for the most part with structurally homogeneous antigens. The problem makes its appearance when a multiplicity of ligands exists within a compartment (as, for example, within a cell membrane fraction) that is used for immunological assay. When a particular tissue fraction adsorbs a relatively large quantity of "normal" globulin (one to ten parts per thousand) one has a difficult time deciding whether the so-called nonspecific effect is a case of nonreactivity with respect to binding sites or whether it involves actual binding of a highly heterogeneous mixture of multiple uninstructed antibodies with an equally heterogeneous mixture of ligands. Since polar forces, hydrogen bonds, and hydrophobic and charge interactions that do not directly involve binding sites may also be involved, and since these may also increase with the heterogeneity of adsorbing ligands, the answer is not immediately forthcoming. The problem will not be compounded in this paper, however, by use of the term "nonspecific"; to the contrary, where substantial "normal" immunoglobulin binding is encountered with wide-ranging compartmental cross-reactivity, the term "nonselective" will be used whether or not binding sites are involved, and the term "nonreactive" will be relegated to those cases in which binding of whatever nature is too weak or too insignificant to be a factor.

The focus of the remainder of this article is on antigenic distribution, not because the subject is important in itself apart from the other two facets of tissue immunology, but because it must be understood fully if antigenic architecture and the extent of reaction are also to be understood fully. The distribution analysis of microbial and cellular antigens is actually one of the oldest continuing immunological activities, arising as it did from the demands of infectious disease control, stimulated later by the problems inherent in blood transfusions, and currently carried along by the mutually exclusive requirements for rejection of malignancies and acceptance of healthy transplanted organs, tissues, and cells. Taking the form of classical typing techniques in whatever era it was or is practiced, the antigenic distribution analysis of red cells, leukocytes, bacteria, viruses, and tumors has been crucial to the successful classification of these antigenic systems. Other newer forms of distribution analysis can be described or devised, however, to widen the scope and to grasp the full potential of the distribution parameter.

Not all fields are compartmentalized to begin with, at least not in a form useful for experimental purposes. In fact, some of the most interesting and challenging of these require deliberate manipulation before the application of analytical antibody reagents. The familiar immunoelectrophoretic profiles of plasma proteins introduced by Williams and Grabar (1955) are a case in point. Another not so obvious example is the compartmentalization of allotypic specificities of the *a* and *b* loci in rabbit γG to Fd and L-chain regions, respectively (Feinstein, Gell, and Kelus, 1963; Gilman, Nisonoff, and Dray, 1964; Stemke, 1964; and Reisfeld, Dray, and Nisonoff, 1965).

It is the purpose of this work to call attention to and to examine critically three additional schemes of distribution analysis, ones with which the author has had some experience. All three have direct application to tissue immunology and all three involve the use of radiolabeled antibodies as an indicator of antigenic distribution. The first is the *in vivo* localization technique; the second is the multicompartment distribution analysis of tissue antigens subsequent to density-gradient ultracentrifugation; and the third is the technique of sequential adsorption analysis.

II. Distribution Analysis with Radioantibodies In Vitro and In Vivo

A. Simple Distribution Analysis *In Vivo* with Radioantibodies

1. Introduction

Nearly a quarter of a century ago Pressman and Keighley (1948) showed for the first time that antibody could be trace-labeled with radioiodine. In the same paper they showed that an antitissue antibody, when injected into the circulatory system of a laboratory animal, would actually localize in its tissues. This was the beginning of distribution analysis *in vivo* with radioantibodies. The work was prompted by the studies of Smadel (1936) on the nephrotoxic activity of antikidney antiserum and was a logical extension, retrospectively, of the reports by Masugi (1933) that had not yet come to the attention of the authors; thus, the kidney-antikidney system became the main target of study. During the next nine years a number of other organs in the rodent—liver, lung, placenta, aorta, lymph node, spleen, pancreas, adrenal, ovary (Pressman, 1957; Bale and Spar, 1957)—became the focal points for the localization of radioantibodies; nevertheless, the kidney remained the model for all normal tissue studies.

Localization of antibodies in tumors became the main thrust of the Pressman–Keighley technique during the decade, 1952–1962. It was explored first by Korngold and Pressman in New York, then by Bale and Spar in Rochester, Wissler and Flax in Chicago, Wong-Chia in Mexico City, and Day and Pressman in Buffalo (reviewed by Day, 1962, 1964, 1965). During the first part of the decade transplanted murine tumors were used, but these were later shown to be unsatisfactory by both the Buffalo and Rochester groups. The antibody that did localize in the transplants was found to be antifibrin, but no true antitissue antibody was ever knowingly observed. The Buffalo group, turning to induced hepatomas in rats, found that true antitissue antibodies would localize therein, and subsequently investigated the system further.

The emphasis in all the early localization work was upon specificity—kidney specificity, lung specificity, tumor specificity. In the present context the sought-for specificity would be called *compartmental,* depending as it did on the natural compartmentalization of the various target tissues as they lay interconnected *in vivo* by the circulatory system. The attainment of localization specificity, as measured by the Pressman–Keighley technique, obviously required measuring other tissue compartments for localizing antibody and hopefully finding them void of adsorbed antibody and free from compartmental cross-reaction. Since, in the assay of all crude antitissue radioantibodies, compartmental cross-reaction was universally encountered, the systematic search for specificity quickly became one of distribution analysis—establishing an initial distribution profile of a given radioantibody preparation and then either comparing it to the profiles of other antitissue antibodies or, after performing appropriate adsorption rituals upon the radioantibody itself, comparing the pre- and postadsorbed distribution profiles. Weighted localization in favor of the target organ was taken as evidence of the presence of specific antibody in the antiserum even when cross-reaction was not completely eliminated. In other words, Landsteiner's definition of specificity—the disproportional action (extent of localization) of a number of similar agents (radioantibody preparations) on a variety of substrata (various tissues) — was invoked.

Pressman and Eisen (1950), for example, reported that they had raised an antilung antiserum in rabbits whose immunoglobulin, when radioiodinated, would localize radioactivity not only in lung tissue but also in kidney, liver, brain, heart, and spleen tissues. In spite of this extensive cross-localization the labeled entity was said to contain antibodies specific for lung. It appeared to the investigators that since antikidney, antibrain, and antiheart radioantibodies did not appear to localize in lung tissue to any greater extent than antiovalbumin radioantibody (even though the antisera did localize in a number of other tissues to a much greater extent), whereas antilung radioantibody did localize in lung tissue as well as elsewhere over and above antiovalbumin, the case for specificity was established. An inspection of the tabulated data in this paper reveals, however, that there actually must have been a significant amount of various antitissue antibodies that localized in lung tissue (e.g., antikidney antibody at the end of six days), thus making it impossible to establish a strong case for antilung specificity on the basis of comparison with other antitissue radioantibody distribution profiles.

Subsequent papers in that early series attempted to resolve the question through comparison of antibody distribution profiles both before and after antibody adsorption with various tissues. Simple adsorption with kidney, as called for in the experimental design, was expected to remove compartmentally cross-reactive antilung antibody that reacted with kidney and to leave behind the compartmentally specific antilung antibody. The result would be a disproportionately affected distribution profile weighted in favor of the lung. Eisen, Sherman, and Pressman (1950) performed this test, felt they had removed more kidney-localizing than lung-localizing activity, and concluded that specific antilung antibody must therefore have been present (Table 1). Recalculation of the data into the accepted form (percentage of the injected radioactive dose remaining in the tissues per gram) reveals that what the authors had taken for induced lung-localizing activity in unadsorbed antilung radioantibody was more likely nonselective radioglobulin with an affinity for lung, activity that was also present in unadsorbed antiovalbumin radioantibody (Table 2). The apparent selective removal of antilung activity by adsorption with lung tissue, over

Table 1. Lung-localizing activity in unadsorbed antilung radioantibody, and its differential removal by adsorption with lung more than with kidney

Radioantibody Treatment	Radioactivity in tissues after three days (cpm/g)	
	Kidney	Lung
Unadsorbed	613	657
Adsorbed with kidney	160	357
Adsorbed with lung	100	150

Data from Eisen, Sherman, and Pressman, 1950.

and above that with that liver and kidney, was not proved, since the same adsorption experiments and subsequent distribution analysis were not carried out with antiovalbumin. The case for nonselective adsorption of the antilung radioglobulin in lung is made the stronger by consideration of the biological half-lives of localized radioantibodies determined by Eisen et al. Antilung antibody that had cross-localized in kidney tissue was found to have a long half-life of 25 days as compared with eight days for antiovalbumin, whereas both globulins disappeared from lung tissue at equal rates with half-lives of six days.

2. Distribution Analysis within a Tissue Compartment

The subtleties of the localization assay, however, require more than the simple control measures suggested above. The dual adsorption of antilung and control radioglobulins by lung tissue would, perhaps,

Table 2. Lung-localizing activity in unadsorbed antilung and unadsorbed antiovalbumin radioantibodies

Radioantibody preparation	Percentage of injected radioactive dose remaining per gram after three days		
	Liver	Kidney	Lung
Antilung	0.076	0.143	0.156
Antilung	0.091	0.159	0.156
Antilung	0.060	0.114	0.105
Antiovalbumin	0.045	0.037	0.111
Antiovalbumin	0.057	0.041	0.119

Recalculated from Eisen, Sherman, and Pressman, 1950.

have resolved the question of whole organ compartmental specificity versus nonselectivity, and seemingly would have satisfied the demands of experimental design, yet it would, by its very nature, have missed a very important point, one that was caught by Tamanoi et al. (1961) and beautifully described. Although, on a total organ basis, antilung and control radioglobulins were found to localize to similar extents in lung tissue in the same gross manner as a decade earlier, the distributions of the two proteins within the lung compartment were considerably different. Immunohistochemical technique revealed that the distribution of control radioglobulin was everywhere diffuse and not selective for any particular area, whereas antilung radioantibody had concentrated along alveolar walls.

Thus, it is not so much the extent to which a particular immunoglobulin localizes in a particular target organ that is interesting, but the manner in which it is distributed within the tissue.

An example from this author's laboratory illustrates the point even more graphically. In preliminary explorations to determine whether human brain tumors would act as zones of localization for radioantibodies (Day et al., 1965), it was recognized that the normal levels of plasma proteins in the tumors would be considerably higher than in normal brain tissue, and that the radioglobulin levels for both antibody and control proteins would also be higher. The first problem was to try to distinguish between tumor-localized radioantibody (specific or cross-reactive) and radioglobulin that was nonselectively localized in the tumors. The problem was further compounded by the fact that the tissues would not effectively be washed free of blood prior to assay; therefore, globulins would be present in an unbound state not only in the extracellular spaces but within the blood vessels as well. Indeed, it was not unexpected that out of seven different cases only one clear-cut case of tumor localization would be observed (over and above control protein) on the basis of the conventional expression for localized antibody (the percentage of the injected radioactive dose). The tissue-blood ratio (percentage dose in 1 g of tissue/percentage dose in 1 ml of blood), which normalizes for differences in disappearance rates of ^{125}I-labeled antibody and ^{131}I-labeled control proteins, although it did improve the positive localization score somewhat, was also far from satisfactory. However, when the biopsied tumor specimens were homogenized, compartmentalized into supernatant fluids and sedimentable portions by centrifugation, and assayed for radioactivity distribution between the two phases, a striking difference between the distribution profiles of radioantibody and radiocontrol was obtained in every single case (Table 3).

The sedimentable portion of a brain-tumor homogenate could be further subdivided into two layers and separated by repeated low-speed centrifugation ($100 \times g$). The bottom stromal layer was collagen-rich; the middle parenchymal layer, collagen-poor; the top supernatant fluid, also collagen-poor. In the case of biopsied specimens, containing localized ^{125}I-antibody and ^{131}I-control globulins, the distribution of radioactivity was established among the three layers and demonstrated that some antibodies favored the stromal (blood vessel) fraction (Table 4), others the parenchymal (Table 5), while control proteins routinely remained primarily in the soluble, protein-rich, supernatant fluids.

To show whether the antitumor antibodies were compartmentally specific for tumor, as opposed to normal tissues, or were actually compartmentally cross-reactive in the human, it was necessary to approach the problem indirectly since, of course, normal tissue levels of trace amounts of radioglobulins would be unknown. The test antibody was divided into two portions, one of which was labeled with ^{125}I, the other with ^{131}I. The ^{125}I-labeled antibody was administered in the usual manner via the internal carotid artery, the ^{131}I-labeled antibody via the brachial vein far removed from the tumor. No clue was offered by the percentage of the injected radioactive dose remaining in the tumor at the time of biopsy, nor was the tissue-blood ratio revealing. The compartmental distribution based upon the simple centrifugation technique, however, told the story (Table 6). Whatever else was true, it was clear that very little of the remotely administered antibody ever reached the tumor and must have been either removed by cross-reaction with normal tissues or (as we now suspect) neutralized by circulating tumor antigens.

The compartmentalization of tissue-localized radioglobulins into the various sedimentable fractions of a tissue homogenate is a hazardous procedure with respect to interpretation unless there is some control, some index, to indicate that the labeled globulin had actually localized *in vivo* before homogenization rather than *in vitro* after homogenization but before laboratory compartmentalization, i.e., centrifugation. This consideration requires yet a different mode of dis-

Table 3. Compartmentalization of *in vivo* localized radioantibodies in biopsies of human brain tumors by low-speed centrifugation of homogenates.

Tumor number	Percentage of injected dose localized in biopsy[a]		Tissue-blood ratio[b]		Percentage of localized dose sedimented[c]	
	^{125}I-antibody	^{131}I-control	^{125}I-antibody	^{131}I-control	^{125}I-antibody	^{131}I-control
9	10.35	1.47	2.22	0.34	ND	ND
28	2.31	2.77	0.90	0.65	58	13
36	0.25	4.67	2.14	0.87	71	9
43	1.63	2.37	0.52	0.57	100	6
56	0.82	0.73	0.63	0.26	100	9

Data from Day et al., 1965.

[a] $10^{-3}\%$ injected dose/g wet wt biopsy.

[b] Percentage of injected dose per gram of biopsy/percentage of injected dose per millileter of blood.

[c] Percentage of the radioactivity in the biopsied specimen that remains with sedimented portion after homogenate centrifugation.

Table 4. The stromal (blood vessel) fraction of human brain tumors as a zone of localization for radioantibodies

Fraction	Compartmentalized quantities			
	Dry wt[a]	Collagen[b]	^{131}I-control[c]	^{125}I-antibody[d]
Supernatant	39	0.0	87	42
Parenchymal	34	0.7	4	2
Stromal	27	99.3	9	56

Data from Day et al., 1965.

[a] 0.837 g total from 3.986 g wet wt.

[b] 17.6 mg total based on hydroxyproline assay.

[c] 2.77 millipercent injected radioactive dose/g wet wt.

[d] 2.31 millipercent injected radioactive dose/g wet wt.

Table 5. The parenchymal (cellular) fraction of human brain tumors as a zone of localization for radioantibodies

Fraction	Tumor No. 56[a]		Tumor No. 43[b]	
	^{131}I-control	^{125}I-antibody	^{131}I-control	^{125}I-antibody
Supernatant	91	0	94	0
Parenchymal	6	78	4	72
Stromal	3	22	1	27

Data from Day et al., 1965.

[a] 0.82 millipercent antibody ánd 0.73 millipercent control per g wet wt.

[b] 1.62 millipercent antibody and 2.37 millipercent control per g wet wt.

Table 6. Adsorption of remotely injected radioantibody before reaching human brain tumor No. 27; a test for compartmental cross-reactivity when only specific biopsied target is available for measurement

Fraction	Injection near target[a] ^{125}I-antibody	Injection remote from target[b] ^{131}I-antibody
Supernatant	0	85
Parenchymal	76	12
Stromal	23	3

Data from Day et al., 1965.

[a] Intracarotid artery; biopsy contained 0.304 millipercent/g wet wt.

[b] brachial vein; biopsy contained 0.342 millipercent/g wet wt.

tribution analysis of which there are many variations. The presence in brain tumors of a plasma gradient (descending from a high value at the point of the entering blood supply down to a low value at the most distal end where invasion of normal brain cortex begins) suggested a particular control for these particular situations. If antibody globulin were present as a nonreacting passive plasma protein before biopsy and were to be adsorbed to tumor tissue only after homogenization, then there would be no change in the distribution profile between sedimentable and nonsedimentable portions as one proceeded along the gradient from one piece of tumor to the next. A decided shift in distribution did, in fact, occur in our studies (Table 7) and assured us that we were not misinterpreting the localization data. In tumor No. 36, the example presented here, the tissue-blood ratio diminished from 2.6 to 0.7 along the plasma gradient, but as it did so the amount of sedimentable antibody radioglobulin increased from 45% to 90% and then decreased again to 72%, this while the sedimentable control protein fluctuated only slightly about a mean value of 9–10%.

The simple examples of gross compartmentalization of localized radioantibody between two or three phases on the basis of sedimentability illustrate the point but do not resolve real questions concerning actual cellular and subcellular elements involved in localization. The approach through multicompartment distribution analysis is required.

Table 7. A test to demonstrate radioantibody adsorption *in vivo* before homogenization as opposed to radioantibody adsorption *in vitro* after homogenization but before centrifugation. Use of the plasma gradient in human brain tumor No. 36.

Plasma gradient[a]	Sedimented radioactivity	
	^{125}I-antibody	^{131}I-control
2.57	45	9
2.48	60	7
2.26	64	8
2.14	67	7
1.92	67	10
1.88	76	8
1.38	90	8
0.93	86	12
0.70	82	8
0.69	72	16

Data from Day et al., 1965.

[a] Indicated by tissue-blood ratio in each small tumor piece; top piece nearest feeding blood vessel, bottom piece most distal to feeding blood vessel and nearest normal brain.

B. Multicompartment Distribution Analysis *In Vitro* and *In Vivo* with Radioantibodies

1. Introduction

What has been gained from our experience with brain tissue, as recounted in this section, is not so specialized that it does not apply to other tissue systems. There are, to be sure, unique situations that have no counterpart, but overall the brain, as a model for general tissue systems, is certainly no less satisfactory than the classical biochemical model, the liver, or the model of early localization studies, the kidney. Moreover, the enormous technical difficulties involved in brain research are not so much a matter of kind but of degree.

2. *The Partitioning Effect*

An earlier technique (Day et al., 1958) for the measurement of radioantibody adsorption *in vitro* by so-called insoluble tumor sediments was applied to brain sediments, but it was soon found that there were unusual properties in the brain adsorption system that required investigation and control before a satisfactory quantitative method could be developed (Day and Lassiter, 1967).

Insoluble hamster brain sediment was operationally defined as that material from a 10% (w/v) brain homogenate at pH 8, 4°C, and 0.15 ionic strength that persistently sedimented at $100 \times g$ in 10 min with repeated washings (about eight times) until the spectrophotometric measurements of the supernatant fluids at 280 mμ became negative for protein. Adsorptions of constant amounts of antibrain and control radioglobulins with varying quantities of insoluble brain sediment at 25°C for 1 hr in a constant volume of suspension medium resulted in what appeared to be a classical adsorption isotherm for radioantibody binding (Figure 1). The sediments, after centrifugation at $1500 \times g$ for 20 min and four centrifugal washings, reached a maximum adsorption value of 6% for the radioantibody, 1% for the radiocontrol, i.e., 5% for selective adsorption due to antibody, and 1% for nonselective uptake. The combination of 25 μg of antibody radioglobulin with 3 mg of insoluble sediment appeared to satisfy the conditions of equivalence.

By using 500 μg of sediment in 600 μl of suspension medium, one knew from the adsorption isotherm of Figure 1 that 3% of the antibody radioglobulin would be removed from 25 μg of the crude whole γG. Presumably 3% additional radioglobulin would remain in the supernatant fluid, representative of the unbound antibody portion. One could also presume that the more radioglobulin that was used, keeping antigen constant, the smaller percentage of it that would be adsorbed in this apparent region of antibody excess. Moreover, adsorption of supernatant fluids by additional sediment should result in uptake of the remaining unbound antibody. On the contrary, a fairly constant level of antibody globulin (3%) was adsorbed regardless of the amount of radioglobulin added, varying from 6 μg to 400 μg, and a uniformly constant level of antibody globulin (1%) was adsorbed from the resultant supernatant fluids in all cases (Figure 2). The result was strikingly analogous to the distribution law in physical chemistry in which the

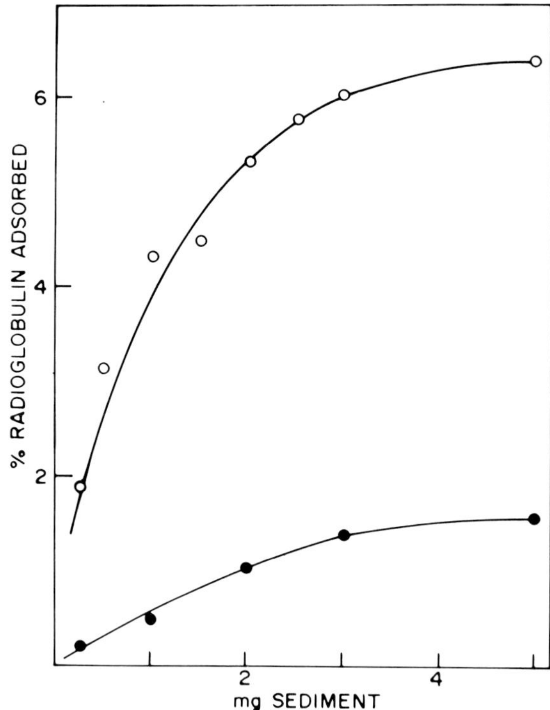

Fig. 1. Adsorption of 25- μg portions of ^{125}I-labeled antibrain antibody globulin *(open circles)* and ^{125}I-labeled normal glogulin *(closed circles)* by varying amounts of brain sediment in volumes of 600 μl. (From Day and Lassiter, 1967.)

partitioning of a solute between two immiscible phases depends on the relative proportions of the two phases to each other but is independent of solute concentration. Assuming the law to be operative in the present instance, the two phases could only be the solid sediment phase and the liquid medium phase. The observed substance subject to partitioning would, of course, be the labeled immunoglobulin, but the only way to account for the effect would be to assume that antigen in the sediment was in reality the partitioned entity, that it was actually being extracted at the same time that antibody was being adsorbed, that the amount of antigen extracted, by distribution law, would depend upon sediment-volume ratios, and that the distribution of labeled antibody between the two phases would reflect the distribution of antigen.

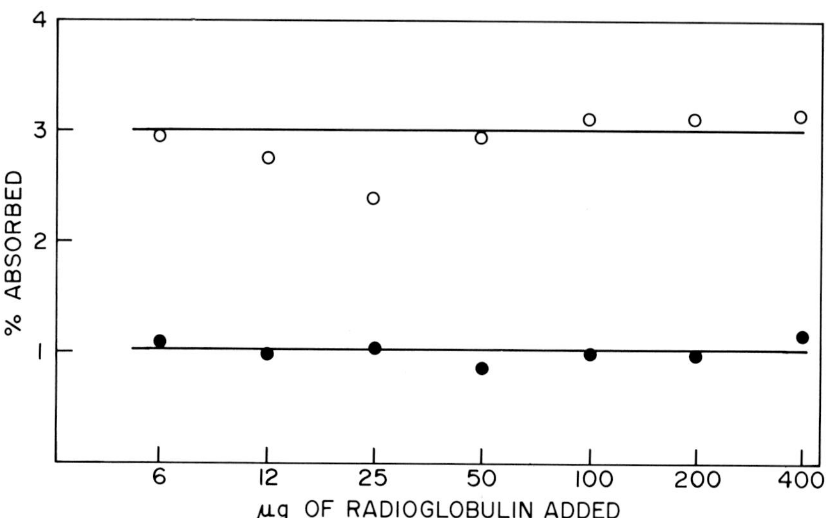

Fig. 2. Adsorption by varying amounts of ^{125}I-labeled antibrain antibody globulin by 500- μg portions of brain sediments in volumes of 600 μl *(open circles)*. Adsorption of supernatant fluids of the first adsorption tests by additional 500- μg portions of brain sediment *(closed circles)*. (From Day and Lassiter, 1967.)

With ^{125}I-antibody kept at 25 μg and brain sediment at 500 μg, the volume of the medium was varied from 75 μl to 1400 μl in the adsorption procedure at 25°C. The four successive washes in each case were made with 1000 μl borate-buffered NaCl at 4°C, pH 8, and ionic strength of 0.15. A peak adsorption of 6.7% was obtained at the smallest volume, a low adsorption of 1.9% at the largest volume (Figure 3). Thus, it was evident that a partitioning was indeed involved. The inverse relationship between sediment and volume was firmly established by the linear relation between the log of the sediment-volume ratio and the percentage of antibody adsorbed (Figure 4).

That the most critical point in the partitioning of antigen occurred during the incubation time of sediment-antibody adsorption rather than during washing was established in a number of ways: the incubation of sediment prior to its use in adsorption resulted in the release of 30% of sediment nitrogen into the supernatant fluid phase; the adsorption of antibody by sediment in a small volume and resuspension in a larger volume also resulted in the loss of adsorbed radioactivity to the su-

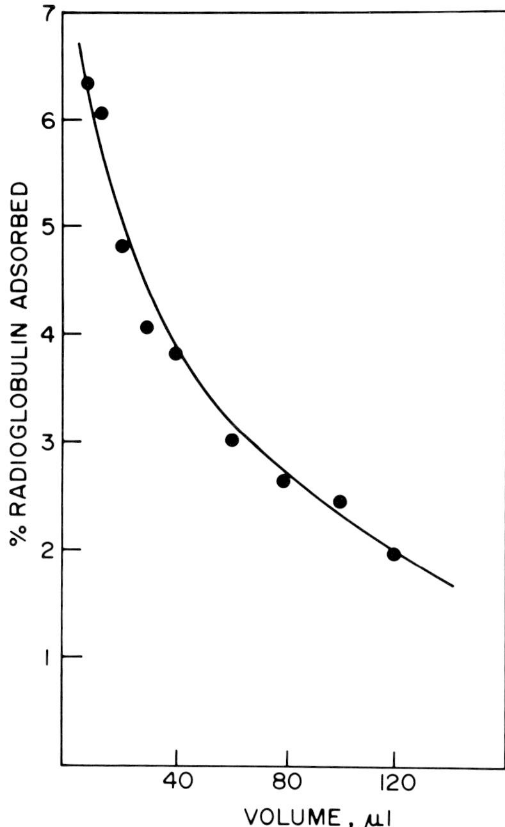

Fig. 3. Adsorption of 25- μg portions of ^{125}I-labeled antibrain antibody globulin by 500- μg amounts of brain sediment in varying volumes. (From Day and Lassiter, 1967.)

pernatant phase (the released antibody in this case was shown to be complexed with antigen and not available for adsorption or for agar gel immunodiffusion); and the distribution analysis of radioglobulin in the initial supernatant fluid and the four wash fluids (in which the sediment-volume ratio was high during incubation and low during washing) showed the usual diminution in serial wash fluid radioactivity (typical of the washing process) rather than maintenance of high wash fluid radioactivity (indicative of extraction).

An attempt was made to determine a partition coefficient for the phenomenon. However, antigenic heterogeneity within the sediment

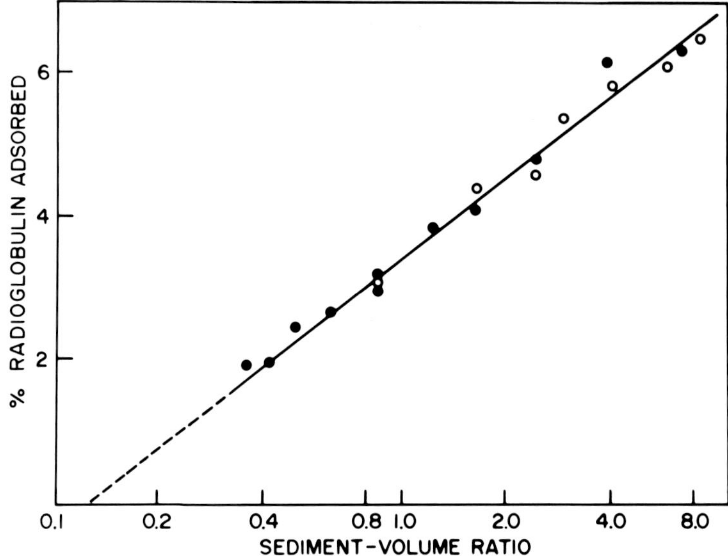

Fig. 4. Adsorption of 25- μg portions of ^{125}I-labeled antibrain antibody globulin as a logarithmic function of the brain sediment-fluid volume ratio (μg/ μl). *Open circles,* data from Figure 1; *closed circles,* data from Figure 3. Line extrapolates to a sediment-volume ratio of 12.5 μg/100 μl for 0% adsorption. (From Day and Lassiter, 1967.)

made precise measurements impossible and estimated values meaningless. Since certain antigenic moieties were more extractable than others, heterogeneity among individual distribution coefficients was to be expected. Nevertheless, all entities remained intact as readily sedimented composite antigen when the sediment-volume ratio was kept high. Now it was apparent that the seemingly antibody excess region, displayed previously by 25 μg of radioglobulin in the presence of 500 μg of brain sediment, was in reality an antigen excess region. (In fact, as subsequently determined by complement isofixation curves of the type described by Rapport and Graf (1967), the composite equivalence point for 25 μg of any of the individual rabbit antibrain radioglobulins was routinely less than 100 μg of brain sediment.) When tested in triplicate at either the 25-μg or the 5-μg level against 500 μg of brain sediment in 150-μl volumes, antibody radioglobulins were found to adsorb to the same extent, 5.4%, and the control radioglobulins at the two levels likewise adsorbed to the same extent, 0.5% (Table 8). Distribution analysis showed that the fourth wash in each test contained negligible amounts of radioactivity and was truly a wash, not an antigen extract. The success of the technique made it possible subsequently to apply sequential adsorption analysis *in vitro* to the analysis of various subcellular fractions of brain and the antibodies against them (cf. Section II, C). The phase-partitioning effect itself also suggested an alternative method of analysis — immunozoning in density gradients and multicompartment distribution analysis of radioglobulins along the gradient.

3. Immunozoning

The approach taken here is not to limit the partitioning effect but rather to take advantage of it and to extend it further (Day and Lassiter, 1969). The quantitative aspects of this particular new method depend on and serve to illustrate the more general concept embodied in multicompartment distribution analysis (MCDA). Radioantibody and brain sediment are reacted together in the typical manner except that they are layered over a sucrose density gradient instead of at the bottom of a tube. After incubation the reaction mixture is centrifuged, the gradient is fractionally separated, and the radioactivity distribution is determined. What portion of radioactivity in each fraction (i.e., compartment) can be taken as antibody and what portion as nonselective immunoglobulin is determined by incorporating normal globulin, with a different radioactive label, into the same reaction mixture. *It is not sufficient to use parallel tubes for the normal globulin distribution analysis, since the interaction of antibody with antigen will change its own density gradient profile in a manner not really parallel to a separate control tube and will produce an unmatched distribution.* Similarly, it is crucial to eliminate $C'1$ components from the immunoglobulins in order to avoid analytical complications arising from the binding of radioactive $C'1q$ to the compartmentalized antigen-antibody complexes.

The paired label (Pressman, Day, and Blau, 1957) and triadic label (Day, Planinsek, and Pressman, 1961) were developed to help

Table 8. Triplicate adsorption analysis of antibrain and normal radioglobulins at two different levels by 500 μg brain sediment in 150 μl[a]

Amount of radioglobulin	Brain fraction containing radioglobulin	Compartmentalization of total radioglobulins during adsorption (%)					
		Normal radioglobulin			Antibrain radioglobulin		
	Supernatant	89.9	92.3	88.1	86.0	85.3	84.8
	First three washes	9.6	7.2	11.4	8.4	9.4	9.5
25 μg level	Fourth wash	0.1	0.1	0.1	0.1	0.2	0.3
	Brain sediment	0.4	0.4	0.4	5.5	5.1	5.4
	Supernatant	89.1	89.6	89.3	85.2	86.4	86.2
	First three washes	10.2	9.7	9.9	8.6	8.0	7.8
5 μg level	Fourth wash	0.2	0.2	0.3	0.3	0.2	0.2
	Brain sediment	0.5	0.5	0.5	5.9	5.4	5.8

Data from Day and Lassiter, 1967.

[a] Adsorption in 13×10 mm tubes, 30 min, room temperature, gentle swirling, 50–50 buffered saline (pH 8)—normal rabbit serum; washings by centrifugation at $1500 \times g$ in 500 μl buffered saline; antibrain radioglobulin labeled with 131 nCi/ μg, normal with 154 nCi/ μg.

correct for the nonselective binding of normal or nonsense immuno-globulins in the adsorption analysis of tissue-localizing radioantibodies. Accordingly, it was held that if antibody globulin was labeled with one iodine isotope and normal globulin with another, the percentage uptake of the antibody radioglobulin could be corrected for the normal globulin in it by subtracting the percentage uptake of the other labeled, strictly normal, globulin. The net value, it was said, could then be attributed completely to antibody itself. Although net values obtained by this simple calculation have often provided fairly close approximations to real values for antibody, they are based on an assumption, neither always in evidence nor always valid, that the ratio of percentage antibody globulin $(Ab + N)$ to percentage normal globulin (N) in a compartment void of reacting antibody is 1.00. Identification of a compartment free from reacted antibody is crucial to MCDA. It is also crucial to the correct mathematical treatment of any paired-label data.

The concepts of simple paired-label analysis on the more extended MCDA depend on one assumption: the distribution of nonselective globulin (n) among compartments is the same whether the entity comes from the antiserum globulin or from the control globulin. The assumption is conservative with respect to antibody adsorption, since it does not allow overestimation. To the extent, however, that a particular control globulin actually contains binding activity, the assumption permits underestimation. Only by experience with a number of control globulins will one know what normally to expect. Given this assumption, consider two globulins, P and Q, in which P contains only nonselective binding components while Q contains selectively binding antibody in addition. P and Q are labeled and mixed, reacted with antigen, and compartmentalized by some procedure that will produce at least one compartment that contains no selectively bound antibody but does contain nonselective components. Let X be the compartment devoid of reacted antibody and let Y represent all other compartments containing reacted antibody. The nonselective distribution coefficient, v, that represents the manner in which nonselective globulin is distributed between X and Y, is obtained from the manner in which P is divided, i.e.,

$$v = P_Y/P_X.$$

The nonselective portion of Q is distributed the same way such that

$$\nu = P_Y/P_X = Q_{YN}/Q_X.$$

It then follows that since

$$Q_{Ab} = Q_Y - Q_{YN}$$

it is also true that

$$Q_{Ab} = Q_Y - \nu Q_X.$$

Since in distribution analysis one deals with the fractional amount of the total that is distributed rather than absolute amounts, one needs a conversion coefficient that can be obtained from the nonselective distribution of the control protein and applied to the distribution of the antibody. The fractional amount of antibody in total Q is given by the ratio Q_{Ab}/Q. Since total Q is the same whether expressed as $Q_{Ab} + Q_N$ or as $Q_X + Q_Y$, it follows that

$$\frac{Q_{AB}}{Q} = \frac{Q_Y}{Q_X + Q_Y} - \frac{\nu Q_X}{Q_X + Q_Y},$$

$$\frac{Q_{AB}}{Q} = \frac{Q_Y}{Q_X + Q_Y} - \frac{(P_Y/P_X)Q_X}{Q_X + Q_Y},$$

$$\frac{Q_{Ab}}{Q} = \frac{Q_Y}{Q_X + Q_Y} - \frac{Q_X}{Q_X + Q_Y} \cdot \frac{P_X + P_Y}{P_X} \cdot \frac{P_Y}{P_X + P_Y},$$

$$\frac{Q_{Ab}}{Q} = \frac{Q_Y}{Q_X + Q_Y} - \eta \frac{P_Y}{P_X + P_Y}.$$

As can be seen, η is a coefficient given by the ratio of the fractional amounts of antiserum globulin and control globulin in the antibody-empty compartment. Through its use the fractional amount (percentage) of nonselective control serum globulin in any antibody compartment can be converted to the fractional amount of nonselective antiserum globulin that is contained in that same antibody compartment. When $\eta = 1.00$, the equation becomes the net value calculation of former paired-label usage, and only when $\eta = 1.00$ is the former method of calculation valid.

Letting the number of compartments containing antibody be multiple (1 through n), the multicompartment distribution analysis profile is given by

$$\frac{Q_{Ab}}{Q} = \frac{Q_1 + Q_2 + \cdots + Q_n}{Q} - \eta \frac{P_1 + P_2 + \cdots + P_n}{P},$$

and the fractional amount of total antibody in any given compartment n is given by

$$\frac{Ab_n}{Q} = \frac{Q_n}{Q} - \frac{\eta P_n}{P}.$$

4. *Immunozoning by Low-Speed Centrifugation after Adsorption* In Vitro

The application of MCDA to the interaction between 25 μg of antibrain radioglobulin (anti-B) and 250 μg of a crude brain sediment (fraction A, isopycnic in 15% sucrose) in the presence of 25 μg of a control radioglobulin is presented in Table 9. The whole mixture, contained in 75 μl, was layered upon a 6-ml sucrose density gradient, incubated in the cold overnight, and centrifuged at $1000 \times g$ for 90 min. The compartment chosen for the antibody void was the top 100 μl which was further diluted to 1 ml with saline and spun at $100,000 \times g$ for 60 min to produce a clear supernatant fluid. The ratio of ^{125}I-globulin to ^{131}I-control in this complex-free soluble fraction was used as the void conversion coefficient, η. The remainder of the gradient was unloaded from the top in ten 500-μl portions to form the

Table 9. Multicompartment distribution analysis of radioantibodies adsorbed *in vitro* to brain fraction A and compartmentalized by low-speed sucrose density centrifugation [a]

Gradient fraction	Percentage of sucrose (w/w) (5°C)	Tube A[b]				Tube B[b]				Tube C[b]			
		$Ab+N$ (^{125}I)	N (^{131}I)	N^d (^{125}I)	Ab (^{125}I)	$Ab+N$ (^{125}I)	N (^{131}I)	N^d (^{125}I)	Ab (^{125}I)	$Ab+N$ (^{125}I)	N (^{131}I)	N^d (^{125}I)	Ab (^{125}I)
1	14.5	55.93	49.09	49.09	0.00	56.86	50.13	50.13	0.00	51.34	45.16	45.16	0.00
2	15.8	30.17	30.83	26.48	4.35	26.96	26.86	23.77	3.09	34.50	34.41	30.35	4.06
3	16.0	5.38	6.35	4.72	1.63	4.75	5.69	4.19	1.50	3.13	3.74	2.75	0.99
4	16.2	2.74	3.36	2.40	0.96	2.76	3.56	2.43	1.13	5.70	6.01	5.01	1.00
5	16.8	1.98	2.95	1.73	1.22	2.97	4.11	2.62	1.49	1.63	2.58	1.43	1.15
6	18.2	0.93	1.43	0.82	0.61	1.49	2.04	1.31	0.73	0.99	1.44	0.87	0.57
7	20.3	1.54	2.86	1.35	1.51	2.70	3.88	2.38	1.50	1.63	3.44	1.43	2.01
8	24.0	0.59	1.15	0.52	0.63	0.37	0.82	0.33	0.49	0.33	0.57	0.29	0.28
9	28.1	0.15	0.36	0.13	0.23	0.37	0.65	0.33	0.32	0.18	0.89	0.16	0.73
10	34.0	0.41	1.39	0.36	1.03	0.55	1.91	0.48	1.43	0.49	1.56	0.43	1.13
11	43.0	0.10	0.13	0.09	0.04	0.10	0.18	0.09	0.09	0.03	0.14	0.03	0.11
12	54.0	0.08	0.10	0.07	0.03	0.12	0.17	0.11	0.06	0.05	0.06	0.04	0.02
Total		100.00	100.00	87.76	12.24	100.00	100.00	88.17	11.83	100.00	100.00	87.95	12.05

Data from Day and Lassiter, 1969.

[a] 25 μg of antibrain (*Ab*) radioglobulin (^{125}I), 25 μg normal (*N*) radioglobulin (^{131}I) and 250 μg brain fraction A in 75 μl layered on gradient, incubated overnight at 4°C, and centrifuged next day at $1000 \times g$ for 90 min.

[b] The letters A, B, and C designate individual tubes in the triplicate analysis.

[c] Fraction 1, 100 μl, diluted to 1 ml, spun 60 min at $100,000 \times g$, used to obtain void conversion coefficient η. Fractions 2 through 11 were 500 μl. Fraction 12 was 975- μl "cushion."

[d] Calculated from $\eta \times {}^{131}I - (N)$: $\eta_a = 49.09/55.93 = 0.8777$; $\eta_b = 50.13/56.86 = 0.8816$; $\eta_c = 45.16/51.34 = 0.8796$.

multicompartmented sediment and a bottom 975-μl portion to form the gradient "cushion." The analysis, performed in triplicate, showed that half of the antibody was confined to the three compartments immediately following the antibody-void compartment. The total antibody contained in all fractions was 12% of the ^{125}I-globulin, a value that was also obtained by the more conventional adsorption procedure.

When the same globulin, anti-B, was reacted with a different brain sediment, fraction C (isopycnic in 25% sucrose), an entirely different profile was obtained (Figure 5). Yet when a mixture of A and C fractions was reacted with anti-B or when A-anti-B and C-anti-B reaction mixtures were mixed and immediately centrifuged, an intermediate distribution profile was obtained. The total antibody adsorbed in all

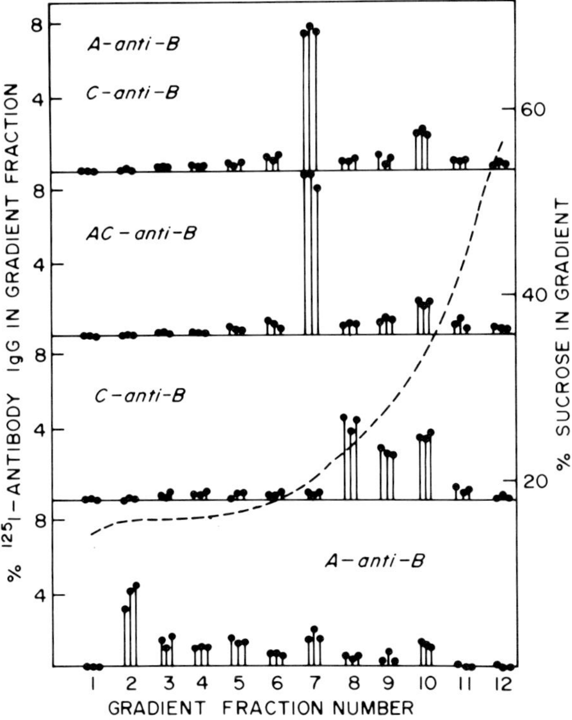

Fig. 5. Density gradient distribution profiles of radioantibodies in aggregates formed between antibrain antibodies and brain fractions. Corrected for nonselective adsorption by the method shown in Table 9. Triplicate analyses are shown. *Dashed line,* the sucrose density gradient for all four assays. (From Day and Lassiter, 1969.)

four types of assays was the same, 12% (Table 10), and was nondis-criminatory. One could conclude that antibodies in the main compartment of A-anti-B were compartmentally cross-reactive with antigens in the main compartment of C-anti-B and *vice versa,* since aggregates representing A-anti-B and C-anti-B formed one main large aggregate of intermediate density in the mixture. One other minor compartment (at 34%) in all four profiles was structurally noncross-reactive with the main compartment (e.g., with the one at 20% in the mixture) and was marked by its own antibody in all four distributions without any shift in density.

The separations that were obtained in this example of MCDA were the result of immunozoning of particles aggregated by antibodies and were obtained by low-speed centrifugation. The densities reached, however, were primarily the isopycnic indices of the particulate matter since the antibodies linking them, although much denser, were only a relatively small portion of the total, 3 μg of γG bound to 250 μg of sediment.

Table 10. Density gradient distribution profiles of aggregates formed between antibrain radioantibodies (anti-B) and brain fractions (A and C)

Densities in sucrose gradient (g/ml at 5°C)	Percentage of ^{125}I-labeled antibrain γG^a in aggregates formed between radioantibodies and brain fractions			
	A-anti-B	C-anti-B	AC-anti-B	A-anti-B + C-anti-B
< 1.062	0.00	0.00	0.00	0.00
1.062–1.065	3.83	0.00	0.00	0.00
1.066–1.070	3.69	0.76	0.54	0.60
1.071–1.089	2.31	0.51	8.99	8.03
1.093–1.127	0.89	6.63	1.06	0.86
1.131–1.209	1.28	3.86	2.03	2.01
> 1.210	0.04	0.16	0.18	0.04
Total	12.04	11.92	12.80	11.54

Data from Day and Lassiter, 1969.

[a] Corrected for presence of nonselective adsorption by multicompartment distribution analysis as in Table 9. The column for A-anti-B is the average of the three [125]I-*Ab* columns in Table 9. The other columns were obtained in the same manner.

5. *Immunozoning by Ultracentrifugation after Adsorption In Vivo*

In the case of adsorption experiments *in vivo* involving the localization of radioantibodies in brain after intravenous injection, the quantity of adsorbed radioantibody is far too small and in the presence of far too much antigen to favor aggregation. Thus, if methods of immunozoning and MCDA are to be used in the study of radioantibody distributions within brain after localization *in vivo,* high-speed centrifugation techniques must be incorporated (Day and Rigsbee, 1969).

Three rat brains (3 g wet wt) containing localized ^{125}I-labeled antibrain antibody (0.84 μg) and ^{131}I-labeled nonselective control globulin (0.11 μg) were homogenized, brought to 30 ml, and injected into the center of a B-XV zonal centrifuge rotor (that was spinning at 3,000 rpm and that was already loaded with a sucrose gradient). A 200-ml gradient overlay of light sucrose was then injected to move the homogenate into position. The rotor was increased to 20,000 rpm, run until a digital integrated $\omega^2 t$ value of 1.51×10^{10} had been reached (1 hr), slowed to 3,000 rpm, and pumped free of its gradient by displacement with 55% sucrose. The gradient, beginning with the lightest material, was passed through a recording spectrophotometer to plot light-scattering values of the compartmentalized brain homogenate before collection in 44 40-ml fractions. Each fraction was measured for density by refractometry and counted for its ^{125}I and ^{131}I radioactivity. The count rates were summed and recalculated in terms of 100%, with each fraction given a percentage of the ^{125}I and ^{131}I. Fraction 6 of the gradient (containing mainly soluble proteins which remained stationary during the centrifugation just beyond the gradient overlay), after dilution with saline, was centrifuged at $200,000 \times g$ for 1 hr to provide an antibody-free supernatant fluid that could be used as an antibody-void compartment. The ratio of percentage of ^{125}I to percentage of ^{131}I in that compartment was taken as the void conversion coefficient η from which the antibody distribution by MCDA was calculated. As shown in Table 11 and Figure 6, there were four major peaks of ^{125}I-antibody: one between 10% and 12% sucrose, one at 21.4% sucrose, one at 45.8% sucrose with a shoulder at 37.4%, and one at 52.6% sucrose. Of the localized γ G, 84.5% was present as antibody and 15.5% as nonselective immunoglobulin. The only peak of consequence in the normal profile was the initial one at 10.5% sucrose; minor peaks (e.g., at 32.6%

Table 11. Multicompartment distribution analysis of radioantibodies adsorbed *in vivo* in rat brain and compartmentalized by sucrose density zonal ultracentrifugation to an $\omega^2 t$ of 1.58×10^{10} radian²/sec

Zonal fraction	Density (g/ml at 5°C)	Relative absorbancy (280 mμ)	Percentage of [131]I — N	Percentage of [125]I — $Ab+N$	Percentage of [125]I — N^a	Percentage of [125]I — Ab^b
4	1.033	0.00	0.0	0.0	0.0	0.0
5	1.034	0.95	13.4	2.1	2.1	0.0
6[c]	1.043	1.47	35.5	13.3	5.5	7.8
7	1.048	1.04	6.8	8.4	1.1	7.3
8	1.051	0.76	1.9	5.4	0.3	5.1
9	1.059	0.19	1.5	3.6	0.2	3.4
10	1.063	0.86	1.4	2.4	0.2	2.2
11	1.068	1.52	1.3	2.3	0.2	2.1
12	1.074	2.61	1.3	2.5	0.2	2.3
13	1.079	4.33	0.6	2.1	0.1	2.0
14	1.087	5.42	1.2	2.2	0.2	2.0
15	1.091	6.84	1.4	9.9	0.2	9.7
16	1.097	6.27	1.5	2.5	0.2	2.3
17	1.102	5.67	2.1	1.3	0.3	1.0
18	1.106	4.52	1.4	1.0	0.2	0.8
19	1.112	4.32	1.3	0.8	0.2	0.6
20	1.115	3.18	0.6	1.2	0.1	1.1
21	1.120	2.80	0.6	0.8	0.1	0.7
22	1.123	2.57	0.6	0.9	0.1	0.8
23	1.127	1.85	1.3	0.9	0.2	0.7
24	1.129	1.76	0.7	1.1	0.1	1.0
25	1.131	1.90	0.6	1.1	0.1	1.0

26	1.132	2.33	0.7	1.2	0.1	1.1
27	1.134	2.42	1.3	1.2	0.2	1.0
28	1.135	6.84	2.0	0.6	0.3	0.3
29	1.137	8.37	4.7	0.8	0.7	0.1
30	1.144	12.03	4.7	0.8	0.7	0.1
31	1.158	4.56	2.6	3.5	0.4	3.1
32	1.186	2.09	2.0	5.3	0.3	5.0
33	1.213	0.38	1.2	10.4	0.2	10.2
34	1.233	0.10	0.6	2.5	0.1	2.4
35	1.238	0.05	0.5	1.3	0.1	1.2
36	1.246	0.00	1.6	0.8	0.3	0.5
37	1.251	0.00	0.6	4.9	0.1	4.8
38	1.255	0.00	0.5	0.9	0.1	0.8
39	1.260	0.00	0.0	0.0	0.0	0.0
40	1.263	0.00	0.0	0.0	0.0	0.0
		100.00	100.0[d]	100.0[e]	15.5	84.5 [f]

From Day and Rigsbee, 1969.

[a] $\eta \times \%\ ^{131}I\text{-}N$.

[b] $\%\ ^{125}I - \eta \times \%\ ^{131}I$.

[c] Centrifugation of fraction 6 at $200,000 \times g$ for 1 hr after dilution resulted in an antibody-void supernatant fluid. Ratio of percentage of ^{125}I to ^{131}I in supernatant was 0.1551. This was used as value for η.

[d] Equivalent to 0.011% injected radioactive dose of ^{131}I (1,039,201 c/10 min in three brains).

[e] Equivalent to 0.084% radioactive dose of ^{125}I (7,633,492 c/10 min in three brains).

[f] 84.5% of 0.084% leaves 0.071% as localizing dose in brain due to antibody and 0.013% as that due to normal globulin.

sucrose) followed the light-scattering profile indicative of nonselective surface adsorption on the subcellular particulate matter. The antibody peaking at 21.4% sucrose (the second peak) coincided with myelin. The first peak was associated with a fraction rich not only in soluble proteins but also in microsomes, synaptic vesicles, light myelin, and unaggregated cell-surface membranes; the third was heavily populated with mitochondrial elements, nuclei, and unidentifiable cell fragments, all contaminated with myelin; and the fourth contained only dense cell debris, collagen-rich material, and red cells. Synaptosomes at fractions 12 and 20, mitochondria at fraction 20, and synaptic membranes at fraction 26 accounted for only a small portion of the total antibody.

Because myelin was known to be a contaminant of nearly all fractions prepared in sucrose density gradients, it was not clear whether the compartmental analysis was indicative of a mixture of compartmentally specific antibodies against a variety of separately compartmentalized and structurally different antigens or of wide compartmental cross-reactivity of a single class of antibody-antigen interactions. In any case the profile was determined to be caused by antibody localized *in vivo* rather than *in vitro* after homogenization. The latter possibility was eliminated when it was found that different immunozoning profiles would be obtained if a brain homogenate was mixed with the original inoculum or with plasma taken from the animals at the time of assay.

Clearly one could conclude that this type of immunozoning would be most effective as soon as a better means of subcellular fractionation of whole brain by density gradient centrifugation was obtained and as soon as one learned how to raise antibodies with compartmental specificity. The method of sequential adsorption analysis, however, was felt to be a better means of evaluating progress in isolative techniques and in antibody production.

C. Sequential Adsorption Analysis

1. Introduction

The method of sequential adsorption analysis finds its origins in the classical work of Landsteiner and van der Scheer (1936) which was designed to contrast two types of cross-reaction. In the one "multiple

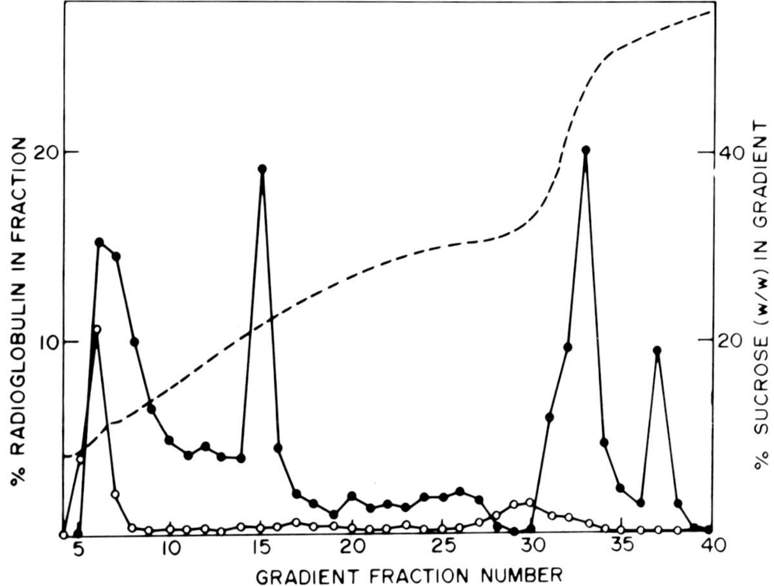

Fig. 6. Zonal ultracentrifuge profile of radioantibody localized in rat brain after intravenous injection. *Open circles,* nonselectively bound portion of antiserum globulin. *Closed circles,* selectively bound portion of antiserum globulin as determined by the method shown in Table 11. *Dashed line,* sucrose gradient. (From Day and Rigsbee, 1969.)

but related antibodies" were developed through the stimulus of a single determinant structure, and in this type "continued adsorption with a reacting heterologous antigen was often seen to exhaust the immune serum completely." In the other multiple antibodies were developed through the stimulus of multiple determinant structures on a given antigen, and in that event continued adsorption with a reacting heterologous antigen that lacks one or more of the multiple determinant structures would not exhaust the serum completely. The first type emphasized the chemistry of a given determinant and its spectrum of chemical analogues, i.e., what has been termed *structural* in this paper. The second type emphasized the distribution of a given set of chemical determinants among a number of different antigens in which any given determinant might be qualitatively present or absent, i.e., what has been termed *compartmental* in this paper. It is a characteristic of any group of homologous antibodies remaining after exhaustive adsorption with heterologous antigen that they are both structurally specific and compartmentally specific for their respective homologous antigenic determinants as distinguished from the heterologous adsorbing antigen. It is *not* necessarily characteristic, nor particularly common, that the cross-reactivity observed by this approach is dually structural and compartmental, since one may be specific and the other cross-reactive or *vice versa* and still be cross-reactive overall at all times. It is also obvious that the sequential adsorption technique makes no statement about degrees of affinity but rather distinguishes qualitatively between the presence and absence of a ligand (and absence means absence within the limits of detection and experimental error). The usefulness of the Landsteiner approach, through sequential adsorption to exhaustion, is its ability to differentiate between two antigenic structures, one of which contains a relatively high concentration of a given determinant or its analogues and the other of which contains little or none.

The present method of sequential adsorption analysis (Mickey et al., 1971; McMillan et al., 1971) makes use of primary binding not only for the adsorption and centrifugal removal of cross-reacting antibodies, but also for the subsequent measurement of the remaining specific ones. The early Landsteiner technique necessarily required a secondary analytical technique such as the precipitin reaction to test for remaining antibodies, and could assess the amount of cross-reacting antibody only by inference. The primary binding of radioantibodies to brain fractions, as developed into a quantitative method in this laboratory and applied to multicompartment distribution analysis, has been particularly well suited to the evaluation of the quantitative progress of the serial adsorption steps. In keeping with previous findings concerning the extractibility of particle protein in large volumes, the ratio of volume to antigen content in any particular adsorption is kept to a minimum (125 μl, 75 μg). As before, pseudoglobulin fractions of antiserum γG are used as the source of radioiodinated antibodies in order to avoid the adsorption of radiolabeled C$'$1q to antigen–antibody complexes.

2. The Method

All analyses are carried out in triplicate. The suspensions of subcellular brain particles (mitochondria, synaptosomes, myelin, synaptic membranes, etc.) in cold borate-buffered NaCl (pH 8, $\Gamma/2 = 0.1$ are measured out in 75-μg (and 75-μl) amounts (in terms of protein) into 13×100 mm culture tubes, centrifuged, and drained. Antibody pseudoglobulin labeled with [125]I (25 μg in 25 μl) and control pseudoglobulin labeled with [131]I (25 μg in 25 μl) are mixed, brought to 125 μl, and added to the first particle sediment in a given sequence. The radioglobulins and subcellular deposit are shaken for 20 min (tubes covered) at ambient room temperature and centrifuged. The supernatant fluids are removed by pipette and transferred to the next subcellular deposit in the sequence, the adsorption procedure is repeated, and so on until the final tubes in the sequence (from 4 to 8 steps later) are used. Meanwhile, each sediment tube in the sequence, after adsorption and removal of the supernatant, is washed three times with 250-μl amounts of ice cold buffer. The washes, the final supernatant fluid in the series, and all the washed sediments are counted for the presence of ^{125}I and [131]I. The percentage of immunoglobulin adsorbed by a tissue fraction at a given step is calculated from a knowledge of the total radioactivity used for adsorption. Since there is a loss of radioactivity at each step of the sequence resulting not only from antibody adsorption but also from nonselective adsorption and from nonreactive physical entrapment, the total radioactivity at each step must be readjusted. The adjustment is allowed since a wide range of antibody concentrations yields the same percentage adsorbed by excess antigen.

3. Nonselective Adsorption

During the first adsorption step "normal" globulins will react with various subcellular brain fractions to the extent of 0.5–2.5% of the total radioactivity. The actual amount varies from one "normal" globulin to the next (Table 12) within this range, and appears to be a characteristic set value for each globulin from one iodination to the next. During the second adsorption an additional 0.1–0.3% will react with brain sediments. In subsequent steps of the sequence the amounts of normal radioglobulin contained in the washed sediments can be accounted for on the basis of physical entrapment of nonreacting globulin. Thus, the lower limits of analytical precision can be set by testing exhaustively adsorbed normal globulins for their uptake in the various types of brain fractions (Table 13).

Because the first and second adsorption steps in a sequence vary somewhat from one normal globulin to the next, it is not known exactly how much of a particular antibody globulin adsorption must be attribut-

Table 12. Sequential adsorption analysis[a] of nonselective "normal" radioglobulins by rat tissue fractions

Step in sequence	Percentage of radioglobulin adsorbed at each step in sequence by brain fraction[b]				
	1	2	3	4	5
1	LM 1.36	BM 1.06	SY 2.24	LM 1.35	SY 0.89
2	LM 0.33	BM 0.24	SY 0.25	LM 0.20	SY 0.11
3	LM 0.21	BM 0.09	LM 0.38	SY 0.16	BM 0.05
4	BM 0.18	LM 0.07	LM 0.21	SY 0.22	BM 0.05
5	—	—	BM 0.16	BM 0.21	MY 0.12
Total	2.08	1.46	3.24	2.14	1.22

Data from Mickey et al., 1971.

[a] 25 μg of ^{131}I-labeled pseudo-γG + 75 μg of tissue fraction in 125 μl in first step supernatant fluids added to 75 μg of tissue fraction at each successive step; adsorptions at room temperature, 20 min.

[b] Average of three values in triplicate analysis; individual values in original paper; LM = liver mitochondria, BM = brain mitochondria, SY = brain synaptosomes, MY = brain myelin.

ed to nonselective adsorption. After the first two adsorptions there is a tenfold increase in precision. Whereas no conclusion should be drawn on antibody adsorptions smaller than 3% of the total radioactivity at the first adsorption and smaller than 0.5% at the next stage or (to be safe) even at the third step, antibody adsorptions greater than 0.3% of the total radioactivity at the fourth or subsequent stages have great significance.

Table 13. Extent of entrapment of nonreactive "normal" radioglobulins after exhaustive preadsorption by rat tissue fractions

Fraction	Percentage of radioglobulin remaining in fraction after four centrifugal washes
Liver mitochondria	0.08 ± 0.03
Brain mitochondria	0.10 ± 0.03
Brain myelin	0.14 ± 0.04
Brain synaptosomes	0.19 ± 0.07
Synaptic membranes	0.10 ± 0.03
Microsomes	0.10 ± 0.03

Data from Mickey et al., 1971.

4. Sequential Adsorption Analysis of Antisynaptosome and Antimyelin Radioantibodies

After a first and second adsorption of an antisynaptosome radio-globulin with liver mitochondria (Table 14), a portion of the globulin was shown to be compartmentally cross-reactive with myelin at the third step and cross-reactive with myelin in diminished amount at the fourth step. Adsorption with synaptosomes at the fifth step showed that a large amount of antibody still remained for reaction with the homologous antigen.

Table 14. Sequential adsorption analysis of ^{125}I-labeled antisynaptosome pseudo-γG by rat tissue fractions

Adsorption sequence		Percentage of radioglobulin adsorbed at each step in sequence by brain fraction[a]				
		Triplicate				
Step	Fraction	a	b	c	Avg.	Net[b]
1	Liver mitochondria	2.4	2.4	2.2	2.3	2.2
2	Liver mitochondria	0.6	0.6	0.5	0.6	0.5
3	Myelin	2.2	2.5	2.4	2.4	2.2
4	Myelin	1.6	1.7	1.6	1.6	1.5
5	Synaptosomes	9.8	10.4	10.0	10.1	9.9
	Total	16.6	17.6	16.7	17.0	16.3

Data from Mickey et al., 1971.

[a] 25 μg of ^{125}I-labeled pseudo-γG + 75 μg of tissue fraction in 125 μl in first step; supernatant fluids added to 75 μg of tissue fractions at each successive step; adsorptions at room temperature, 20 min.

[b] Corrected for entrapped globulins as given in Table 13.

After a first and second adsorption of antimyelin radioglobulin with synaptosomes and a third and fourth with brain mitochondria (Table 15), a significant amount of antibody remained for reaction with homologous myelin antigen at the fifth step.

These two assays and several others of similar nature were used to demonstrate that our improved procedures for synaptosome and myelin isolation from adult rat brain (Day et al., 1971; Mickey et al., 1971) resulted in the separation of relatively clean neuronal and

Table 15. Sequential adsorption analysis of ^{125}I-labeled antimyelin pseudo-γG by rat tissue fractions

| Adsorption sequence | | Percentage of radioglobulin adsorbed at each step in sequence by brain fraction[a] | | | | |
| | | Triplicate | | | | |
Step	Fraction	a	b	c	Avg.	Net[b]
1	Synaptosomes	7.7	6.9	7.3	7.3	7.1
2	Synaptosomes	2.9	2.4	2.7	2.7	2.5
3	Brain mitochondria	0.8	0.9	1.0	0.9	0.8
4	Brain mitochondria	1.0	0.6	0.8	0.8	0.7
5	Myelin	2.3	2.5	2.5	2.4	2.3
	Total	14.7	13.3	14.3	14.1	13.4

Data from McMillan et al., 1971

[a] See footnote *a*, Table 14.

[b] Corrected for entrapped globulin as given in Table 13.

glial-type fractions. After sequential adsorption to remove compartmentally cross-reactive entities, compartmental specificity was demonstrated.

Brain mitochondria could be distinguished immunochemically from liver mitochondria (Table 16) and also from synaptosomes (Table 17), although in the latter case the compartmental cross-reactivity was almost overwhelming. Synaptosomes could also be distinguished from isolated synaptic membranes and from brain mitochondria (Table 18), a finding that possibly suggested a conformational-type determinant in synaptosomes that was destroyed once synaptic membranes were prepared.

The cross-reactivity among purified myelins from a number of species could also be measured by the sequential adsorption technique. After an antirat-myelin radioglobulin had been adsorbed twice with rat liver mitochondria to remove nonselective immunoglobulins and heterologous antibodies against general species-type antigens, it was adsorbed twice with nonhomologous myelin from a given species other than rat and then was adsorbed three times with rat brain myelin. The results (Table 19) followed the expected evolutionary distance among

Table 16. Sequential adsorption analysis of ^{125}I-labeled antiserum pseudoglobulins raised to rat liver and brain mitochondria

Step in sequence	Net percentage of radioglobulin adsorbed in each step[a]	
	Anti-LM	Anti-BM
1	BM 3.47	LM 5.77
2	BM 0.99	LM 0.84
3	BM 0.63	LM 0.46
4	LM 1.12	BM 8.51
Total	6.21	15.58

Data from Mickey et al., 1971.

[a] Triplicate analysis averaged, net values corrected for entrapped globulins as in Tables 14 and 15; see reference for individual values. BM = brain mitochondria, LM = liver mitochondria.

Table 17. Sequential adsorption analysis of ^{125}I-labeled antibrain-mitochondria pseudo-γG by rat tissue fractions

Step in sequence	Net percentage of radioglobulin adsorbed at each step[a]	
	Anti-BM (113-8)	Anti-BM (113-8)
1	SY 8.8	LM 4.5
2	SY 2.5	LM 0.5
3	LM 2.0	SY 5.7
4	LM 0.4	SY 1.8
5	BM 1.6	BM 1.9
Total	15.3	14.4

Data from Mickey et al., 1971.

[a] Triplicate analysis averaged, net values corrected for entrapped globulins as in Tables 14 and 15; see reference for individual values. BM = brain mitochondria, LM = liver mitochondria, SY = synaptosomes.

Table 18. Sequential adsorption analysis of ^{125}I-labeled antisynaptosome pseudo- γG by rat brain fractions

Step in sequence	Net percentage of radioglobulin adsorbed at each step[a]	
	Anti-SY (131-8) (8-week antiserum)	Anti-SY (131-4) (4-week antiserum)
1	SM 8.7	SM 3.5
2	SM 5.5	SM 1.5
3	BM 6.6	BM 2.7
4	BM 2.0	BM 0.9
5	SY 4.5	SY 2.0
Total	27.3	10.6

Data from Mickey et al., 1971.

[a] Triplicate analysis averaged, net values corrected for entrapped globulins as in Tables 14 and 15; see text for individual values. SM = synaptic membranes, SY = synaptosomes, BM = brain mitochondria.

species; myelins from bullfrog and chicken brain were least cross-reactive and those from hamster and mouse were most cross-reactive. More reactive than chicken or frog myelin was the myelin from the immunized species, rabbit, which had a 50% cross-reactivity with rabbit antirat myelin.

Of course, we can now design radioantibodies with a degree of compartmental specificity higher than that of the crude radioantibodies used in the multicompartment distribution analysis shown in Figure 5. However, we must first cross one last hurdle in separation technique—the problem of the heterogeneous small membrane fraction (microsomes). Microsomes, for example, cross-react completely with myelin (Table 20). This is not surprising since glial-cell membranes and myelin fragments are known to appear in that fraction. The problem will be to design gradients such that these membrane fractions can be separated into compartments free from synaptic vesicles, endoplasmic reticulum, and other small particles. In light of the continued difficulty in compartmentalizing subfractions of brain tissue completely, the radioantibody zonal profile of Figure 6 is the more remarkable. The

Table 19. Sequential adsorption analysis of ^{125}I-labeled antirat-myelin pseudo- γG by myelins of various species after a double adsorption with liver mitochondria

Adsorption sequence	Average net percentage of globulin adsorbed at each step[a]				
	None	Bullfrog	Chicken	Rabbit	Guinea pig
3. Nonhomologous myelin	—	1.8	2.7	4.2	3.6
4. Nonhomologous myelin	—	0.5	1.0	0.8	1.4
5. Homologous rat myelin	6.4	5.2	4.5	3.4	3.2
6. Homologous rat myelin	2.3	1.8	1.3	1.1	1.4
7. Homologous rat myelin	1.3	0.7	0.5	0.5	0.4
Total nonhomologous	—	2.3	3.7	5.0	5.0
Total rat myelin	10.0	7.7	6.3	5.0	5.0
	Dog	Human	Neonatal rat	Hamster	Mouse
3. Nonhomologous myelin	3.9	4.4	3.9	5.1	5.8
4. Nonhomologous myelin	1.4	1.5	2.2	2.2	1.4
5. Homologous rat myelin	3.0	2.8	2.4	1.6	1.5
6. Homologous rat myelin	1.2	0.8	1.0	0.9	0.9
7. Homologous rat myelin	0.5	0.5	0.5	0.2	0.4
Total nonhomologous	5.3	5.9	6.1	7.3	7.2
Total rat myelin	4.7	4.1	3.9	2.7	2.8

Data from McMillan et al., 1971.

[a] Triplicate analysis averaged, net values corrected for entrapped globulins as in Tables 14 and 15; data normalized to a total of 10.0% adsorbed in steps 3 through 7; average total adsorption of all 30 assays (10 triplicates) was 9.65% in steps 3 through 7.

Table 20. Sequential adsorption analysis of ^{125}I-labeled antirat-myelin pseudo-γG by rat brain microsomes and myelin after a double adsorption with liver mitochondria

Adsorption sequence	Average net percentage of globulin adsorbed at each step[a]					
	Anti-MY 411		Anti-MY 411		Anti-MY 411	
3	MIC	7.7	MY	6.1	SY	2.8
4	MIC	1.9	MY	2.0	SY	0.8
5	MY	0.4	MY	0.8	MIC	4.2
6	–	–	MIC	1.1	MIC	1.8
7	–	–	–	–	MY	0.4
Total		10.0		10.0		10.0

Data from McMillan et al., 1971.

[a] Triplicate analysis averaged, net values corrected for entrapped globulins as in Tables 14 and 15; data normalized to a total of 10.0% adsorbed in steps 3 through 7; average total adsorption overall was 9.05% for the three different assays.

myelin-localized antibody peak was readily distinguished in spite of the compartmental cross-reactivity between myelin and the small particle fraction.

D. The Kinetics of Radioantibody Localization *In Vivo*

1. Introduction

The kinetics of *in vivo* localization with respect to both the rate of localization of injected antibody and the disappearance rate of antibody once localized suggest additional ways in which compartmentalization can be viewed and distribution analysis can be applied.

2. Rate of Localization

In the measurement of the rate of localization of antikidney radio-antibody in kidney and liver (Blau et al., 1957) the rate of blood flow through the organs and the efficiency with which the organs removed the radioantibody from the circulation upon each pass were important factors. An equation for multicomponent localizing entities was envisioned, and the analysis of experimentally derived curves for kidney and liver was made accordingly.

Each localizing radioantibody component, $a, b, c, \ldots n$, that reached a target organ was visualized as requiring several passes before it would be adsorbed *in vivo* 100%. As long as the concentration of such components was kept considerably below the amount needed for saturation of available ligands in the target organ, the adsorption efficiency for each component, $k_a, k_b, k_c, \ldots, k_n$, could be considered constant. With knowledge of the fraction, f, of the total blood volume that flowed through the organ per minute and of the time, t, at which measurements were made after injection, the percentage of the initial localizing activity still remaining in the circulation, %ILA, could be compartmented as follows:

$$\%\text{ILA} = A \exp\left(-k_a ft\right) + B \exp\left(-k_b ft\right)$$
$$+ C \exp\left(-k_c ft\right) + \ldots + N \exp\left(-k_n ft\right).$$

The coefficients $A, B, C, \ldots, N$ would be the initial percentage of each component in the injected dose such that

$$A + B + C + \cdots + N = 100\%.$$

For one particular antikidney radioglobulin the curves (Figures 7 and 8) suggested a two-component system in both kidney and liver, and the two-component equations that best fitted the data were:

$$\text{kidney:} \quad \%\text{ILA} = 79 \exp\left(-0.17t\right) + 21 \exp\left(-0.007t\right),$$
$$\text{liver:} \quad \%\text{ILA} = 80 \exp\left(-0.35t\right) + 20 \exp\left(-0.021t\right).$$

Analysis of the curves according to the factors listed above revealed that there were two major classes of kidney-localizing components and two major classes of liver-localizing components:

kidney: component a_K, 79% of the kidney-localizing antibody that is adsorbed with an efficiency of 70% as it flows through the kidney; component b_K, 21% of the kidney-localizing antibody that is adsorbed with an efficiency of 3%;

liver: component a_L, 80% of the localizing antibody that is adsorbed with an efficiency of 90% as it flows through the liver; component b_L, 20% of the localizing antibody that is adsorbed with an efficiency of 6%.

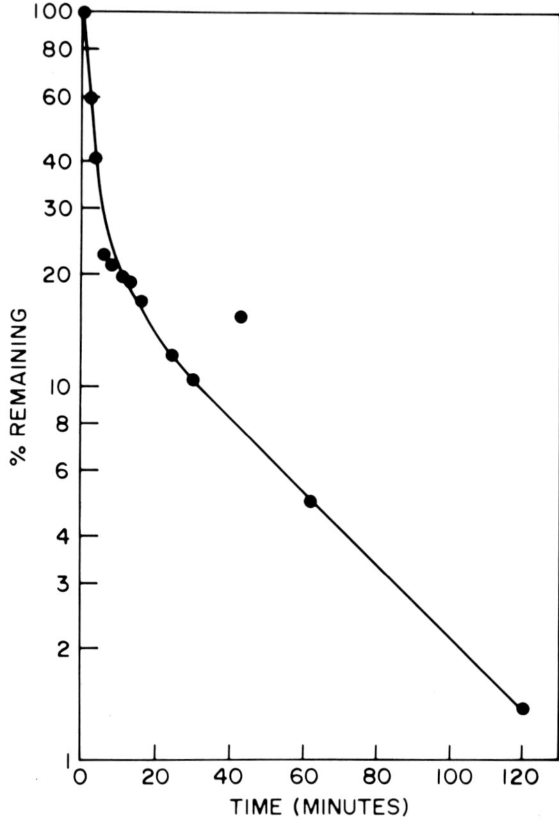

Fig. 7. Rate of localization of liver-localizing radioantibodies from an antikidney serum after intravenous injection in rats. (From Blau, Day, and Pressman, 1957.)

It was established that the curves were not dose dependent and, therefore, that the adsorption efficiencies could be considered constant. The first of the two classes of antigens in each organ was obviously a vascular component in relatively high concentration in direct contact with the blood. The second was thought to be either a different vascular antigen in very low concentration or a tissue antigen somewhat removed from the vascular bed.

Where competition exists among tissues for localization of antibodies in a mixture it appears that the rates of localization in the various tissues must be known in order for us to provide a more complete picture of the observed compartmental cross-reactions.

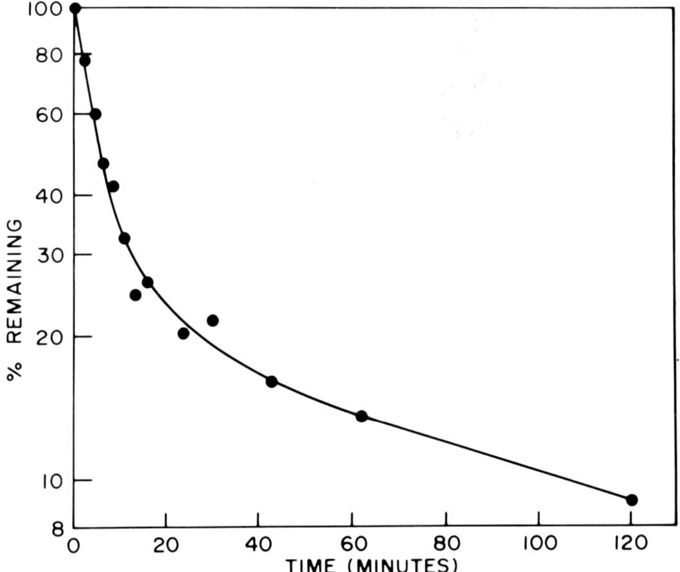

Fig. 8. Rate of localization of kidney-localizing radioantibodies from an antikidney serum after intravenous injection in rats. (From Blau, Day, and Pressman, 1957.)

3. Stability of Radioantibodies Once Localized

Radioactivity in kidneys of mice that had received radioiodinated antikidney antibodies was reported to have the extremely long biological half-life of 20 days, as compared with 2.3 days in blood (Pressman, 1949). The data, when reevaluated by the method of least squares, give the somewhat shortened half-life of 16 days, but there is no question about the apparent stability of the localized antibody. Antirat-kidney antibodies labeled with radioactive $[^{131}I]$-p-iodobenzoyl groups disappeared from kidney even more slowly with a half-life of 24 days as compared with five days for a $[^{14}C]$-p-iodobenzoylated normal globulin (Blau et al., 1958). Antikidney antibody that had cross-localized in liver had an initial rapid decay in liver with a half-life of only three days, and a subsequent slower decay, after ten days, with a half-life of 20 days (Pressman, 1949). In the experiments of Eisen et al. (1950), antilung antibody that had cross-localized in kidney was found to have a long half-life of 25 days in kidney, as compared with eight days for an antiovalbumin preparation, whereas both globulins disappeared from lung at equal rates with half of each gone in six days. From liver and blood the two radioglobulins disappeared at nearly equal rates also (12 and 10 days in the former, five and four days in the latter). On the basis of disappearance rates it was apparent that the supposed lung-localizing antibodies in these experiments were in essence no different from nonselective control globulins. Seegal (1962) found that injected antiplacental antibody in normal female rats was bound to and retained in kidney glomeruli for at least ten months, thus creating a nidus of foreign protein which could act as a continuing stimulus for chronic kidney disease. Day (1965) observed that while liver-localized and hepatoma-localized antibodies did not remain long in those target organs, cross-localized antibodies in kidney appeared to have extreme stability with a half-life in the rat that extrapolated to three years. The data were explained, however, as reflecting an initial kidney-localized radioantibody, gradually diminishing, that was continually augmented by radioantibody coming in from other tissues in the form of antibody-antigen complexes. The stability was taken to be more apparent than real with respect to the initial localizing components.

4. Negative Localization

The kidney model would suggest that all localization of antibodies in tissues is positive, that is, measurable as a positive value over and above control protein. With the advance of time in that model the localization appears to become increasingly positive, as compared with nonselective radioglobulins, and takes on an aura of extreme stability.

The phenomenon of negative localization would hold that the disappearance rate of antitissue antibody, once localized in the target organ, would be faster than the disappearance rate of nonselective control globulin that was localized such that, in time, there would be a lower percentage of the injected antibody in the organ than of control globulin. Such a phenomenon was encountered in the experiments of Day and Appel (1970) in which the biologic half-lives of antisynapse radioantibodies were measured in brain, liver, kidney, and spleen. The principles of multicompartment distribution analysis were used in the study, the first step being that of establishing a compartment free of bound antibody. In fact, five were found—lung, testes, heart, thymus, and blood—leaving brain, liver, kidney, and spleen as the four principal targets of localization.

Measurements that were made between the third and

Table 21. Biologic half-lives of localized antisynapse antibodies in brain and other organs as compared with those of normal immunoglobulins resident in tissues between the third and twenty-seventh days after intravenous injection

Perfused tissues containing radioglobulins[a]	Percentage of injected dose extrapolated back to zero time		Biologic half-lives (days) of localized immunoglobulins	
	Normal portion [b] (Anti-SY 77)	Antibody portion[b] (Anti-SY 77)	Normal portion (Anti-SY 77)	Antibody portion (Anti-SY 77)
Lu-Te-He-Tm	0.940	0.000	13.8	—
Li-Ki-Sp-Br	0.900	0.876	13.5	10.4
Liver	0.572	0.580	13.4	12.0
Kidney	2.221	0.117	14.2	9.2
Spleen	0.096	0.147	13.8	5.8
Brain	0.011	0.032	13.8	7.4

Data from Day and Appel, 1970.

[a] Lu-Te-He-Tm: Lung, testes, heart, thymus contained no localized antibody. Li-Ki-Sp-Br: liver, kidney, spleen, brain contained localized antibody.

[b] Multicompartment distribution analysis was used to calculate normal and antibody portions in the tissue.

twenty-seventh day after intravenous injection (Table 21) showed that antisynapse radioantibodies disappeared faster from the four tissues than did nonselective radioglobulins; moreover, they revealed that the disappearance rate of the nonselective control was relatively uniform in all tissues and the blood (half-lives, 13.3–14.2 days), whereas the disappearance rate of the localized antisynapse radioantibodies was varied: a half-life of 7.4 days in brain, 5.8 in spleen, 9.2 in kidney, 12.0 in liver. The removal of localized antibody, particularly from brain and spleen, at such faster rates suggests a mechanism not too different from that of the nephrotoxic syndrome (Burkholder, 1961): (a) localization of antibody, (b) fixation of complement, (c) cell damage, (d) loss of both antibody and antigen. The localization of antibody might in some instances be only fleeting and transient and remain undetectable; in other instances, it would be stable long enough to be discerned by localization-type radioassays. Localizing radioantibodies with ability to enter into complement fixation reactions (as the ones in these experiments were) would be expected to display the characteristics of negative localization. Only those radioantibodies of immunoglobulin classes not reactive with complement or in too low a concentration, or those whose complement-binding sites had been destroyed by iodination (and which, in any case, would not be immunogenic after localization), would be expected to display relatively long biologic half-lives. Negative localization would appear to be commensurate with the more usual immunologic phenomena *in vivo*.

Literature Cited

Bale, W. F., and I. L. Spar. 1957. Studies directed toward the use of antibodies as carriers of radioactivity for therapy. Adv. Biol. Med. Phys. 5: 285–356.

Blau, M., E. D. Day, and D. Pressman. 1957. The rate of localization of anti-rat kidney antibodies. J. Immunol. 79: 330–333.

Blau, M., A. C. Johnson, and D. Pressman. 1958. *p*-Iodobenzoyl groups as a paired label for *in vivo* protein-distribution studies: specific localization of anti-tissue antibodies. Int. J. App. Radiat. Isotopes. 3:217–225.

Boyd, W. C. 1962. Introduction to Immunochemical Specificity. Interscience, New York.

Burkholder, P. M. 1961. Complement fixation in diseased tissues. I. Fixation of guinea pig complement in sections of kidney from humans with membranous glomerulonephritis and rats injected with anti-rat kidney serum. J. Exp. Med. 114: 605–616.

Day, E. D. 1962. The vascular efficiency of tumors, pp. 671–679. *In* M. J. Brennan and W. L. Simpson (eds.), Biological Interactions in Normal and Neoplastic Growth. Little, Brown, Boston.

Day, E.D. 1964. Vascular relationships of tumor and host. Prog. Exp. Tum. Res. 4: 57–97.

Day, E. D. 1965. The Immunochemistry of Cancer. Charles C Thomas, Springfield, Ill.

Day, E. D., and S. H. Appel. 1970. The biologic half-life of brain-localized antisynapse radioantibodies. J. Immunol. 104: 710–717.

Day, E. D., G. W. Barnes, J. H. Planinsek, and D. Pressman. 1958. Improved methods for the purification of tumor-localizing antibodies. J. Nat. Cancer Inst. 20: 1123–1139.

Day, E. D., and S. Lassiter. 1967. The *in vitro* absorption of antibrain radioantibodies with brain sediments: some unusual properties and a quantitative method. J. Immunol. 98: 56–61.

Day, E. D., and S. Lassiter. 1969. Multi-compartment distribution analysis of antibrain radioantibodies in density gradients. J. Immunol. 103: 550–555.

Day, E. D., S. Lassiter, B. Woodhall, J. L. Mahaley, and M. S. Mahaley, Jr. 1965. The localization of radioantibodies in human brain tumors. I. Preliminary exploration. Cancer Res. 25: 773–778.

Day, E. D., P. N. McMillan, D. D. Mickey, and S. H. Appel. 1971. Zonal centrifuge profiles of rat brain homogenates: instability in sucrose, stability in iso-osmotic Ficoll-sucrose. Anal. Biochem. 39: 29–45.

Day, E. D., J. A. Planinsek, and D. Pressman. 1961. Triadic labeling with I^{130}, I^{131}, and I^{133} for controlled determinations of tumor-localizing antibodies. J. Nat. Cancer Inst. 26: 1321–1333.

Day, E. D., and L. C. Rigsbee. 1969. Distribution analysis of brain-localized radioantibodies after zonal ultracentrifugation in a sucrose density-gradient. J. Immunol. 103:556–558.

Eisen, H. N., B. Sherman, and D. Pressman. 1950. The zone of localization of antibodies. IX. The properties of anti-rat-lung serum. J. Immunol. 65: 543–558.

Feinstein, A., P. G. H. Gell, and A. S. Kelus. 1963. Immunochemical analysis of rabbit gamma-globulin allotypes. Nature 200: 653–654.

Gilman, A. M., A. Nisonoff, and S. Dray. 1964. Symmetrical distribution of genetic markers in individual rabbit gamma globulin molecules. Immunochemistry 1: 109–120.

Haimovich, J., R. Tarrab, A. Sulica, and M. Sela. 1970. Antibodies of different specificities in normal rabbit sera. J. Immunol. 104: 1033–1034.

Kabat, E. A. 1961. Kabat and Mayer's Experimental Immunochemistry, 2nd ed. Charles C Thomas, Springfield, Ill.

Landsteiner, K. 1962. The Specificity of Serological Reactions, republication of the 2nd English edition of 1945. Dover, New York.

Landsteiner, K., and J. van der Scheer. 1936. On cross reactions of immune sera to azoproteins. J. Exp. Med. 63: 325–339.

Masugi, M. 1933. Uber das Wesen der spezifischen Veränderungen der Niere und der Lieber durch das Nephrotoxin bzw. das Hepatotoxin. Zugleich ein Beitrag zur

Pathogenese der Glomerulonephritis und der eklamptischen Leberkrankung. Beitr. Pathol. Anat. Allgem. Pathol. 91: 82–112.

McMillan, P. N., D. D. Mickey, B. Kaufman, and E. D. Day. 1971. The specificity and cross-reactivity of antimyelin antibodies as determined by sequential adsorption analysis. J. Immunol. 107:1611–1617.

Mickey, D. D., P. N. McMillan, S. H. Appel, and E. D. Day. 1971. The specificity and cross-reactivity of antisynaptosome antibodies as determined by sequential adsorption analysis. J. Immunol. 107:1599–1610.

Pressman, D. 1949. The zone of localization of antibodies. IV. The *in vivo* disposition of anti-mouse-kidney serum and anti-mouse-plasma serum as determined by radio-active tracers. J. Immunol. 63: 375–388.

Pressman, D. 1957. Current status of the tissue localization of I^{131}-labeled antitissue antibodies. Ann. N. Y. Acad. Sci. 70: 72–81.

Pressman, D., E. D. Day, and M. Blau. 1957. The use of paired labeling in the determination of tumor-localizing antibodies. Cancer Res. 17: 845–850.

Pressman, D., and H. N. Eisen. 1950. Specific localization of anti-rat-lung serum in the lung. Proc. Soc. Exp. Biol. Med. 73: 143–146.

Pressman, D., and G. Keighley. 1948. The zone of activity of antibodies as determined by the use of radioactive tracers; the zone of activity of nephritoxic antikidney serum. J. Immunol. 59: 141–146.

Rapport, M. M., and L. Graf. 1967. Preparation and testing of lipids for immunological study. Meth. Immunol. Immunochem. 1:187–196.

Reisfeld, R. A., S. Dray, and A. Nisonoff. 1965. Differences in amino acid composition of γG-immunoglobulin. Light polypeptide chains controlled by allelic genes. Immunochemistry 2: 155–167.

Seegal, B. 1962. Effects of antiplacenta serum. pp. 215–230. *In* A. Tyler and K. A. Laurence (eds.), Proc. Conference on Immuno-Reproduction. Population Council.

Smadel, J. E. 1936. Experimental nephritis in rats induced by injection of anti-kidney serum. I. Preparation and immunological studies of nephrotoxin. J. Exp. Med. 64: 921–942.

Stemke, G. W. 1964. Allotypic specificities of A- and B-chains of rabbit gamma globulin. Science 145: 403–405.

Tamanoi, I., Y. Yagi, R. Hiramoto, and D. Pressman. 1961. Lung localizing antibodies in anti-lung and anti-kidney serum. Proc. Soc. Exp. Biol. Med. 106: 661–663.

Williams, C. A., Jr., and P. Grabar. 1955. Immunoelectrophoretic studies on serum proteins. I. The antigens of human serum. J. Immunol. 74: 158–168.

Author's address: Dr. Eugene D. Day, Box 3045, Duke University Medical Center, Durham, North Carolina 27710 (U.S.A.).

Comparative Immunochemistry of IgA

J. P. VAERMAN

Department of Experimental Medicine, University of Louvain, Brussels, Belgium

Contents

I. Introduction 93
II. Identification of IgA in Nonhuman Vertebrates 94
  A. Criteria of Identification.. 94
  B. Critical Review of Proteins Identified as IgA in Animals 96
    1. Primates.. 96
    2. Carnivora 96
      a. The Dog.. 96
      b. The Cat 97
      c. The Mink.. 97
      d. The Sea Lion 97
    3. Ungulates 97
      a. Artiodactyls... 97
        (i) Ruminants: The Bovine, the Goat, the Sheep 97
        (ii) Suidae: The Pig.. 99
      b. Perissodactyls: The Horse 100
      c. Proboscideans: The Elephant 101
    4. Lagomorphs: The Rabbit 101
    5. Rodents 103
      a. The Mouse... 103
      b. The Rat 103
      c. The Guinea Pig.. 104
      d. The Hamster... 105
    6. Cetacea: The Dolphin 105
    7. Insectivora 105
      a. The Hedgehog 105
      b. The Mole.. 105
    8. Marsupials and Monotremes 106
    9. Chordata Other Than Mammals 106
      a. Birds 106
        (i) The Chicken 106
        (ii) The Duck 106
      b. Reptiles, Amphibians, and Fishes 107
  C. Conclusion 107

92   J. P. Vaerman

III. Physical Properties of IgA	107
A. Introduction	107
B. Properties Related to Electrical Charge	109
1. Electrophoretic Mobility	109
2. Ion Exchange Chromatography	110
C. Properties Related to Molecular Size	110
D. Other Physical Parameters	112
E. Electron Microscopy	113
IV. Chemical Properties of IgA	116
A. Composition in Amino Acids and Carbohydrates	116
B. Constitutive Polypeptide Chains of IgA	117
1. Light Chains	117
2. α-Chains	120
a. Human α-Chains	120
b. Dog α-Chains	122
c. Bovine α-Chains	123
d. Sheep α-Chains	123
e. Rabbit α-Chains	123
f. Mouse α-Chains	124
3. The Secretory Component (SC)	125
a. Human SC	125
b. Canine SC	129
c. SC in Ruminants	130
d. SC in Pigs	132
e. SC in Horses	133
f. Rabbit SC	133
g. SC in Rodents	134
4. J-Chains	134
a. Human J-Chains	134
b. Canine J-Chains	136
c. Bovine J-Chains	136
d. Sheep J-Chains	136
e. Pig J-Chains	136
f. Rabbit J-Chains	136
g. Mouse J-Chains	138
h. J-Chains in Birds, Amphibians, and Fishes	138
i. Conclusion	138
C. Sensitivity to Mild Reducing Agents	139
D. Proteolytic Fragmentation	139
1. Human IgA	139
2. Dog IgA	140
3. Rabbit IgA	140
4. Mouse IgA	141
V. Biological Properties of IgA	141
A. Concentration in Serum and Secretions	141

1. Human IgA ... 141
2. IgA from Animals ... 142
   a. Dog IgA ... 142
   b. IgA from Ruminants ... 142
   c. Pig IgA ... 143
   d. Horse IgA ... 143
   e. Rabbit IgA ... 150
   f. Mouse IgA ... 150
B. Synthesis, Catabolism, and Secretion ... 150
  1. Human IgA ... 150
  2. Dog IgA ... 152
  3. Cat IgA ... 153
  4. IgA in Ruminants ... 153
  5. Pig IgA ... 154
  6. Horse IgA ... 154
  7. Rabbit IgA ... 155
  8. Mouse IgA ... 155
  9. Rat IgA ... 156
 10. Hamster IgA ... 156
 11. Guinea Pig IgA ... 157
 12. Hedgehog IgA ... 157
 13. Chicken IgA ... 157
C. Complement Fixation. Opsonization ... 157
D. Precipitation, Agglutination, Valence, Affinity ... 158
  1. Human IgA ... 158
  2. Dog IgA ... 159
  3. Rabbit IgA ... 159
  4. Mouse IgA ... 160
Literature Cited ... 161

I. Introduction

Immunoglobulin A (IgA) was originally described (Williams, 1954) as a precipitin arc, called βx, in the complex immunoelectrophoretic pattern of human serum. Its name was changed to β_{2A} by Burtin et al. (1957) and finally to γ_{1A} (Heremans, 1960) and γA or IgA (W.H.O., 1964), after Heremans and Schultze (1959) had purified it and shown it to be antigenically related to the two other immunoglobulins known at that time, IgG and IgM.

Interest in IgA immunoglobulins has considerably increased with the discovery by Tomasi and Zigelbaum (1963) that IgA represented the principal immunoglobulin in human exocrine secretions, where it differs from serum IgA by its molecular size and antigenic properties. The concept of a human secretory immunological system, different and independent from the serum immunological system and based principally on the presence of secretory IgA (Tomasi et al., 1965), has gained wide acceptance and has been the subject of considerable investigation and speculation. Much of the information available on this topic is condensed in a few comprehensive sources (Tomasi and Bienenstock, 1968; Heremans, 1968; Conference on the Secretory Immunologic System, 1971; Heremans and Vaerman, 1971; Hanson and Brandtzaeg, in press).

The aim of the present article is to review those species of animals in which IgA has been identified and to compare the immunochemical properties of IgA in these species to those of human IgA. The search for literature related to this review was ended by November 1971.

II. Identification of IgA in Nonhuman Vertebrates

A. Criteria of Identification

In a previous study (Vaerman, 1970), we made a tentative classification of criteria for the identification of proteins homologous to human IgA in different animal species. These criteria were classified as first-, second-, and third-order criteria in the order of what we believed to be decreasing reliability, and a justification for this classification was also presented.

First-order criteria consist of: (1) amino acid sequence similarities between stretches of sufficient length from constant regions of heavy chains (peptide map homologies were considered to be much less reliable); (2) immunological cross-reactions between human and animal α-chains.

As second-order criteria, we consider a set of properties which have, so far, been found associated essentially with immunoglobulins clearly identified as IgA. These second-order criteria included: (1) the specific intimate association of very large numbers of IgA-producing cells, as compared to other Ig-producing cells, with mucosal or glandular surfaces, particularly those of the intestinal tract; (2) the occurrence, in several external secretions, of a secretory component (SC), either bound to IgA to form secretory IgA (SIgA) or in the free form (FSC); (3) the absence of disulfide bridges linking L- to H-chains, as found in most Caucasian IgA_2 molecules; (4) a selective concentration in several exocrine secretions, resulting for IgA in the highest secretion-serum concentration ratio among the various immunoglobulin classes, but not necessarily in the highest absolute concentration.

Third-order criteria include several physicochemical and biological properties which, though found in human IgA, are not restricted to this immunoglobulin class. Such criteria have not infrequently led to what has later proved to be misidentifications, or to very poorly supported identifications. Among these physicochemical properties are: (1) a heterogeneous molecular size (between 7 S and 19 S as judged by gel filtration or by a sedimentation rate); (2) intermediate susceptibility to sulfhydryl reduction; (3) a large carbohydrate content; (4) a fast electrophoretic mobility or retarded elution from DEAE-ion exchangers, both properties being indicative of a high net negative charge; (5) a relatively high solubility in the presence of zinc ions. Among the biological properties are: (6) the predominance of the immunoglobulin in one or several exocrine secretions, particularly colostrum; (7) an inability to fix complement, unless by the bypass reaction; (8) an inability to induce direct or reverse passive cutaneous anaphylaxis in guinea pig skin; (9) the absence of transplacental transference.

Even the combination of several third-order criteria does not furnish a reliable basis for the unequivocal identification of IgA. It should be realized that this classification is somewhat arbitrary and provisional, and will probably have to be revised in the light of future information. The following examples will illustrate this point, particularly with regard to second-order criteria.

(1) Large numbers of IgM-producing cells may occur in the intestinal mucosa of individuals lacking IgA (Crabbé, 1967; Brandtzaeg, Fjellanger, and Gjeruldsen, 1968). Furthermore, the abomasal and intestinal mucosa of parasitized sheep have been reported to contain larger numbers of IgG_1 cells than of IgA cells (Curtain and Anderson, 1971); (2) secretory component, under particular conditions, can be found bound to IgM (Thompson, 1970; Mach, 1970; Rádl et al., 1971); (3) the immunoglobulins of a primitive chordate, the lamprey, have their light chains noncovalently bound to their heavy chains

(Marchalonis and Edelman, 1968). Furthermore, a human IgG_1 myeloma protein, having an extensive H-chain deletion, has been shown to have the majority of its light chains in the form of disulfide-linked dimers noncovalently bound to the H-chains (Deutsch and Suzuki, 1971): (4) IgE has also been shown to have a high secretion-serum ratio (Ishizaka and Newcomb, 1970; Ishizaka et al., 1971). Also, in IgA-deficient persons, IgM may become the predominant immunoglobulin in secretions (Crabbé, 1967; Brandtzaeg, Fjellanger, and Gjeruldsen, 1968).

B. Critical Review of Proteins Identified as IgA in Animals

1. Primates

Immunological cross-reactions between IgA from humans and primates have been found by numerous investigators (Picard, Heremans, and Vandebroek, 1962a,b; Felsenfeld et al., 1966, 1968a,b; Wang et al., 1968; Acharya, Poulik, and Goodman, 1968; Monte and Arbesman, 1969; Bauer, 1970a,b; Wicher and Arbesman, 1971). This is not surprising since apes and monkeys are so closely related to man. In addition, numerous IgA-type plasma cells have been observed in their intestinal mucosae (Felsenfeld, Greer, and Jiřička, 1968; Felsenfeld et al., 1968a; Wicher and Arbesman, 1971). Evidence for a high secretion-serum ratio was obtained for saliva, stomach and jejunal contents, stools, and bile (Felsenfeld, Greer, and Felsenfeld, 1967; Keclik et al., 1970).

IgA is thus identified beyond doubt in several primates on the basis of first- and second-order criteria.

2. Carnivora

a. The Dog

Third-order criteria only were given by several workers to tentatively identify canine IgA (Okoshi, Tomoda, and Makimura, 1967; Patterson, Roberts, and Pruzansky, 1968; Rockey and Schwartzmann, 1967). Since those early reports, however, cross-reactions with antihuman IgA have repeatedly been described (Vaerman and Heremans, 1968; Schwartzmann, Halliwell, and Rockey, 1970; Ricks, Roberts, and Patterson, 1970; Hurvitz et al., 1971; Orlans and Feinstein, 1971). The predominance of IgA cells in the intestinal mucosa (Vaerman and

Heremans, 1969a), a high secretion-serum concentration ratio (Johnson and Vaughan, 1967; Vaerman and Heremans, 1969b; Reynolds and Johnson, 1970a,b,c; Lieberman et al., 1970), the occurrence of a secretory component (Johnson and Vaughan, 1967; Ricks et al., 1970; Vaerman, 1971; Reynolds and Johnson, 1971), and of molecules with noncovalently bound light chains (Vaerman, 1970; Reynolds and Johnson, 1971), are all second-order criteria which confirm, if necessary, the correct identification of IgA in the canine species.

b. The Cat

On the basis of a vague resemblance to the human immunoelectrophoretic pattern, Okoshi et al. (1968) suggested the existence of IgA in the cat. Immunological cross-reaction of a feline protein with human IgA (Vaerman, Heremans, and Van Kerckhoven, 1969; Orlans and Feinstein, 1971), a high secretion-serum concentration ratio, as well as abundant IgA-type plasma cells in the intestinal mucosa (Vaerman, 1970), have established the identification of IgA in this species by first- and second-order criteria.

c. The Mink

Only third-order criteria, namely immunoelectrophoretic resemblances, are available for this species (Porter and Dixon, 1966; Williams, Russel, and Kenyon, 1966), whose IgA therefore remains unidentified.

d. The Sea Lion

Immunological cross-reactions between human or bovine IgA and sea lion IgA have established its exact identification (Nash and Mach, 1971; Orlans and Feinstein, 1971). In addition, human FSC was shown to combine *in vitro* with sea lion serum IgA (Nash and Mach, 1971).

3. *Ungulates*

a. Artiodactyls

(i) Ruminants: The Bovine, the Goat, the Sheep

The Bovine — The presence of a precipitin arc of γ_1-mobility, solubility in the presence of zinc ions, and molecular size and/or abundance in lacteal and/or salivary secretions were the third-order criteria used by numerous investigators to suggest the existence of bovine "IgA" (Murphy et al., 1964; Murphy, Osebold, and Aalund, 1965; Blanc, 1964; Sullivan and Tomasi, 1964; Mansa, 1965; Rice, Tailyour, and Cochrane, 1966; Nansen and Nielsen, 1966; Morris, 1967; Sullivan et al., 1969; Jacks and Glantz, 1970; Penhale and Christie, 1969; Faust and Tengerdy, 1970). However, these data have now been completed by serological cross-reactions with antihuman IgA (Vaerman et al., 1969; Mach and Pahud, 1971; Hurlimann and Darling, 1971; Orlans and Feinstein, 1971). In addition, both bovine IgA-bound SC and free SC have been identified (Mach, Pahud, and Isliker, 1969; Mach and Pahud, 1971; Porter and Noakes, 1970; Butler, Groves, and Coulson, 1970; Butler, 1971). A high secretion-serum concentration ratio (Mach, Pahud, and Isliker, 1969; Vaerman, 1970; Mach and Pahud, 1971; Porter and Noakes, 1970; Butler et al., 1972) and abundant IgA-type plasmocytes in the intestinal mucosa (Yurchak, Butler, and Tomasi, 1971) provide additional confirmation of the exact identification of bovine IgA.

The Goat—Cross-reactions with human IgA (Vaerman et al., 1969; Pahud and Mach, 1970; Orlans and Feinstein, 1971), a high secretion-serum concentration ratio (Vaerman, 1970; Pahud and Mach, 1970), the demonstration of free and bound SC (Pahud and Mach, 1970) and of large numbers of IgA cells in intestinal mucosae (Vaerman, 1970; Yurchak et al., 1971) form a strong basis for the exact identification of goat IgA.

The Sheep—Early workers on sheep immunoglobulins have often suggested the existence of sheep "IgA," but this identification rested only on third-order criteria, and primarily on immunoelectrophoretic resemblances (Silverstein et al., 1963; Chordi and Kagan, 1964; Aalund, Osebold, and Murphy, 1965; Pan et al., 1968; Outerridge, Mackenzie, and Lascelles, 1968; McDowell and Lascelles, 1969; Heimer, Clark, and Maurer, 1969; Jonas, 1969; Hudson, Bandy, and Kitts, 1970; Lascelles and McDowell, 1970). In a detailed study, Sullivan et al. (1969) stated that, as for the cow, they could not find any definite evidence for the existence of "IgA" in sheep colostrum, saliva, and tears, although they did not exclude the possibility of its presence in very small amounts. In contrast, Heimer, Jones, and Maurer (1969) claimed to have identified two "IgA" subclasses in sheep colostrum. One, called "IgA$_2$", had a sedimentation coefficient close to 15 S (not extrapolated), and was said to contain "SC" and noncovalently bound light chains. The other, called "IgA$_1$", had a sedimentation coefficient close to 10 S, was not associated with "SC", and did not release light chains in dissociating solvents. Some care should be exercised in interpreting the findings of the latter authors since their "IgA$_2$" was obtained in pure form in the void volume of a Sephadex G-200 column. No allusion to the existence of IgM in that fraction was made, although IgM has been repeatedly found in large amounts in such a fraction (Pahud and Mach, 1970; Vaerman, 1970).

Unequivocal identification of sheep IgA was obtained (Vaerman, et al., 1969; Pahud and Mach, 1970; Hurlimann and Darling, 1971; Orlans and Feinstein, 1971) by means of immunological cross-reactions between human and sheep IgA. Also, free and bound SC were clearly identified in the sheep (Pahud and Mach, 1970); the secretion-serum concentration ratio in this species was the highest for IgA in many different secretions (Vaerman, 1970; Pahud and Mach, 1970) and the normal intestinal mucosae were shown to be populated with large numbers of IgA-producing cells (Vaerman, 1970; Lee and Lascelles, 1970; Curtain and Anderson, 1971). On the basis of these first- and second-order criteria, one may consider that sheep IgA is identified with reasonable certainty. One may add that cross-reactions for IgA and SC have been easily demonstrated between ruminants (Pahud and Mach, 1970), as well as for IgM, IgG$_1$ and IgG$_2$ (Pahud and Mach, 1970; Aalund, 1968; Feinstein and Hobart, 1969).

(ii) Suidae: The Pig

Many identifications of "IgA" in pigs have been proposed on the sole basis of third-order criteria, such as immunoelectrophoretic similarities to human IgA, or molecular size characteristics (Kim, Bradley, and Watson, 1966; Rejnek, Kostka, and Trávniček, 1966; Tormo et al., 1967; Mattheus and Korn, 1967; Mattheus, Korn, and Jakubik, 1970; Baumstark, 1968; Karlsson, 1966a,b,c; Surján, 1969a,b; Brummerstedt-Hansen, 1967; Bourne, 1969a; Metzger and Fougereau, 1968).

Cross-reactions between human and porcine IgA have now been demonstrated (Vaerman et al., 1969; Vaerman and Heremans, 1970a; Richardson and Kelleher, 1970; Hurlimann and Darling, 1971; Orlans and Feinstein, 1971; Atkins, Schofield, and Reeder, 1971). In addition, numerous IgA plasma cells populated the lamina propria of the porcine intestinal mucosa (Vaerman, 1970; Allen and Porter, 1970; Bourne, Pickup, and Steele, unpublished). A high secretion-serum concentration ratio in many secretions (Vaerman, Arbuckle, and Heremans, 1970; Vaerman, 1970; Porter, 1969a,b; Porter and Allen, 1969; Porter, 1971; Bourne, Pickup, and Honour, 1971), and the observation of free and bound forms of the porcine SC (Bourne, 1969b; Bourne et al., 1971; Porter and Allen, 1970; Porter, 1971; Vaerman, 1971) clearly confirm the correctness of the identification.

b. Perissodactyls: The Horse

Several workers were struck by the resemblance of the immunoelectrophoretic pattern of the equine T-globulin with that of human IgA (Schwick and Schultze, 1960; Heremans, Vaerman, and Vaerman, 1963; Rockey, Klinman, and Karush, 1964), and suggested an homology between T-globulin and human IgA. This view was largely accepted (Hill and Cebra, 1965; Raynaud, Iscaki, and Mangalo, 1965; Acharya and Rao, 1966; Sardesai and Rao, 1968), and was seemingly supported by the lack of complement fixation by antibodies of T-globulin class (Lavergne, Raynaud, and Iscaki, 1966), as well as by their high carbohydrate content (Klinman et al., 1966). However, Weir, Porter, and Givol (1966) discovered the existence of twelve identical amino acid positions in C-terminal octodecapeptides of horse IgG, IgT, rabbit IgG, and human IgG_1 and IgG_3; whereupon they proposed the designation IgG(T) for equine T-globulin. In addition, Rockey (1967) described antigenic determinants common to the Fc fragment of $IgG_{a,b,c}$ and the protein they called "IgA." The homology between human IgA and equine IgT was therefore considered highly improbable. Audibert and Sandor (1968) purified, from lacteal secretions, a γ_1-protein immunologically distinct from IgG, IgT, and IgM, which was rich in carbohydrate and resistant, to some extent, to precipitation by zinc ions. They suggested that this was the equine homologue of human IgA, but still only on the basis of third-order criteria. However, Genco, Yecies, and Karush (1969) and Rouse and Ingram (1970) stated that there appeared to be little or no secretory "IgA" in equine parotid fluid and colostrum, whereas $IgA_{a,b,c}$, IgG(T), and IgM were found in comparable ratios in colostrum and serum.

The identification of IgA has eventually been achieved by immunological cross-reaction with antihuman IgA (Vaerman et al., 1969; Vaerman, Querinjean, and Heremans, 1971; Pahud and Mach, 1972; Orlans and Feinstein, 1971). Its association with intestinal mucosa (Vaerman et al., 1971), the occurrence of free and bound SC (Pahud and Mach, 1972) and of noncovalently bound light chains (Vaerman et al., 1971), as well as the exceptionally high secretion-serum concentration ratio of this protein (Vaerman et al., 1971); Pahud and Mach, 1972) have confirmed its exact identification as equine IgA. Although not reported in the literature, zebra IgA, donkey IgA, mule IgA, and hinny IgA extensively cross-reacted with equine IgA, a finding already observed with equine $IgG_{a,b}$, IgG_c (γ_1), IgT, and IgM (Allen and Vaerman, unpublished data; Helms and Allen, 1971).

c. Proboscideans: The Elephant

Cross-reaction of human and elephant IgA has permitted the identification of IgA in this species (Orlans and Feinstein, 1971).

4. Lagomorphs: The Rabbit

Several authors have identified rabbit "IgA" on the sole basis of third-order criteria, i.e., electrophoretic mobility, molecular size, carbohydrate content, and abundance in colostrum (Feinstein, 1963; Onoue, Yagi, and Pressman, 1964, 1966; Cebra and Robbins, 1966; Sell, 1967). Fortunately, several second-order criteria have been brought to light, such as the abundance of IgA cells in the intestinal mucosa (Crandall, Cebra, and Crandall, 1967; O'Daly and Cebra, 1968; Cebra, 1969; O'Daly, Craig, and Cebra, 1971; Craig and Cebra, 1971) and the occurrence, in SIgA, of a small amount of noncovalently bound light chains (Cebra and Small, 1967).

Small polypeptide chains were dissociated from rabbit colostral SIgA by gel filtration in 5 M guanidine containing iodoacetamide. This material consisted of light chain dimers and a polypeptide (mol wt about 50,000), called "T-chains," which displayed a characteristic fast anodal mobility upon acrylamide gel electrophoresis in alkaline urea after complete reduction and alkylation (Cebra and Small, 1967). An antiserum against purified "T-chains," when properly absorbed, reacted with "T-chains" and SIgA, but not with α-chains, light chains, or IgG. Fluorescein-labeled "anti-T" did not stain rabbit plasma cells, but stained epithelial cells in intestinal and mammary glands (O'Daly and Cebra, 1968), as antihuman-SC would (Tourville et al., 1968).

A similar "T-like" polypeptide was obtained upon alkaline urea gel electrophoresis of totally reduced and alkylated human SIgA (Rejnek, Kostka, and Kotynek, 1966; Cederblad, Johansson, and Rymo, 1966; Hanson and Johansson, 1967; Tomasi and Bienenstock, 1968). Since at that time, human SIgA was assumed to contain only three polypeptide chains, i.e., α-chains, light chains, and SC, the homology of the rabbit "T-chains" with human SC seemed evident. No direct experimental proof, however, was available to test whether "T-chains," as defined by alkaline urea gel electrophoresis, did react with "anti-T." Indeed, to observe the characteristic electrophoretic mobility of the "T-chains," complete reduction and alkylation of "T-chains" seemed necessary; a treatment assumed to destroy their antigenicity. Thus, it was never proved that "anti-T" actually reacted with "T-chains," as defined by electrophoresis, or with a contaminant present in the guanidine-dissociated material and accompanying these "T-chains" on DEAE-cellulose (O'Daly and Cebra, 1968).

One has to assume that this contaminant was the true SC, distinct from light chains and "T-chains," and that "anti-T" was, in fact, antirabbit SC. Recent data (Halpern and Koshland, 1970; O'Daly and Cebra, 1971a,b,c) have confirmed this explanation and have clearly shown that "T-chains" correspond to a fourth polypeptide chain of SIgA, now known as J-chain, completely different, both antigenically and electrophoretically, from the true rabbit SC. In addition, free SC was identified in, and purified from, rabbit colostrum, and was shown to have a molecular weight and a carbohydrate and amino acid composition different from those of the J-chain (O'Daly and Cebra, 1971c). Surprisingly, the electrophoretic mobilities in alkaline urea gels of J-chains, on the one hand, and SC dissociated from SIgA and totally reduced and alkylated on the other hand, were at the anodal and cathodal extremes of the pattern, respectively. Fluorescent antisera specific for the native forms of J-chain and SC, do not cross-react and stain plasma cells and epithelial cells, respectively.

The demonstration of a true SC in rabbit colostrum and SIgA supports the previous identification of rabbit IgA, which has now been confirmed by immunological cross-reactions between human and rabbit IgA using chicken antisera against human IgA (Orlans and Feinstein, 1971).

5. Rodents

a. The Mouse

Until 1967, it could be said that the identification of mouse IgA was supported only by third-order criteria (Fahey, 1961a,b; Rask-Nielsen et al., 1961; Clausen and Heremans, 1960; Arnason, de Vaux St-Cyr, and Shaffner, 1964; Arnason, Salomon, and Grabar, 1964; Fahey, Wunderlich, and Mishell, 1964; Fahey and Barth, 1965; Bazin, 1966, 1967a,b). However, the occurrence, in mice, of spontaneous and induced transplantable tumors producing homogeneous immunoglobulins (myeloma proteins), many of which closely resembled human myeloma IgA, and obviously represented the true IgA of the mouse, has allowed the dismissal of some of the former candidates to this title (Heremans and Clausen, 1960; Rask-Nielsen et al., 1961; Arnason et al., 1964a,b), as being a mere subclass of IgG (γ_1 or IgF).

In 1968, Crabbé et al. demonstrated the presence of very large numbers of IgA-containing cells in the intestinal mucosa of adult conventional mice. In addition, some evidence for the existence of a mouse SC has been obtained (Asofsky and Hylton, 1968; Nash et al., 1970; Benveniste, Lespinats, and Salomon, 1971). Most of the IgA myeloma proteins of mice have noncovalently bound light chains (Abel and Grey, 1968; Seki, Appella, and Itano, 1968; Grey, Sher, and Shalitin, 1970). Finally, the C-terminal tripeptides of mouse and human α-chains have been shown to be identical (Abel and Grey, 1967). This, however, does not constitute a first-order criterion, since the same C-terminal tripeptide was found in human μ-chains (Prahl, Abel, and Grey, 1971). Homologies need to be compared on much larger stretches of sequence.

Recently, Orlans and Feinstein (1971) obtained a cross-reaction between human and mouse IgA, using chicken antisera, thereby confirming the previous identification of mouse IgA.

b. The Rat

For many years, the identification of rat IgA has been supported only by third-order criteria (Arnason, de Vaux St-Cyr, and Relyveld, 1964; Binaghi and Sarandon de Merlo, 1966; Jones and Ogilvie, 1967; Aschkenasy, de Vaux St-Cyr; and Courcon, 1967; Bloch and Wilson, 1968; Bloch, Morse, and Austen, 1968; Banowitz and Ishizaka, 1967;

Wiedermann, Auerswald, and Denk, 1968). Since rat IgA myeloma proteins were not available at that time, the identification of rat IgA was far from established until 1969.

Cross-reactions have now been obtained between rat and mouse IgA, using antisera to mouse IgA as well as antisera to rat IgA (Nash et al., 1969; Hurlimann and Darling, 1971). The presence of very large numbers of IgA-containing cells in the rat's intestinal mucosa, as well as the finding of a very high secretion-serum concentration ratio for rat IgA (Bistany and Tomasi, 1970; Stechschulte and Austen, 1970), have aided in establishing its identification. Most of the previously proposed rat "IgAs" have, in fact, turned out to be a fast-moving subclass of IgG. Some evidence was presented to identify the rat secretory component (Hurlimann and Darling, 1971). Confirmation is needed on this point. Recently, transplantable tumors, producing homogeneous IgA globulins have been found in the rat (Bazin et al., 1972; Nash, Deckers and Heremans, 1971). Such proteins will doubtlessly promote progress in structural studies on rat IgA.

The correct identification of rat IgA may now be considered achieved, since Orlans and Feinstein (1971) obtained a cross-reaction between human and rat IgA.

c. The Guinea Pig

Most tentative identifications of guinea pig "IgA," all based on immunoelectrophoretic resemblances or molecular size characteristics (Olson and Wostmann, 1964; Havez, Bonte, and Moschetto, 1965; Rothman, 1966; Ashimura and Koyama, 1967), proposed as "IgA" what was, in fact, the "7 S γ_1-globulin" described by Benacerraf et al. (1963). That this "7 S γ_1" was not the homologue of human IgA was evident from its low carbohydrate content, transference to the fetus, and peptide mapping in comparison with "7 S γ_2" (Bloch et al., 1963; Oettgen, Binaghi and Benacerraf, 1965; Lamm, Lisowska-Bernstein, and Nussenzweig, 1967).

There exists in guinea pigs a γ_1 immunoglobulin, abundant in tears and colostrum, which may correspond to IgA, judging from its high secretion-serum concentration ratio (Hathaway and Peters, 1969). Direct identification of guinea pig serum IgA was eventually obtained through cross-reactions with human IgA (Orlans and Feinstein, 1971).

Further criteria for guinea pig IgA (Vaerman and Heremans, 1972) are its association with intestinal mucosa plasma cells, highest secretion-serum concentration ratio, and evidence for free and bound SC.

d. The Hamster

Hamster IgA was identified (Bienenstock, 1970; Bienenstock and Bloch, 1970; Dolezel and Bienenstock, 1970; Haakenstad and Coe, 1971) by its high secretion-serum concentration ratio and its association with immunocytes in the intestinal mucosa. Evidence for SC has not yet been reported. A transplantable plasmocytoma, known as KG-13 (Mohr and Dontenwill, 1964), synthesizes an immunoglobulin which may, by third-order criteria only, be proposed as homologous to human IgA. Cross-reactions with human IgA are not yet obtained, but hamster and rat or mouse serum IgA do cross-react (Bienenstock and Bazin, personal communications).

6. Cetacea: The Dolphin

Identification of IgA in dolphins was achieved by means of immunological cross-reactions with antihuman and antibovine IgA antisera (Nash and Mach, 1971). Dolphin serum IgA (and, to some extent IgM) combined *in vitro* with human FSC, a finding which provides a second-order criterion for the identification of IgA, as outlined by Mach (1970).

7. Insectivora

a. The Hedgehog

Tentative identifications of European hedgehog IgA (Picard et al., 1967; Larsen and Tönder, 1967) were initially based on mere immunoelectrophoretic similarities to human IgA. However, hedgehog IgA has now been shown to cross-react with human IgA (Vaerman et al., 1969; Orlans and Feinstein, 1971). Association of IgA with intestinal tract plasma cells and highest secretion-serum concentration ratio further confirmed this identification (Vaerman and Heremans, 1971).

b. The Mole

Orlans and Feinstein (1971) recently observed cross-reactions between human and mole serum IgA using chicken antisera.

8. Marsupials and Monotremes

Studies on the immunoglobulins of opossums and echidnas (Rowlands and Dudley, 1968; Rowlands, 1970; Diener, Wistar, and Ealey, 1967; Jordan and Morgan, 1969), have not specifically dealt with the identification of IgA in these species. However, the articles on echidna mention what may be considered as third-order criteria for the existence of IgA, e.g., a high concentration in milk, molecular size higher than 7 S, and a precipitin arc of γ_1 mobility upon immunoelectrophoresis.

9. Chordata Other Than Mammals

a. Birds

(i) The Chicken

Previous identifications of chicken "IgA" were all supported only by third-order criteria. Again the most commonly employed criterion was the similarity in immunoelectrophoretic pattern (Benedict, Hersch, and Larson, 1963; Patterson, Suszko, and Pruzansky, 1965; Delhanty and Solomon, 1966; Dreesman et al., 1965; Ivanyi, Valentova, and Cerny, 1966; Tenenhouse and Deutsch, 1966; Orlans, 1968; Kono et al., 1969). A recent report on the immunoglobulins in secretions of the fowl (Leslie, Wilson, and Clem, 1971) concluded that the chicken had the same predominant immunoglobulin, IgG, in serum and secretions (seminal plasma, tracheobronchial, and duodenal and crop washes). A 10.8 S component present in seminal plasma was thought to be a nonimmunoglobulin component or a dimer of IgG. Recently, however, Lebacq-Verheyden, Vaerman, and Heremans (1972) described a possible homologue (Iga) of mammalian IgA in chicken serum and secretions. It was clearly distinct from IgM and IgG (or IgY; Leslie and Clem, 1969) and displayed the highest secretion-serum concentration ratio in bile and intestinal secretions. The same group also observed the large predominance of "IgA" containing cells in the intestinal mucosa (Lebacq-Verheyden et al., 1972). Although further criteria are desirable, the identification of the chicken "Iga" as the true homologue of human IgA seems to rest on solid grounds.

(ii) The Duck

A few attempts to identify duck "IgA" (Grey 1963; Kaminski,

1965; Ligouzat and Kaminski, 1965) were all based on only third-order criteria and in fact leave this identification very doubtful.

b. Reptiles, Amphibians, and Fishes

We are not aware that in animals from these orders any immunoglobulin has ever been proposed to represent the homologue of human IgA. However, Grey (1969) pointed out the striking similarity between the structure of the lamprey immunoglobulins, whose disulfide dimers of light chains were not covalently linked to the heavy chains, on one hand, and the structure of human IgA_2 and mouse IgA myeloma proteins, on the other hand. In addition, the 14 S and 7 S forms of lamprey immunoglobulins were as immunologically identical with respect to each other as are the monomers and polymers of IgA (Apicella and Allen, 1970).

C. Conclusion

IgA has been reasonably identified in at least 19 animal species (Table 1). The use of chicken antisera for detecting cross-reactions between human and other mammalian IgA is to be highly recommended, since this type of reagent seems to be unusually successful in picking up cross-reactions between mammalian IgA proteins from various sources (Orlans and Feinstein, 1971).

Whenever cross-reaction or sequential data are unavailable, criteria of "second-order" should be looked for eagerly, since they have more fiducial value than any of the "third-order" criteria, even if several of these are available.

III. Physical Properties of IgA

A. Introduction

Physical properties of IgA can be measured on the purified protein, but may also be deduced from studies on body fluids by following the behavior of IgA during the various fractionation procedures by means of specific antisera. The former measurements are not necessarily more informative, since some native properties of the protein

Table 1. Identification of IgA in various species

| Species | First-order criteria | | Second-order criteria | | | |
	Sequence of amino acids	Immunological cross-reactions	Association with intestinal mucosa plasma cells	Highest secretion-serum concentration ratio in several secretions	Secretory component	Noncovalently linked L-chains
Primates	−	+	+	+	−	−
Dog	−	+	+	+	+	+
Cat	−	+	+	+	−	−
Seal	−	+	−	−	+?[a]	−
Cow	−	+	+	+	+	−
Sheep	−	+	+	+	+	+
Goat	−	+	+	+	+	−
Elephant	−	+	−	−	−	−
Pig	−	+	+	+	+	+?[b]
Horse	−	+	+	+	+	+
Rabbit	−	+	+	+	+	+
Mouse	+?[c]	+	+	+	+?[d]	+
Rat	−	+	+	+	−	−
Hamster	−	+?[e]	+	+	−	−
Guinea pig	−	+	+	+	+	−
Dolphin	−	+	−	−	+?[a]	−
Hedgehog	−	+	+	+	−	−
Mole	−	+	−	−	−	−
Chicken	−	−	+	+	−	−

[a] Binding of human FSC by seal or dolphin serum IgA (Nash and Mach, 1971).

[b] Noncovalently bound L-chains only identified by acid-urea starch gel electrophoresis (Vaerman, 1970).

[c] Only 3 C-terminal amino acids in common with human α-, but also with μ-chains (Abel and Grey, 1967).

[d] Needs confirmation (Asofsky and Hylton, 1968; Benveniste et al., 1971).

[e] Cross-reaction with rat and mouse IgA (Bienenstock and Bazin, personal communications).

may be modified by the isolation procedure which, in addition, may operate a selection among different subfractions of IgA.

Normal human serum IgA has been purified by a variety of physicochemical procedures, which have been reviewed (Vaerman, 1970), and by methods involving the use of specific anti-α-chain antisera (Anderson, Zschocke, and Bach, 1970; Mestecky, Kulhavy, and Kraus, 1971a). Serum IgA has been purified from normal serum in primates (Felsenfeld et al., 1966), dogs (Reynolds and Johnson, 1971), bovine (Butler and Maxwell, 1971), pigs (Bourne, 1969b), mice (Grey, Sher, and Shalitin, 1970), and hamsters (Bienenstock, 1970).

IgA myeloma proteins from humans, dogs, and mice are usually much easier to purify, by virtue of their high concentrations and relative homogeneity. A combination of salting-out, gel filtration, ion exchange chromatography, and/or preparative zone electrophoresis generally results in a reasonable immunochemical purity.

Secretory IgA was purified from a variety of human exocrine secretions including lacteal, salivary, nasal, bronchial, urinary, and intestinal secretions (Tomasi and Bienenstock, 1968; Rossen et al., 1966; Masson and Heremans, 1966; Bienenstock and Tomasi, 1968; Bull, Bienenstock and Tomasi, 1971). In nonhuman species, secretory IgA has been purified from canine milk (Vaerman and Heremans, 1970b; Reynolds and Johnson, 1970b) and feces (Reynolds and Johnson, 1970a), bovine lacteal (Mach et al., 1969; Porter and Noakes, 1970; Butler and Maxwell, 1971), salivary (Mach and Pahud, 1971) and nasal secretions (Morein, 1970), ovine and caprine colostrum (Pahud and Mach, 1970; Heimer et al., 1969), equine colostrum (Vaerman, 1970; Pahud and Mach, 1972), porcine lacteal (Porter, 1969a; Bourne, 1969a; Vaerman, 1970; Richardson and Kelleher, 1970) and intestinal secretions (Bourne et al., 1971), rabbit colostrum (Cebra and Robbins, 1966), hamster colostrum (Bienenstock, 1970), guinea pig milk (Vaerman and Heremans, 1972), and chicken bile (Lebacq-Verheyden et al., in preparation).

B. Properties Related to Electrical Charge

1. Electrophoretic mobility

The absolute figure for the electrophoretic mobility of normal human serum IgA, in Michaelis buffer (pH 8.6) is 2.2 ($\times 10^{-5}$ cm^2 ·

$V^{-1} \cdot sec^{-1}$), with a range of 1.2 to 3.6 (Heremans, 1960). Such absolute values offer less interest than does the mobility of IgA relative to that of other immunoglobulins within each species. Much overlapping between these mobilities is unavoidable if one considers the large degree of electrophoretic heterogeneity for every immunoglobulin class in normal serum. Anodal mobilities of IgA, relative to those of other immunoglobulin classes, in several species, are listed in Table 2. These values were inferred mainly from immunoelectrophoretic data. The modal anodal electrophoretic mobility is not always higher for IgA than for other Ig classes.

IgA myeloma proteins often display less electrophoretic homogeneity than do myeloma proteins of other classes, even in media without molecular sieve effect. Complexes of IgA with albumin, heterogeneity in molecular size, and, possibly, sialic acid content (Vaerman, 1970) are factors which might be responsible for this effect.

In humans, the anodal electrophoretic mobility of SIgA in milk, saliva (Tomasi et al., 1965), bile (Dive, 1970), and intestinal secretions (Bull et al., 1971) is slightly slower than that of serum IgA. A similar trend is seen in SIgA from dogs (Vaerman and Heremans, 1968a; Reynolds and Johnson, 1971), goats (Vaerman, 1970), horses (Vaerman et al., 1971), mice (Fahey and Barth, 1965), and rats (Bistany and Tomasi, 1970; Stechschulte and Austen, 1970).

2. Ion Exchange Chromatography

Like human IgA, IgA from various other mammals is eluted from DEAE ion exchangers at ionic strengths higher than those required to elute the bulk of the various IgG subclasses, and slightly lower than required for elution of the major part of IgM. Considerable overlapping between IgA and the other classes occurs, particularly in those species in which IgG subclasses with a fast anodal mobility are found, such as IgG_1 ("IgG_a") in the dog and IgT in the horse (Vaerman, 1970).

C. Properties Related to Molecular Size

Molecular size measurements or estimates may be obtained by analytic ultracentrifugation of purified IgA as well as by comparative

Table 2. Electrophoretic mobility of serum IgA relative to other serum immunoglobulins in various species

Species	Relative anodal mobilities					Reference
Human	IgA	$>$ IgM	$>$ IgG			Heremans (1960)
Primates	IgA	$>$ IgM	$>$ IgG			Picard et al. (1962a, b)
Dog	IgG$_1$ (IgGd)	$>$ IgM	$>$ IgA	$>$ IgG$_{2c}$ (IgGc)	$>$ IgG$_{2ab}$ (IgGab)	Johnson and Vaughan (1967); Vaerman and Heremans (1969)
Cat	IgM	$>$ IgA	$>$ IgG$_1$	$>$ IgG$_2$		Vaerman (1970)
Seal	IgM	$>$ IgA	$>$ IgG			Nash and Mach (1971)
Cow	IgM	$>$ IgA^a	$>$ IgG$_1$	$>$ IgG$_2$		Mach et al. (1969); Vaerman (1970)
Sheep	IgM	$>$ IgA^a	$>$ IgG$_1$	$>$ IgG$_2$		Pahud and Mach (1970); Vaerman (1970)
Goat	IgM	$>$ IgA^a	$>$ IgG$_1$	$>$ IgG$_2$		Pahud and Mach (1970); Vaerman (1970)
Pig	IgA	$>$ IgM	$>$ IgG$_1$	$>$ IgG$_2$		Porter (1969a); Vaerman et al. (1970)
Horse	IgT	$>$ IgM	$>$ IgA	$>$ IgG$_c$ (γ1)	$>$ IgG$_{ab}$	Vaerman et al. (1971)
Rabbit	IgA	$>$ IgM	$>$ IgG			Cebra and Robbins (1966)
Mouse	IgA	$>$ IgM	$>$ IgG$_1$ (IgF)	$>$ IgG$_2$ (IgG + IgH)		Fahey et al. (1964)
Rat	IgA	$>$ IgM	$>$ IgG$_1$	$>$ IgG$_2$		Nash et al. (1969)
Hamster	IgA	$>$ IgM	$>$ IgG$_1$	$>$ IgG$_2$		Bienenstock (1970)
Guinea pig	IgA	$>$ IgM	$>$ IgG$_1$	$>$ IgG$_2$		Vaerman and Heremans (1972)
Dolphin	IgM	$>$ IgA	$>$ IgG			Nash and Mach (1971)
Hedgehog	IgA	$>$ IgG$_1$	$>$ IgM	$>$ IgG$_2$		Vaerman and Heremans (1971)
Chicken	"Iga"	$>$ IgM	$>$ IgG (IgY)			Labacq-Verheyden et al. (1972)

^{a} Secretory IgA.

sedimentation in sucrose density gradients, by the comparison of positions of elution from Sephadex (or similar molecular sieve) columns, or by the comparison of electrophoretic mobilities in acrylamide gels of different concentration or those containing detergents. Molecular weight estimates may also be deduced from amino acid and carbohydrate composition.

Data on the molecular size of human and animal IgA in serum and secretions are listed in Table 3.

In most species, except humans and probably primates, serum IgA contains a larger proportion of dimers than monomers. In some species, only traces of monomeric IgA are found in serum. For the cow, rat, and hamster, the data are conflicting, perhaps because of environmental, strain, and age differences. Secretory IgA has an average size slightly larger than that of serum dimer IgA in most species. Small amounts of poorly defined higher polymers of IgA are usually found in secretions, occasionally together with traces of monomers, except in the human, where 7 S monomeric IgA may reach 10–20% of total IgA in secretions (Tomasi et al., 1965). It would be interesting to know whether the apparently privileged proportion of monomers in human serum IgA applies to other primates.

Diffusion coefficients ($D_{20, w} \times 10^{-7}$ cm$^2 \cdot$ sec^{-1}) are 3.0–3.6 and 2.6–2.9 for 7 S human serum and secretory IgA, respectively (Hurlimann, Waldesbühl, and Zuber, 1969; Kobayashi, 1971; Grey, Abel, and Zimmerman, 1971).

D. Other Physical Parameters

Extinction coefficients and partial specific volumes have been reported for IgA, in a few species, and are listed in Table 4.

Studies on optical rotation have revealed the absence of α-helix structure in human serum and secretory IgA (Tomasi and Bienenstock, 1968). Optical rotatory dispersion curves on human and canine IgA myeloma proteins disclosed the absence of Cotton effects at 240 nm. This effect is typical for IgG of various species, and is also present in Fab$_\alpha$ (Dorrington and Rockey, 1968).

E. Electron Microscopy

The structure of the IgG antibody molecule has been elegantly unraveled by Valentine and Green (1967). The IgG molecule is represented as a Y-shaped structure, whose two arms are Fab fragments (30–35 × 70 Å), with the tail corresponding to the Fc fragment (40 × 70 Å).

Electron micrographs have been obtained from human myeloma and secretory IgA, rabbit secretory IgA, and a mouse IgA myeloma protein having anti-DNP antibody activity (Svehag and Bloth, 1970; Bloth and Svehag, 1971; Munn, Feinstein, and Munro, 1971; Dourmashkin, Virella, and Parkhouse, 1971; Green, Dourmashkin, and Parkhouse, 1971; Parkhouse, Virella, and Dourmashkin, 1971).

The basic monomeric unit of IgA is comparable to the IgG molecule and has the same measurements (two Fab of 35 × 70 Å, one Fc of 40 × 65–70 Å). This monomeric unit is similar, whether it comes from secretory IgA or from dimeric IgA myeloma proteins of murine or human origin. The dimers (secretory IgA and myeloma proteins) are double Y-structures, joined by the ends of their Fc fragments. Flexibility is found both at the hinge regions (Fab-Fc joint) and at the Fc-Fc intersubunit joint. There is only a suspicion of a slightly (5–15 Å) larger length for the double Fc fragment of dimeric SIgA as compared to that of the serum myeloma dimeric IgA, suggesting a compact form for SC. Oligomers larger than dimers are structures assembled radially via their Fc fragments.

Mouse dimeric IgA myeloma protein (MOPC-315) was studied in the presence of mono- or bifunctional DNP haptens, as well as of DNP-ferritin. With the latter, the two free arms of IgA were distinctly shown to be the antigen-binding fragments (Fab). With monofunctional hapten, the appearance of the double Y was unchanged, but in the presence of bifunctional haptens, very particular structures, called "ladders" or "double bars," were seen. These occurred with the dimeric as well as the monomeric form of MOPC-315 protein. These double bars represented hapten-linked tetrads of dimers, or of monomers, in which the four pairs of Fab fragments were closely packed by virtue of hapten-binding and protein-protein interactions between hapten-linked molecules, possibly via their Fc fragments. "Double bars" could not be

Table 3. Molecular size of IgA in various species

Origin of IgA	Sedimentation coefficient(s)[a]	Elution zone(s) from Sephadex G-200[b]	Molecular weight estimation(s)	Gross proportions of monomer (M), dimer (D), and higher polymers (P)		
				M	D	P
Normal human serum IgA	6.3–7.0 S	7 S	162,000	+ +[c]	+	( )
Human myeloma IgA	7,10,13,15,17 S	From 7 S to excluded	Variable	Variable		
Human myeloma IgA	or 7,9,11,13,15 S					
Human secretory IgA	10.9–11.7 S	10–11 S	375,000–394,000	+	+ +	+
Canine normal serum IgA	10 S	10–11 S	280,000–310,000	( )	+ +	
Canine myeloma IgA	9.8–11 S	10–11 S	376,000	+	+ +	+
Canine secretory IgA	11.7–11.8 S	10–11 S	357,000–392,000	( )	+ +	+
Cat normal serum IgA		10–11 S		( )	+ +	
Sea lion serum IgA		10–11 S			+ +	
Bovine serum IgA[d]	6.7 S	7 S		+ +		
Bovine serum IgA[d]		10–11 S	350,000		+ +	
Bovine secretory IgA	10.8–11.2 S	10–11 S	406,000		+ +	+
Sheep serum IgA		10–11 S	330,000		+ +	
Sheep secretory IgA		10–11 S	420,000		+ +	+
Sheep secretory "IgA$_2$"[e]	15 S	Excluded				+ +
Sheep secretory "IgA$_1$"[e]	10.8 S	10–11 S			+ +	
Goat serum IgA		10–11 S	330,000		+ +	
Goat secretory IgA		10–11 S	420,000	( )	+ +	+
Porcine serum IgA	9.3–10.0 S	10–11 S		+	+ +	
Porcine secretory IgA	8.6–10 S and	10–11 S		( )	+ +	+
Porcine secretory IgA	10.6–11.2 S					

Source	S^a	Elution^b	MW	^{c}	^{c}	^{c}
Equine serum IgA		10–11 S	340,000	+	++	
Equine secretory IgA		10–11 S	400,000	( )	++	+
Rabbit secretory IgA	10.8 S	10–11 S	370,000–415,000		++	+
Mouse normal serum IgA	9 S	10–11 S		+	++	+
Mouse myeloma IgA	7,9,11,13 S or	From 7 S to excluded	Variable	Variable		
Mouse myeloma IgA	7,10,13,15 S					
Mouse myeloma IgA	3.9 S	Albumin	61,000	"Half-molecules"		
Mouse secretory IgA	11 S				++	
Rat normal serum IgA^d	7 S	7 S		++		+
Rat normal serum IgA^d		10–11 S			++	
Rat secretory IgA	10.9 S	10–11 S		( )	++	+
Hamster serum IgA	7 S	7 S		++	+ or +	
Hamster secretory IgA	15.2 S?	10–11 S			++ or ++	
Guinea pig serum IgA		7 S and 10–11 S		+	++	
Guinea pig secretory IgA	10.96 S	10–11 S		( )	++	+
Dolphin serum IgA		10–11 S		+	++	
Hedgehog serum IgA		10–11 S and 7 S		++	++	
Fowl serum "Iga"^{f}	15 S(?)	Almost excluded		+		++
Fowl secretory "Iga"^{f}	15 S	Excluded		( )	+	++

^{a} Sedimentation coefficient of main IgA component.

^{b} Zone of elution of predominant IgA component from Sephadex G-200; excluded = void volume; 7 S = slightly before IgG; 10–11 S = just behind IgM or blue dextran.

^{c} ++ = Important proportion; + = small proportion; ( ) = trace.

^{d} Conflicting data for bovine and rat serum IgA.

^{e} Questionable identification of "IgA$_2$" and "IgA$_1$."

^{f} Preliminary unpublished data.

Table 4. Extinction coefficients and partial specific volumes

Origin of IgA	Extinction coefficient ($E_{1\%,\ 1\ cm}^{280\ nm}$)	Partial specific volume ($\bar{v}$)	Reference
Human normal serum	13.4		Schultze and Heremans (1966)
	14.2		Vaerman et al. (1965)
	13.4	0.725	Grey et al. (1971)
		0.729	Tomasi and Bienenstock (1968)
Human secretory IgA	13.9	0.723	Tomasi and Bienenstock (1968)
	12.37		Newcomb et al. (1968)
		0.72	Axelsson et al. (1966)
		0.74	Hong et al. (1966)
		0.727	Kobayashi (1971)
Canine normal serum IgA	14.8	0.731–0.743	Reynolds and Johnson (1971)
Canine secretory IgA	11.80	0.728–0.735	Reynolds and Johnson (1971)
Bovine secretory IgA	13.7		Butler et al. (1972)
Porcine IgA	13.9		Curtis and Bourne (1971)
Rabbit secretory IgA	13.5	0.703	Cebra and Small (1967)
		0.685[a]	Cebra and Small (1967)
Mouse myeloma (MOPC315)			
Polymeric IgA	14.0–14.2[b]		Eisen et al. (1968)
Monomeric IgA	12.5[b]		Eisen et al. (1968)

[a] In 5 M guanidine.

[b] Extinction measured at 278 nm.

obtained with bifunctional hapten and $F(ab\ ')_{2\alpha}$ but a considerable drop in affinity for the bifunctional hapten occurred, as compared to the monomer and dimer.

These data are illustrated in Figure 1. So far, there is no indication of the localization of SC or J-chain (see below).

IV. *Chemical Properties of IgA*

A. Composition in Amino Acids and Carbohydrates

As such, amino acid and carbohydrate composition (Table 5) are merely of relative interest, particularly when derived from the very heterogeneous population represented by normal serum or secretory

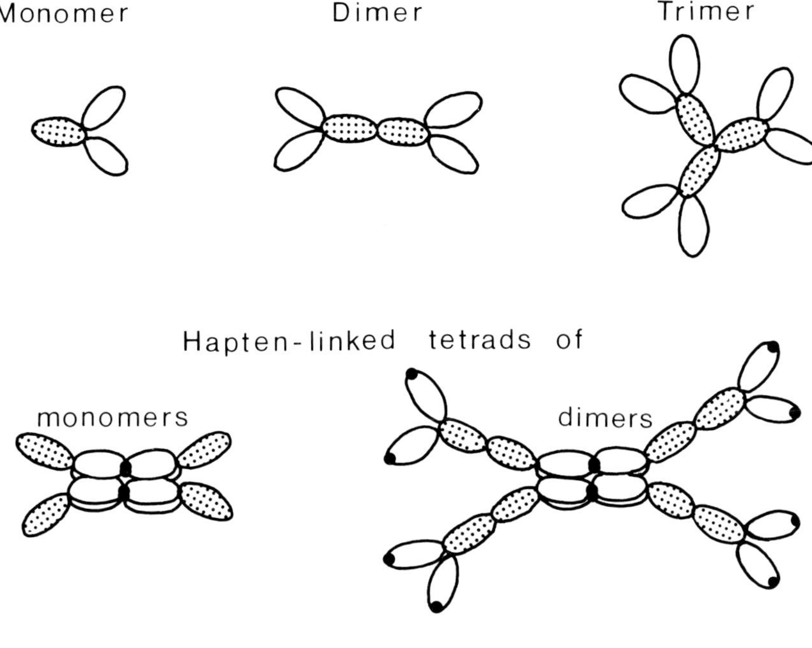

Fig. 1. Schematic models of IgA molecules according to electron micrographs. (From Green et al., 1971, and Dourmashkin et al., 1971).

IgA (Heimburger et al., 1964; Tomasi and Bienenstock, 1968; Axelsson, Johansson, and Rymo, 1966; Kobayashi, 1971).

In animals, only the composition of normal rabbit secretory IgA is available so far (Cebra and Robbins, 1966).

Amino acid compositions of IgA myeloma proteins have been published for humans (Bernier et al., 1965) and dogs (α-chains; Hurvitz, Kehoe, and Capra, 1971).

B. Constitutive Polypeptide Chains of IgA

1. Light Chains

Since they are common to all immunoglobulin classes, light chains need not receive special attention in this review. In human and rabbit SIgA, the light chains of the two monomeric units of the molecule have

Table 5. Carbohydrate composition of IgA (%)

Origin of IgA	Hexose	Hexosamine	Fucose	Sialic acid	Total	Reference
Normal human serum IgA	4.75	3.75	0.22	1.74	10.66	Heremans (1960)
Normal human serum IgA	5.5	–	–	–	–	Franklin (1962)
Normal human serum IgA	3.2	2.9	0.22	1.8	8.12	Heimburger et al. (1964)
Normal human serum IgA	3.4–3.7	3.9–4.3	–	1.7	–	Vaerman et al. (1965)
Normal human serum IgA	5.0	–	–	1.8	–	Tomasi and Bienenstock (1968)
Human myeloma IgA	3.6	–	–	–	–	Laurell and Heremans (1961)
Human myeloma IgA	6.65	2.7	–	–	–	Cummings and Franklin (1965)
Human myeloma IgA	5.1–5.3	5.1–4.5	–	2.2–1.5	–	Vaerman et al. (1965)
Human myeloma IgA	2.7–2.56	1.97–1.95	0.14–0.29	0.60–1.15	5.41–5.95	Clamp and Putnam (1967)
Human myeloma IgA	3.02	2.48	0.21	1.01	6.72	Dawson and Clamp (1968)
Human myeloma IgA	2.5–17.0	0.72–3.6	0.18–0.76	0.4–2.0	7.0–19.84	Wang and Fudenberg (1970)
Human secretory IgA	5.35	2.5	–	1.32	–	Montreuil et al. (1960)
Human secretory IgA	5.0	3.2	0.8	1.0	10.0	Muh (1966)
Human secretory IgA	5.0	4.3	2.8	0.4	12.5	Havez et al. (1966)
Human secretory IgA	4.77	4.10	0.73	0.65	10.25	Hanson and Johansson (1967)

						Reference
Human secretory IgA	6.2	—	—	0.65	—	Tomasi and Bienenstock (1968)
Canine myeloma IgA	4.5	2.21	0.66	0.48	7.85	Hurvitz et al. (1971)
Bovine secretory IgA	5.6	—	—	—	—	Mach et al. (1969)
Bovine secretory IgA	—	—	—	—	8.0	Butler et al. (1970)
Bovine secretory IgA	—	—	—	—	5.5	Butler (1971)
Sheep secretory "IgA$_2$"	4.2	3.9	—	—	—	Heimer et al. (1969)
Sheep secretory "IgA$_1$"	4.1	3.2	—	—	—	Heimer et al. (1969)
Sheep secretory IgA	—	—	—	—	7.5–8.5	MacDowell and Lascelles (1970)
Equine secretory IgA	Similar to human IgA	—	—	—	—	Audibert and Sandor (1968)
Rabbit secretory IgA	3.2	3.2	—	—	—	Cebra and Robbins (1966)
Mouse myeloma IgA	2.0–4.0	—	—	—	—	Fahey (1961)
Mouse myeloma IgA	6.7	—	—	—	—	Rask-Nielsen et al. (1961)

been found to be identical with respect to κ-λ type (Bienenstock and Straus, 1970; Small, Curry, and Waldman, 1971), and allotype (Lawton and Mage, 1969), respectively. This suggests that the SIgA molecules are synthesized as dimers, and do not result from random dimerization of monomers, before the SC is coupled to them.

Some myeloma IgA proteins cannot be typed serologically with respect to the κ-λ system of light chains, unless their light chains are first dissociated from the molecule by reduction and alkylation (Osterland and Chaplin, 1966; Hashimoto et al., 1970).

The special disulfide-linked dimer configuration of L-chains (L-SS-L), which is found in most IgA_2 molecules, is by no means an exclusive property of IgA, since it may also occur in certain forms of IgG (Grey, 1969b; Deutsch and Suzuki, 1971).

2. α-Chains

a. Human α-Chains

α-Chains are the characteristic heavy chains of IgA, supporting the class-specific antigenic determinants and the high carbohydrate content of IgA (Cohen, 1963; Carbonara and Heremans, 1963). The mobility of α-chains in acid urea starch gel electrophoresis lies between that of the γ-chains and that of the μ-chains (at least, after reduction and alkylation, which is usually the first step leading to their separation).

Two antigenically distinct subclasses of IgA molecules, differing by their α-chains, have been called IgA_1 and IgA_2 (Kunkel and Prendergast, 1966; Feinstein and Franklin, 1966; Vaerman and Heremans, 1966). IgA_2 molecules are present in much smaller concentrations than IgA_1 in all normal sera. IgA_2 myeloma proteins also occur much less frequently than IgA_1 and are frequently of high anodal mobility (Grey et al., 1968; Vaerman, Heremans, and Laurell, 1968). The molecular weights of α_1-chains and α_2-chains are similar, between 52,000 and 58,000 (Dorrington and Rockey, 1970; Abel and Grey, 1971; Montgomery, Dorrington, and Rockey, 1969). This molecular weight is not different from that of γ-chains, if the necessary allowance is made for the carbohydrate, but is distinctly smaller than that of μ-chains by about 11,000 (Grey, Abel, and Zimmerman, 1971). The α-chain, like the γ-chain, may be divided into four regions. The N-terminal fourth of the α-chain is the variable region ($V_{H\alpha}$), which appears to be shared with other immunoglobulin classes, and which may belong to any of the four V_H subgroups now identified among the heavy chain variable regions (Köhler et al., 1970; Wang et al., 1970). The three remaining fourths of the α-chain ($C1\alpha$, $C2\alpha$, $C3\alpha$) are the constant sequence regions, $C3\alpha$ being the one that carries the C-terminal amino acid.

Major differences appear to exist between IgA_1 and IgA_2 proteins. There is an absence of the H-L disulfide bonds in most IgA_2 proteins. Their light chains are noncovalently bound in the form of L-SS-L dimers (Grey et al., 1968). Analysis of a sufficient number of IgA_2 myeloma proteins has revealed that the absence of H-L disulfide bond is limited to those proteins that carry the Am2(+)-allotype marker (Kunkel et al., 1969; Vyas and Fudenberg, 1969). This marker occurs with great frequency in Caucasians, but not in Negroes. A few IgA_2 myeloma globulins, which have been found to bear the Am2(−)-marker (Jerry, Kunkel, and Grey, 1970), do have H-L disulfide bonds, which are located in the same peptide of the α_2-chain as the H-L bond of α_1-chains (Mihaesco, Seligmann, and Frangione, 1971).

Other differences between α_1-chains and α_2-chains relate to their carbohydrate and cysteine content. All α_1-chains contain galactosamine and glucosamine, and possess 16–17 cysteines, seven of which are labile; α_2-chains contain only glucosamine, and possess only 14–16 cysteines, with five of them labile (Abel and Grey, 1969; Grey, Abel, and Zimmerman, 1971). The "hinge" region of γ_1-chains is characteristically rich in proline and contains the cysteine residues involved in H-L and H-H disulfide bonds (Steiner and Porter, 1967). A "hinge" peptide isolated from α_1-chains has been shown to contain galactosamine, besides two cysteine residues probably involved in H-H bonds, but to lack the cysteine of the H-L bond. A similar peptide from an α_2-chain lacked galactosamine and 12 amino acids, among which were serine, threonine, and one cysteine (Abel and Grey, 1971). Four cyanogen bromide fragments have been characterized from an α_1-chain (Abel, 1971; Abel, personal communication), as well as three peptides from another α_1-chain: the "hinge" peptide, the H-L peptide, and the C-terminal octapeptide (Wolfenstein, Frangione, and Franklin, 1971; Frangione et al., 1971).

The C-terminal octapeptide is identical in α_1-chains and

α_2-chains. In both cases there was a tendency to spontaneous (proteolytic?) loss of the C-terminal tyrosine. Although it was thought previously (Abel and Grey, 1967; Vaerman, 1970) that the penultimate C-terminal cysteine was involved in H-H disulfide bonds responsible for the intersubunit linkage of IgA polymers, this residue seems more likely to correspond to a labile intrachain bond (Prahl, Abel, and Grey, 1971).

The N-terminus of α-chains is either glutamic acid or its cyclic form, pyrrolidone carboxylic (pyroglutamic) acid (Wang, Goodman, and Fudenberg, 1969; Montgomery, Bello, and Rockey, 1970; Köhler et al., 1970; Kaplan et al., 1971), independently of the α-chain subclass or allotype.

The noncovalent forces linking light chains to α_2-chains are stronger than those which operate between α_1-chains and light chains. This suggests evolutive pressure to select those H-chains that could form stronger noncovalent bonds with L-chains to compensate for the lack of H-L disulfide bond (Zimmerman and Grey, 1971). In *in vitro* studies on noncovalent reassociation, α-chains specifically recombined with α-chains, not with γ-chains (Grey, Abel, and Zimmerman, 1971).

In the so-called α-chain disease (α-CD) (Seligmann et al., 1969; Seligmann, Mihaesco, and Frangione, 1971), diffusely proliferating intestinal or broncho-pulmonary (Stoop et al., 1971) lymphoid plasma cells synthesize a protein similar to the Fc fragment of α-chain, lacking any light chain, rich in carbohydrate, and showing a strong tendency to polymerize. All α-CD proteins thus far studied belonged to the α_1-subclass and lacked a large part of the Fd region ($V_H + C1\alpha$), including the H-L peptide. Their molecular weights varied between 34,500 and 42,000 (Dorrington, Mihaesco, and Seligmann, 1970; Seligmann et al., 1971). The N-terminal amino acids (Val and Ileu) did not correspond to any of the unblocked V_H subgroups. Attempts at analyzing these proteins with the sequenator were unrewarding, marked heterogeneity being manifest after a few steps. The hypothesis of the origin of these α-CD proteins is that of a primary deletion, followed and obscured by secondary proteolysis (Seligmann et al., 1971).

b. Dog α-Chains

α-Chains with molecular weights of 57,000–60,500 have been isolated by classical methods from normal and myeloma serum IgA, and from colostral IgA (Reynolds and Johnson, 1971; Hurvitz et al., 1971).

When alkylated colostral IgA was submitted to gel filtration in 5 M guanidine, about 10% of the OD units were dissociated from the rest of the molecule, and some of this material was identified as light chains (Reynolds and Johnson, 1971). Acidic urea starch gel immunoelectrophoresis of unreduced canine milk IgA also revealed a release of light chains (Vaerman, 1970). Both results suggest that some canine α-chains must lack the cysteine involved in the H-L disulfide bridge.

c. Bovine α-Chains

The molecular weights of bovine α-chains, estimated by electrophoresis of reduced and alkylated bovine SIgA in acrylamide gels with detergents, were 59,000–63,000. No release of light chains from SIgA could be obtained using only dissociating solvents. The existence of some 15 S SIgA polymers in tears and nasal secretions and their disappearance in concentrated urea suggests that noncovalent forces, possibly between α-chains, are important in maintaining their polymeric structure (Butler, 1971).

d. Sheep α-Chains

Sheep α-chains isolated from "IgA_1" and "IgA_2" are reported to have molecular weights of about 63,500 (Heimer et al., 1969). However, the correct identification of these "IgA" immunoglobulins is, as stated above, questionable.

Release of light chain dimers of "IgA_2" by 4 M urea in 0.1 M acetic acid suggests the presence of some α_2-like chains in this species (Heimer et al., 1969).

e. Rabbit α-Chains

The molecular weight of α-chains from colostral IgA, prepared by preparative electrophoresis in alkaline urea gels of acrylamide, is 54,000 (O'Daly and Cebra, 1971c). An earlier value of 64,000 (Cebra and Small, 1967) was caused by contamination of α-chains with SC.

Amino acid compositions and hexosamine contents have been reported (O'Daly and Cebra, 1971c). In 5 M guanidine, 11 S colostral IgA is depolymerized to 7 S units, with release of SC and light chains, suggesting the existence of some α_2-like chains (Cebra and Small, 1967). When guanidine is removed, a 10.4 S molecule (and a 14.5 S component + aggregates) is reconstituted (60%) in the absence of the dissociated material (Lawton, Asofsky, and Mage, 1970a), indicating strong noncovalent interactions between the monomeric IgA subunits, probably via their α-chains. The roles of SC and J-chains in this respect are unclear.

f. Mouse α-Chains

α-Chains from several IgA myeloma proteins have been purified and are being characterized. The vast majority of BALB/c mouse α-chains are α_2-like (Abel and Grey, 1968; Seki, Appella and Itano, 1968; Grey, Sher, and Shalitin, 1970). Their molecular weight is 53,500–55,000. Carbohydrate, without galactosamine, as in human α_2-chains, is found in both Fab and Fc fragments, suggesting the existence of at least two glycopeptides. There are 13–15 cysteine residues in mouse α-chains, 5 of which are labile and 8–10 of which are stable. Disulfide bridges between heavy chains are confined to the Fc region. Preliminary models of α-chains have been presented (Seki et al., 1968; Grey et al., 1970).

A variant of mouse IgA represented by the "two-chain 3.9 S myeloma proteins" (Lieberman et al., 1968) consists of only part of one heavy chain, disulfide-linked to one light chain. The molecular weight of these α-chains is 40,000–46,000 (Seki et al., 1968; Mushinski, 1971). The C-terminal amino acid of the α-chain of one 3.9 S IgA was glutamine (instead of tyrosine), and there would be no cysteine among the 30–35 residues from the C-terminus. Five peptides common to all normal α-chains are lacking in α-chains from 3.9 S IgA. They are all located in the Fc of normal α-chains, suggesting a deletion in this fragment. However, these five peptides account for only 24 of the ~80 residues missing in the 3.9 S α-chains. These proteins are apparently not degradation products, and all of the six two-chain IgA myeloma proteins thus far known possessed idiotypic antigenic determinants, suggesting that the V_H region was always preserved. Such proteins could result from a deletion, possibly involving the Fd-Fc junction, leading to removal of a large stretch of polypeptide containing cysteine residues, followed by a rearrangement of the remaining heavy chain cysteines. Such a deletion could favor H-L disulfide bond formation, and impair disulfide linking of H-chain pairs. It could also explain the lack of sensitivity of these α-chains toward papain.

Another hypothesis is that the 7 S and larger polymeric IgA myeloma proteins with α_2-like chains, on one hand, and the 3.9 S proteins, on the other hand, represent different subclasses of mouse IgA (Mushinski, 1971), and hence correspond to products from different gene loci.

If IgA_2 is the sole or predominant subclass of IgA in mice, the presence of H-L disulfide bonds might reflect a mutation that introduced a critical cysteine residue into the amino acid sequence of the α-chains. It may be added that IgA myeloma proteins of NZB mice have been reported to possess the H-L bond, and that hybrids between BALB/c and NZB appear heterogeneous (heterozygous?) in this respect (Warner and Marcha, 1972).

3. *The Secretory Component (SC)*

a. Human SC

SC is a glycoprotein from secretions, which occurs both in association with two 7 S IgA molecules, as in SIgA, and in the free form (FSC). It is responsible for most of the additional antigenic determinants found on SIgA and absent from serum IgA. It can be isolated from SIgA after splitting of the disulfide bonds (Tomasi and Bienenstock, 1968; Kobayashi, 1971; Mestecky et al., 1972; Newcomb et al., 1968; Brantzaeg, 1970a), or directly from secretions (Brandtzaeg, 1970a; van Munster, Stoelinga, and Poels-Zanders, 1971; Mach, 1970; Kobayashi, 1971). Molecular weight estimates vary from 50,000 to 120,000, depending on the technique of measurement (Table 6), but values in the 60,000–80,000 range are now considered the most reliable.

Amino acid and carbohydrate compositions of SC have been reported (Tomasi and Bienenstock, 1968; Kobayashi, 1971). Estimates of its total carbohydrate range from 9.5% to 15.6%. The anodal electrophoretic mobility of FSC is somewhat variable, but always faster than that of SIgA. FSC probably consists of a single polypeptide chain, since no subunits have been found so far, even after reduction in 6 M guanidine (Tomasi and Bienenstock, 1968; Mach, 1970).

Table 6. Molecular weight of SC from various species

	Molecular weight	Method	Reference
Human dSC[a]	50,000	Ultracentrifugation	Hong, Pollara, and Good (1966)
Human dSC	54,000	Gel filtration	Hurlimann et al. (1969)
Human dSC	58,000	Ultracentrifugation	Tomasi and Bienenstock (1968)
Human dSC	60,000	Ultracentrifugation	Tomasi and Calvanico (1969)
Human FSC[b]	74,000	Ultracentrifugation	van Munster et al. (1971)
Human FSC	75,000	Ultracentrifugation	Kobayashi (1971)
Human dSC	76,000	Gel filtration	Newcomb et al. (1968)
Human FSC	80,000	**Gel filtration**	Brandtzaeg (1970)
Human FSC	85,000	**SDS-acrylamide gel** electrophoresis	Mach (1970)
Human FSC	90,000	Gel filtration	**van Munster et al. (1969)**
Human dSC	90,000–97,000	SDS-acrylamide gel electrophoresis	**Mestecky et al. (1972)**
Canine dSC	50,000	Gel filtration	Reynolds and Johnson (1971)
Bovine FSC	75,000	SDS-acrylamide gel electrophoresis	Mach (1970)
Bovine FSC	48,000	Amino acid composition	**Butler, Coulson, and Groves** (1968)

Bovine FSC	69,000–75,000	Gel filtration	Butler (1971)
Bovine FSC	86,000	Ultracentrifugation	Butler (1971)
Sheep FSC	85,000	Gel filtration	Pahud and Mach (1972)
Goat FSC	85,000	Gel filtration	Pahud and Mach (1970)
Porcine FSC	—	4 S	Porter (in press)
Equine FSC	80,000	Gel filtration	Pahud and Mach (1972)
Rabbit dSC	60,000	Ultracentrifugation	O'Daly and Cebra (1971a, c)
Rabbit FSC	60,000	Ultracentrifugation	O'Daly and Cebra (1971b)
Mouse FSC	—	4 S	Asofsky and Hylton (1968)
Guinea pig FSC	Similar to human	Gel filtration	Vaerman and Heremans (1972)

[a] dSC = secretory component dissociated from SIgA.

[b] FSC = free secretory component.

Several kinds of antigenic determinants have been identified in SC (Brandtzaeg, 1970a). Two determinants, called "A_1" and "A_2," are accessible both in free and in bound SC, "A_1" being susceptible to reduction. Native FSC has a determinant, called "I," which is highly sensitive to reduction, and inaccessible ("I") when SC is bound to SIgA, unless SIgA is first denatured by acid or urea (Brandtzaeg, 1970b). In addition, the presence of SC in SIgA creates a configurational determinant on the latter, which is absent from FSC. None of these determinants is found in serum IgA, except in a trace fraction, which seems to have all the properties of SIgA from secretions (Thompson, Asquith, and Cooke, 1969; Waldman et al., 1970; Thompson and Asquith, 1970; Brandtzaeg, 1971a).

The dissociation of appreciable amounts of SC from SIgA requires the preliminary rupture of disulfide bridges, preferably by means of 0.05 M dithiothreitol, 0.075 M mercaptoethanol, or cysteine (Brandtzaeg, 1970a). Nevertheless, even without reduction, small amounts of SC can be released (Tomasi and Bienenstock, 1968; Hanson and Johansson, 1967; Mestecky et al., 1972) by 1 M acetic or propionic acid, 8 M urea, or 5–6 M guanidine. SC probably binds to the Fc region of the α-chains, since α-CD proteins obtained from the intestinal fluid have been found to contain bound SC (Seligmann et al., 1969). It has been suggested that the fraction of SC that is released from SIgA without disulfide splitting may originate from $SIgA_2$ molecules (Grey et al., 1968); the latter could have some SC with the "I" determinant in the accessible form.

Jerry (1971) has observed increasing inhibition of the urea-induced release of dimeric light chains from IgA_2 myeloma proteins, by increasing amounts of FSC. This inhibition was blocked by iodoacetic acid, which seems to delineate a role for disulfide bridge formation or exchange. The inhibition could also be exerted on $F(ab')_2$ fragments of IgA_2 molecules. This is difficult to visualize, considering the binding of FSC to the Fc fragment in SIgA.

The *in vitro* reaction of SC with serum proteins has been studied repeatedly, both with SC obtained from SIgA after reduction and alkylation (Tomasi and Bienenstock, 1968), and with FSC (Mach 1970; Rádl et al., 1971; Brandtzaeg, 1971). The binding of FSC occurs specifically with polymeric IgA, whether from normal secretions or myeloma sera, but not with monomeric serum IgA. IgM (or possibly only the IgM polymers larger than 19 S) can also bind SC *in vitro*, but to a smaller extent (Thompson, 1970; Brandtzaeg, 1971; Rádl, 1971; Mach, 1970). It is relevant to this discussion that both IgA and IgM are known to engage in disulfide complexes with albumin (Heremans, 1960; Mannik, 1967; Vaerman, 1970). Artificial polymers of myeloma IgA obtained by reduction and reoxidation (Abel and Grey, 1968) do not bind ^{125}I-labeled SC. However, Brandtzaeg (1971) reported an increase in binding after reduction and reoxidation of mixtures of serum IgA and SC.

The recombination yields of Mach and Brandtzaeg were, however, largely different. Discrepancies clearly persist, but experimental conditions, as well as IgA subclass and molecular size, should be better defined. It was suggested that labeling of FSC with ^{125}I could make it "sticky" (Tomasi, unpublished). The new SC-IgA bond formed *in vitro* is resistant (80%) to 6 M guanidine and sensitive to reduction, thus implicating the participation of disulfide bridges (Mach, 1970). The *in vitro* formed SIgA molecules are, antigenically, partly similar to native SIgA, partly to denatured SIgA, with their "I" determinant accessible (Brandtzaeg, 1971b). In addition, it is not known whether reduced and reoxidized polymers contain the so-called polymeric antigenic determinant (Brandtzaeg, 1970a; Apicella and Allen, 1970) and the J-chain, which might be required to bind SC.

b. Canine SC

In the dog additional antigenic determinants have been identified (Figure 2) on SIgA that are absent in serum IgA (Johnson and Vaughan, 1967; Ricks et al., 1970; Reynolds and Johnson, 1971; Vaerman, unpublished). FSC having an α_2-globulin mobility on electrophoresis and a molecular size (Table 6) between those of IgG and albumin on gel filtration was found in canine colostrum, milk, tears, tracheal secretions, saliva, bile, and urine (Ricks et al., 1970; Vaerman, unpublished). An antiserum against FSC detected the "I" inaccessible determinant of FSC, which was hidden in SIgA, allowing the identification of FSC in small amounts even in the presence of SIgA (Vaerman, unpublished). Also traces of SIgA could be detected (Figure 3) in serum, as reported for the human. Some SC dissociates from canine SIgA in the presence of concentrated guanidine and is attached to the Fc fragment of SIgA (Reynolds and Johnson, 1971).

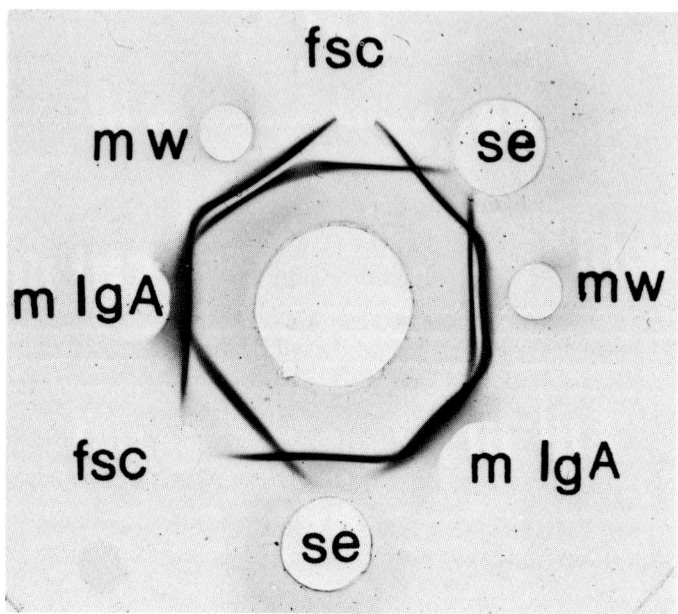

Fig. 2. Demonstration of canine secretory component. The central well received anti-SIgA from canine milk, absorbed with IgG. Peripheral wells: fsc = purified free secretory component from canine milk; se = canine serum; mw = canine milk whey; mIgA = purified SIgA from canine milk.

c. SC in Ruminants

SC has been identified, bound to SIgA and/or in free form, in ruminant colostrum, milk, saliva, tears, nasal secretions, urine, seminal fluid, and intestinal secretions. Ruminant FSC is a protein of β_2-γ_1 mobility, slightly faster than SIgA, with a molecular weight (Table 6) estimated at 75,000–85,000 (Mach, Pahud, and Isliker, 1969; Mach, 1970; Pahud and Mach, 1970; Porter and Noakes, 1970; Butler, 1971). Small amounts of SIgA were found in bovine serum, as well as in sheep and goat serum. Antisera against FSC have demonstrated the inaccessible determinant of SC in SIgA (Butler, 1971). The secretory components of these three ruminants cross-react among each other. Confusion between SC and J-chain in sheep probably led Heimer et al. (1969) to report a molecular weight of 26,500 for their sheep "SC." ^{125}I-labeled bovine FSC binds *in vitro* to IgA polymers and to IgM from the serum of many species, including the human, in a way similar to that reported for human FSC. Bovine FSC also appears to consist of a single polypeptide chain (Mach, 1970).

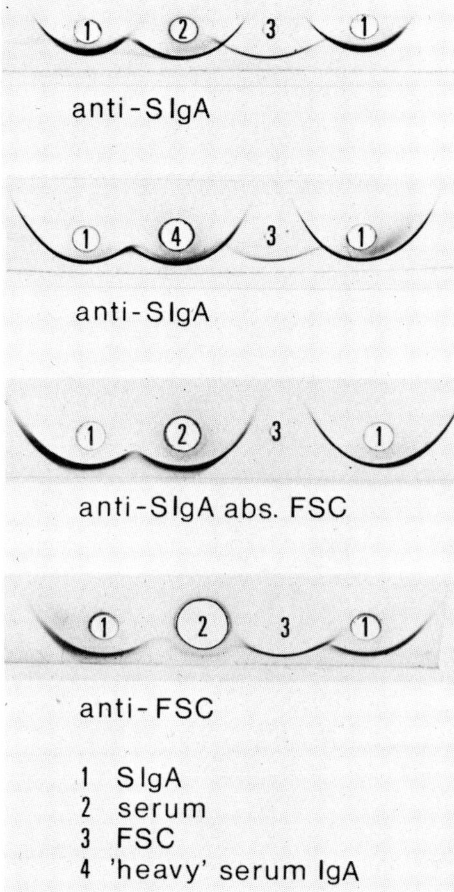

Fig. 3. Occurrence of SIgA in canine serum and of inaccessible determinants of canine SC in canine SIgA. The double precipitin line between anti-SIgA and 4, and reaction of 2 with anti-FSC demonstrate SIgA in canine serum. The spur of 3 over 1 with anti-FSC demonstrates antigenic determinants of FSC inaccessible in SIgA.

In concentrated urea or guanidine, part of the SC of bovine SIgA is released without reduction. A spontaneous partial release of SC from bovine SIgA has also been observed upon storage in aqueous solution at 4°C. Noncovalent forces are thus participating in the binding of SC to SIgA (Butler, 1971). The carbohydrate content of bovine SC was 5%, with 3.1% hexosamine.

d. SC in Pigs

The bound and free forms of pig SC have been identified by

Table 7. Sensitivity of various IgA polymers to partial reduction

Origin of IgA polymers	Conditions of reduction	Depolymerization	Reference
Normal human serum	0.1 M ME[a], 2 hr, 20°C	+	Vaerman et al. (1965)
Human myeloma	0.1 M ME, 16 hr	+	Fahey (1963)
Human SIgA	0.4 M ME, 48 hr	−[b]	Tomasi et al. (1965)
Human SIgA	0.005 M DTT[c], 1 hr	−	Newcomb et al. (1968)
Human SIgA	0.05 M DTT, 1 hr	+	Newcomb et al. (1968)
Canine normal serum	0.05 M DTT	+	Reynolds and Johnson (1971)
Canine normal serum	0.1 M ME, 2 hr, 20°C	+	Vaerman and Heremans (1969b)
Canine myeloma	0.1 M ME, 2 hr, 20°C	+	Rockey and Schwartzman (1967)
Canine SIgA	0.05 M DTT	+	Reynolds and Johnson (1971)
Canine SIgA	0.1 M ME, 2 hr, 20°C	+	Vaerman and Heremans (1969b)
Porcine SIgA	0.2 M ME, 24 hr, 20°C	+	Richardson and Kelleher (1970)
Rabbit SIgA	0.1 M ME, 1 hr	−	Cebra and Robbins (1966)
Mouse myeloma	0.1 M ME, 16 hr	+	Fahey (1961)
Rat serum	0.1 M ME, 2 hr, 20°C	+	Bistany and Tomasi (1970)
Rat SIgA	0.2 M ME, 2 hr, 20°C	−	Bistany and Tomasi (1970)
Hamster serum	0.1 M ME, 2 hr, 20°C	+	Haakenstad and Coe (1971)
Hamster SIgA	0.1 M ME, 2 hr, 20°C	−	Bienenstock (1970)

[a] ME = 2-Mercaptoethanol.

[b] Depolymerization did occur if reduction was followed by alkylation.

[c] DTT = dithiothreitol.

immunological reactions, but the properties of pig SC are as yet unknown (Bourne, 1969b; Bourne et al., 1971; Porter and Allen, 1970).

e. SC in Horses

Pahud and Mach (1972), using antihorse SIgA antiserum, obtained a typical spurring of equine SIgA over serum IgA. FSC was identified in milk, saliva, lacrimal, and nasal secretions as a protein with β_2 electrophoretic mobility and a molecular weight of around 80,000 (Table 6). In addition, ^{125}I-labeled human FSC was shown to bind *in vitro* to the dimer form of serum IgA but not to the monomer form, suggesting a similar binding for equine SC.

f. Rabbit SC

Rabbit SC may be dissociated from SIgA without reduction by 5 M guanidine (Cebra and Small, 1967; O'Daly and Cebra, 1971a) or detergents (Halpern and Koshland, 1970). The classical spur of SIgA over serum IgA was only demonstrated once, by mixing antisera with α-chain and SC specificity, respectively (Lawton et al., 1970a). Native and fully reduced and alkylated SC have been purified from SIgA, and FSC was isolated from colostrum (O'Daly and Cebra, 1971a,b). Dissociated SC (dSC), fully reduced and alkylated, was identified on acrylamide gel electrophoresis in alkaline urea as corresponding to the band with the slowest anodal mobility that was given by whole SIgA fully reduced and alkylated. This was not the case for FSC isolated from colostrum. However, dSC and FSC were antigenically identical, using anti-dSC antiserum. Similarly, their molecular weights (60,000; Table 6) were identical and both consisted of single polypeptide chains. Their amino acid and carbohydrate compositions were similar (O'Daly and Cebra, 1971a,b,c). It is now realized that the first peak of gel filtration, in dissociating solvents, of fully reduced and alkylated rabbit SIgA contains both α-chains and SC, which are now recognized as distinct polypeptides.

In vitro binding of ^{125}I-labeled dSC with guanidine-dissociated SIgA (SIgA minus SC), to an extent of approximately 60%, and with the papain fragment $(Fc)_{2\alpha}$, has been demonstrated (Lawton et al., 1970a; Lawton, 1971). *In vitro* binding of ^{125}I-labeled FSC with dissociated SIgA has also been achieved with a yield of about 40%; the fraction which did not combine was antigenically identical to the original FSC, and did not bind up renewed addition of dissociated IgA. The SIgA molecules formed *in vitro* were again dissociable (90%) by 5 M guanidine, which confirms the noncovalent nature of this linkage (O'Daly and Cebra, 1971b).

An allotypic marker of the rabbit SC molecule, known as the *f*-specificity, has now been identified (Conway, Dray, and Lichter, 1969). Allotypic markers of rabbit IgA governed by the *f*-locus are absent from IgG and IgM and are independent of the *a*- and *b*-gene loci. Five specificities, f_1 through f_5, are inherited in three phenogroups, and are found in both serum and secretory IgA. About 69% of rabbit IgA molecules bear specificities controlled by all three loci; *a, b,* and *f* (Lichter et al., 1970). The same applies to a 5 S pepsin fragment of SIgA. These *f*-markers have been identified in a mixture of α-chains and SC, as well as on purified SC (Lichter, unpublished). These findings would imply the presence of SC in serum IgA, contrary to earlier assumptions (Lawton et al., 1970a). In addition, they imply that SC is fixed to the Fab fragment, and not to $(Fc)_{2\alpha}$, as initially proposed by Lawton (1971).

g. SC in Rodents

There are practically no data on SC in rodents. In mice, FSC synthesized *in vitro* by mammary gland cultures of germ-free animals was shown to coprecipitate with exogenous mouse serum IgA, using antisera to mouse α-chains. While this "FSC" sedimented at about 4 S in density gradients (Table 6), the coprecipitating protein in a similar culture from coventional mice sedimented entirely at 11 S (Asofsky and Hylton, 1968).

In the guinea pig, FSC of milk had a slightly faster anodal mobility than SIgA and was eluted from Sephadex G-200 (Table 6) at a position similar to that of the FSC from other species (Vaerman and Heremans, 1972).

4. *J-Chains*

a. Human J-Chains

A new polypeptide chain, called the J-chain, has been identified in human polymeric IgA myeloma proteins, SIgA, and IgM from patients with Waldenström's macroglobulinemia, but not in IgG or 7 S monomeric IgA (Halpern and Koshland, 1970; Mestecky, Zikán, and Butler, 1971).

J-chains are best detected by submitting the totally reduced and alkylated protein, or its light chain fraction, to acrylamide or starch-gel electrophoresis in concentrated (6–10 M) urea at alkaline pH (8–9.5). J-chains have a much faster anodal mobility in this medium than any of the several light chain populations.

S-sulfonation, in ammonium chloride buffer, pH 8.6, containing cupric ions (Franěk and Zikán, 1964) and reduction with mercaptoethanol in pH 8.5 buffer without urea, followed by alkylation, will also release the J-chain (Cederblad et al., 1966; Hanson and Johansson, 1967; Tomasi and Bienenstock, 1968; Rejnek et al., 1966; Mestecky, et al., 1971b; Mestecky, Kulhavy, and Kraus, 1972a).

No J-chain could be dissociated from SIgA by 5 M guanidine or 1 M acetic acid (Mestecky et al., 1972a) in contrast to SC and light chains, which were released in small amounts.

Human J-chain was purified from the light chain fraction of S-sulfonated SIgA or IgM by means of chromatography on DEAE-Sephadex in 8 M urea. It was immunogenic in rabbits, and a specific antiserum could be obtained which reacted with J-chain, but not with SC, α-chains, or L-chains (Mestecky et al., 1971); conversely, J-chain did not react with specific anti-α-chain, anti-L-chain, or anti-SC.

The molecular weight of J-chain was 23,000–26,000, as estimated by gel filtration and acrylamide gel electrophoresis in detergent (Halpern and Koshland, 1970; Mestecky et al., 1971).

The molecular weights of J-chains from SIgA, polymer serum IgA, and IgM are identical, as are their antigenic properites and chemical composition. Anti-J-antiserum does not precipitate with native SIgA or IgM, but the precipitin reaction between anti-J-antiserum and J-chains can be inhibited partially by SIgA and IgM, although to different extents (Morrison and Koshland, 1972), suggesting a different configuration in the respective molecules.

The amino acid composition of J-chains is remarkable in that there is no tryptophan, but a high content of aspartic acid and cysteine, as well as of arginine and isoleucine. Aspartic acid and glutamic acid are the N- and C-terminals, respectively. The extinction coefficient, $E_{1\%}^{280}$, is given as 6.35. Total carbohydrate amounts to 7.6%, with 3 mannose, 2 galactose, 1 fucose, 3–4 glucosamine, and 1 sialic acid residue per molecule of J-chain (Mestecky et al., 1972b; Niedermeier, Tomana and Mestecky, 1972). In SIgA and IgM, the J-chain is attached to the Fc fragment obtained by trypsin digestion at 60°C (Mestecky, Kulhavy, and Kraus, 1971b).

There is only one J-chain and one SC per SIgA molecule, whose formula can therefore be written as $(\alpha_2 L_2)_2 J_1 (SC)_1$ (Mestecky et al., 1972b).

One of six patients with IgA myeloma had free J-chains in his urine, together with a Bence–Jones protein (Tomasi, unpublished).

b. Canine J-Chains

The J-chain has been identified in normal dog serum IgA as well as in SIgA (Figure 4) (Vaerman, unpublished) by its characteristic electrophoretic mobility. It is also present in canine IgA myeloma proteins (Hurvitz et al., 1971). It was claimed that canine J-chains can turn monomeric canine IgA into dimers and tetramers (Capra, unpublished).

c. Bovine J-Chains

When reduced and alkylated bovine SIgA was electrophoresed in acrylamide gel containing detergent, a polypeptide was detected with an estimated molecular weight of approximately 19,000. It was thought to represent the bovine homologue of the J-chain (Butler, 1971).

d. Sheep J-Chains

J-chains were identified in electrophoretic patterns of totally reduced and alkylated "IgA_2" (Heimer et al., 1969). However, it is not evident whether these J-chains originated from IgA or from IgM molecules, as already discussed.

e. Pig J-Chains

J-chains from porcine SIgA have been identified (Zikán, unpublished) by their electrophoretic mobility in alkaline gels containing urea.

f. Rabbit J-Chains

Rabbit J-chains from SIgA were first misidentified as SC and were called "T-chains" (see above) (Cebra and Robbins, 1966). Recently,

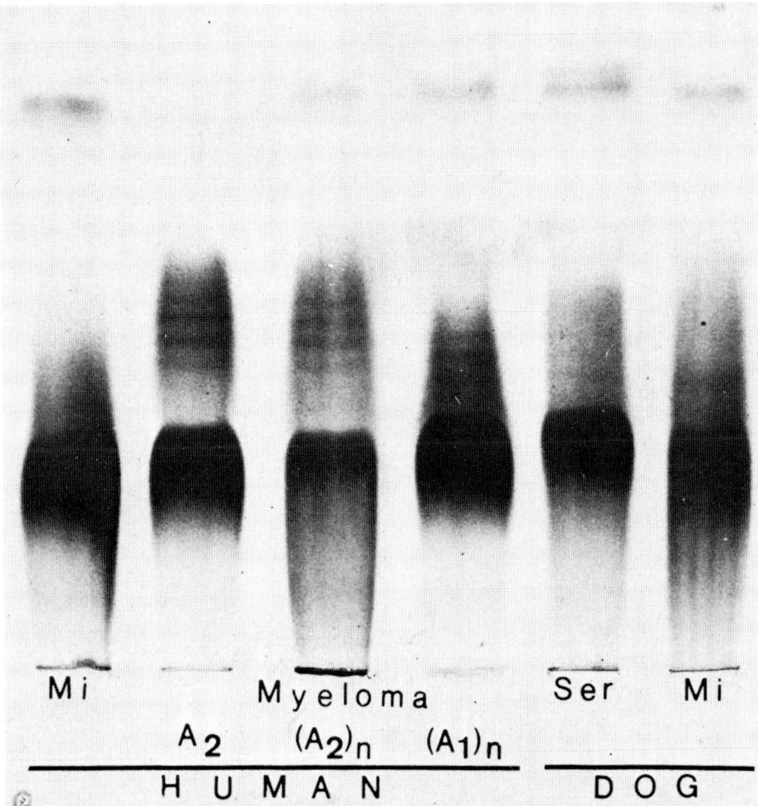

Fig. 4. Detection of J-chains in canine serum and secretory IgA. Human milk (Mi) IgA and monomeric and polymeric forms of myeloma proteins of A_2 and A_1 subclasses are compared to canine serum (Ser) and milk (Mi) IgA, by acrylamide gel electrophoresis in 8 M urea, pH 8.5. All samples were fully reduced and aklylated. Anode upwards. Note the absence of J-chains in monomeric human IgA.

J-chains have been purified in native form by preparative acrylamide gel electrophoresis in alkaline urea, after partial reduction (0.01 M dithiothreitol) and alkylation of colostral SIgA. A specific goat antiserum was obtained against J-chains, which gave no reaction with α-chains, L-chains, and SC. Conversely, J-chains were not precipitated by antisera to α-chains, light chains or SC (O'Daly and Cebra, 1971a). This antiserum to J-chains did precipitate rabbit SIgA, unlike what was found in the human.

The molecular weight of J-chains was estimated to be 23,000 by gel filtration (Halpern and Koshland, 1970) and 22,500 by electrophoresis in acrylamide gel with detergent (O'Daly and Cebra, 1971a,c). By sedimentation equilibrium, a value of 15,000 was obtained (O'Daly and Cebra, 1971c).

The last-mentioned value seems more reliable than those obtained by gel filtration or acrylamide gel electrophoresis. The latter have been shown (Schubert, 1970) to give higher values for polypeptide chains with attached carbohydrate than for the same polypeptide chains without carbohydrate, and the differences in molecular weights were much larger than what could be accounted for by the carbohydrate.

The amino acid composition of J-chains (O'Daly and Cebra, 1971c) resembles that of human J-chains, notably with regard to a high content of aspartic acid, cysteine, arginine, and isoleucine. J-chains contain about five and two residues of glucosamine and galactosamine per 15,000 daltons, respectively.

Rabbit and human J-chains appear to cross-react (Koshland, unpublished).

On the whole, it seems that the formula $(\alpha_2 L_2)_2 J_1(SC)_1$ proposed for human SIgA is also applicable to rabbit SIgA (O'Daly and Cebra, 1971c).

g. Mouse J-Chains

In the mouse, J-chains have been identified by electrophoretic analysis of polymeric IgA myeloma proteins (Koshland, unpublished).

h. J-Chains in Birds, Amphibians, and Fishes

J-chains have been identified by their electrophoretic mobility in the "macroglobulin" fraction from immune sera of pheasants, toads, and catfish (Weinheimer, Mestecky, and Acton, 1971). Whether these "macroglobulins" consisted only of IgM or of a mixture of IgM and "IgA" is unknown.

i. Conclusion

The J-chain is a well individualized polypeptide chain of polymeric IgA and IgM immunoglobulins. Its hypothetic function (Halpern and Koshland, 1970) of joining (J) the monomeric subunits by disulfide bonds remains to be proved. Disulfide bridges need to be broken before J-chains can be set free. The antigenic reactivity of the J-chain in the polymeric Ig molecule seems to be decreased by steric hindrance, at least in the human. Whether J-chains have anything to do with the polymer specificity reported by Brandtzaeg (1970), for SIgA, and by Apicella and Allen (1970), for polymeric IgA myeloma proteins, remains to be verified. One is also tempted to speculate on a possible role of the J-chain in the binding of SC to human SIgA.

C. Sensitivity to Mild Reducing Agents

A fraction of normal human serum IgA and many human IgA myeloma proteins consist of disulfide-linked polymers (from two to five) of a 7 S monomeric subunit, which are easily depolymerized by mild reducing agents such as 0.1 M mercaptoethanol in neutral buffers (Fahey, 1962, 1963a; Ballieux, Imhof, and Niehaus, 1961; Vaerman et al., 1965) but not by dissociating solvents such as concentrated solutions of acetic acid, propionic acid, urea, guanidine, or detergents.

Human secretory IgA is also largely a dimer, but it seems that mild reduction by itself is not sufficient to depolymerize an important proportion of SIgA. Assistance from dissociating agents is required here, suggesting that noncovalent interactions must help in stabilizing the dimeric structure of SIgA, possibly via the SC and the J-chain (Tomasi et al., 1965; Axelsson et al., 1966; Hurlimann et al., 1969; Hanson and Johansson, 1967; Newcomb et al., 1968; Brandtzaeg, 1970; Kobayashi, 1971; Mestecky, Kulhavy, and Kraus, 1972).

The behavior of serum and secretory IgA polymers of various species in the presence of mild reducing agents is listed in Table 7. Serum IgA polymers are always efficiently depolymerized, whereas secretory IgA displays species variation in this respect.

D. Proteolytic Fragmentation

1. Human IgA

Fragmentation of serum and/or secretory IgA has been attempted with papain (Heremans, 1960; Franklin, 1962; Deutsch, 1963; Bernier et al., 1965; Cederblad et al., 1966; Tomasi and Calvanico, 1968; Steinbuch, Reuge, and Audran, 1969), pepsin (Ballieux, Stoop, and

Zegers, 1968; Mul and Ballieux, 1968; Wilson and Williams, 1969; Wilson, 1971; Shuster, 1971), trypsin (Cederblad et al., 1966; Brown, Newcomb, and Ishizaka, 1970; Tomasi and Calvanico, 1968), chymotrypsin, and intestinal juice (Brown et al., 1970; Tomasi and Calvanico, 1968).

The major point emerging from these studies is that Fab_α-like fragments are not difficult to obtain, in contrast to Fc_α-like fragments, which are more likely to become digested to small peptides. Fc_α can be obtained by reduction with sodium borohydride (Yakulis, Costea, and Heller, 1969) or, as shown recently, by trypsin digestion at 60°C (Mestecky, Kulhavy, and Kraus, 1971b). Fc_α fragments are involved in the subunit disulfide linkage(s) of IgA polymers (Ballieux et al., 1968).

Two groups of IgA myeloma proteins, with different sensitivities to peptic digestion, were reported to be (Schuster, 1971) or not to be (Wilson and Williams, 1969) related to the IgA subclass. IgA_2 is believed to be from three to four times more efficiently digested after one hour than is IgA_1.

Secretory IgA, on the whole, appeared mildly (Wilson and Williams, 1969) or strongly (Tomasi and Calvanico, 1968; Brown et al., 1970; Shuster, 1971) more resistant to digestion than serum IgA, but this resistance was never absolute. Self-protective activity of colostral SIgA against tryptic digestion needs confirmation with respect to technical problems and controls (Shim et al., 1969). Colostral IgA was reported to form complexes with trypsin and chymotrypsin, in which significant inhibition of esterolytic activity could be demonstrated (Counitchansky, Berthillier, and Got, 1970). These observations require confirmation, especially in view of the questionable purity of the colostral SIgA employed.

2. Dog IgA

Incubation with trypsin for 30 min at 56°C, after very mild reduction and alkylation (Plaut and Tomasi, 1970), digested one-third of canine colostral IgA (Reynolds and Johnson, 1971) to Fab- and Fc-like fragments with characteristic antigenic and electrophoretic properties.

3. Rabbit IgA

Colostral IgA has been digested with papain, trypsin, and pepsin

(Lawton 1971; Masuda, Kuribayashi, and Hanaoka, 1969; Steward, 1971). Characteristic Fc_α and $(Fc)_{2\alpha}$ were obtained in small yields, and only in the absence of reducing agents; $F(ab')_{2\alpha}$ and Fab_α were not difficult to obtain.

A large fraction of SIgA resisted enzymatic digestion by these enzymes, but removal of SC with 5 M guanidine led to marked increase in enzymatic breakdown (Steward, 1971). However, this was not confirmed by Lawton (1971).

4. Mouse IgA

Fab and Fc fragments, with typical antigenic and electrophoretic properties, are readily obtained by papain digestion of mouse IgA myeloma proteins (Askonas and Fahey, 1962; Fahey, 1963b; Grey, Sher, and Shalitin, 1970). However, the so-called "two-chain" 3.9 S IgA myeloma proteins (Lieberman, Mushinski, and Potter, 1968; Seki, Appella, and Itano, 1969; Mushinski, 1971) were shown to be resistant to papain.

V. Biological Properties of IgA

A. Concentration in Serum and Secretions

1. Human IgA

The mean concentration of IgA in serum of 462 blood donors of both sexes, from 20 to 61 years of age, was estimated to be 2.63 mg/ml $\pm$ 1.13 (SD). Age groups of from 20 to 40 and from 41 to 61 had mean levels of 2.26 and 2.58 mg/ml, respectively; while this difference was of only borderline significance, males had a significantly higher mean level (2.49 mg/ml) than females (2.15 mg/ml). These absolute values were determined by single radial immunodiffusion, using a standard preparation having a polymer content very similar to that of normal serum IgA (Vaerman, 1970). Between about one-fifth and one-tenth of serum IgA is of the IgA_2 variety, but this proportion may be higher in secretions (Grey et al., 1968). In newborns the concentration of serum IgA is very low, of the order of 8 μg/ml (1.5–21.5)

(Faulkner and Borella, 1970) and it takes from 10 to 15 years to reach adult levels. The pathology associated with a deficiency or total lack of IgA in serum and secretions has been reviewed (Ammann and Hong, 1971a,b,c).

The selective concentration of IgA in secretions and the technical problems encountered in quantitating SIgA have been dealt with in several reviews on the secretory IgA system. We will give only a few quantitative data, taken from Hanson and Brandtzaeg (in press), to illustrate the very high secretion-serum ratio of IgA as compared to that of IgM or IgG (Table 8). It should be noted that in humans IgA is the predominant immunoglobulin in colostrum, and this situation prevails throughout lactation (Ammann and Stiehm, 1966).

2. IgA from Animals

Quantitative data on concentrations of immunoglobulins in serum and secretions are listed in Table 8 for several species.

a. Dog IgA

Immunoglobulins have been followed in canine milk during lactation (Vaerman and Heremans, 1969b; Reynolds and Johnson, 1970c). In absolute levels IgG was largely predominant in colostrum, but within a few days levels of IgG became negligible, whereas IgA remained at higher concentrations in milk than in serum. In mature milk, IgA is the predominant immunoglobulin. Puppies are born without IgA in their sera and no IgA is detectable in dog serum until two months of age (Reynolds et al., 1971). It is not known whether, in the suckling puppy, IgA and other immunoglobulins of canine colostrum are readily absorbed from the gut during the first hours after birth, as they are in newborn ruminants, pigs, and horses. Absorption of serum antibodies against *Salmonella* from the gut has been demonstrated to cease after 36 hr post-partum (Gillette and Filkins, 1966; Filkins and Gillette, 1966), but no mention was made of the immunoglobulin class of these antibodies.

b. IgA of Ruminants

In colostrum and milk of these species IgG_1 is the predominant immunoglobulin throughout lactation and IgA represents a quantitatively minor component. However, IgA is the predominant immunoglobulin of several other secretions. In serum IgA appears as a minor or even a trace component, and it may contain an appreciable proportion of SIgA. IgA is readily and nonselectively absorbed by newborn suckling calves, as are all other proteins; their serum IgA levels are higher than in adults.

Butler et al. (1972) determined the concentrations of IgA and IgG_1 in sera, lacteal, lacrimal, and salivary secretions of six cows from six weeks before to four weeks after parturition. Serum IgA increased before and decreased after calving, in contrast to serum IgG_1. In lacteal secretions both IgA and IgG_1 levels dropped sharply at parturition, whereas in saliva only IgA decreased. There was no significant change in tears during this study. The rise and fall in serum IgA before and after calving, respectively, closely paralleled the rise and fall in SIgA found in serum at the same time.

c. Pig IgA

IgA, although present in a much larger concentration in porcine colostrum than in serum, is not the predominant immunoglobulin of this secretion: IgG is. The IgG levels in milk drop sharply during the first few days of lactation, and IgA rapidly becomes the predominant milk immunoglobulin. The newborn piglet is practically devoid of serum immunoglobulins. Colostral IgA is readily absorbed, as are other immunoglobulins, by the suckling piglet during the first 24–36 hr of life. The serum levels of IgA, IgM, and IgG in piglets have been studied longitudinally (Curtis and Bourne, 1971; Porter and Hill, 1970). Germ free pigs are devoid of IgA in their sera at one month of age. Conventional pigs at the same age have 31 ± 4.6 mg IgA/100 ml of serum (Porter and Kenworthy, 1970). Supralethal γ-irradiation of adult pigs significantly increases (140%) the serum level of IgA within two days after irradiation, whereas IgG and IgM do not change significantly (Bazin et al., 1971a).

d. Horse IgA

In equine colostrum the predominant immunoglobulins are IgG_{ab} and IgT (Genco et al., 1969; Rouse and Ingram, 1970; Vaerman et al., 1971; Pahud and Mach, 1972), and they occur in higher concentrations in colostrum than in serum. IgA follows the same pattern, although it is not a major immunoglobulin in colostrum. However, after a

Table 8. Concentrations of IgA in serum and secretions

Species	Biological fluid	Absolute concentrations (mg/100 ml)					
				IgG			
		IgA	IgM	G_{2ab}	G_2	G_{2c}	G_1 (or T)
Human	Serum	328	132		1,230		
	Colostrum	1,234	61		10		
	Whole saliva	30.4	0.6		4.9		
	Jejunal secretions	27.6	–		34		
	Colonic secretions	82.7	–		86		
Primates	Serum	70	125		905		
Patas	Serum	179	370		870		
	Bile	5.2	<3		11.5		
Cercopithe-cus	Serum	416	105		1,082		
	Saliva	12	<3		<5		
	Stomach content	28	<3		<5		
	Jejunal content	16	<3		66		
Dog							
Pure bred	Serum	83	156	512		113	300
Mongrel	Serum	25	–	1,172		–	–
	Serum	79	145	771		112	562
	Colostrum	313	217	670		89	694
	Fecal extract	302	91	56		48	348
	Colostrum	–	–	–		–	–
	Milk day 6	–	–	–		–	–
	Milk day 30	–	–	–		–	–
	Saliva	–	–	–		–	–
	Tears	–	–	–		–	–
	Tracheal pouch secretions	–	–		–		
	Hepatic bile	–	–	–		–	–
	Intestinal secretions	–	–	–		–	–
Cat	Bile	–	–		–		
	Saliva	–	–		–		
	Tears	–	–		–		
Bovine	Serum	30	250		790		1,050
	Serum	78	–		–		–
	Lacrimal secretions	260	0.6		12		30
	Lacrimal secretions	–	–		–		–
	Nasal secretions	195	Traces		2.5		4
	Saliva	56	1		1		3
	Saliva	–	–		–		–
	Seminal fluid	13	Traces		11		13
	Intestinal secretions	24	Traces		6		25
	Bile	8	5		9		10
	Bile	–	–		–		–
	Urine	0.07	Traces		0.1		0.08

| | | Secretion-serum concentration ratios (× 10³) | | | | |
| | | IgG | | | | |
IgA	IgM	G_{2ab}	G_2	G_{2c}	G_1 (or T)	Reference
–	–		–			Hanson and Brandtzaeg
3,762	462		8			(in press)
93	4.5		4			
84.1	–		27.6			
252	–		69.9			
–	–		–			Keclik et al. (1970);
–	–		–			Felsenfeld et al. (1967,
29	<8.1		13.2			1968)
–	–		–			
28.8	<28.6		4.6			
67.3	<28.6		4.6			
38.5	<28.6		10.6			
–	–	–		–	–	Vaerman and Heremans (1969,
–	–	–		–	–	1970); Reynolds and
–	–	–		–	–	Johnson (1970c); Lieber-
3,962	1,497	869		795	1,237	man et al. (1970);
3,823	628	72.6		429	619	Reynolds et al. (1971)
14,041	455	1,833		1,311	1,095	
4,734	344	261		504	178	
6,041	537	10		76	10	
67.2	<0.17	0.09		1.2	<0.57	
285	2.9	2.4		5.7	0.4	
4,000	125		15			
10,179	128	25		131	36	
3,618	115	60		2,224	<18	
485	638(?)		0.3			Vaerman (1970)
15.6	<0.8		0.8			
23	1.2		0.03			
–	–		–		–	Vaerman (1970); Mach and
–	–		–		–	Pahud (1971); Porter
8,667	2.4		15.2		28.6	(1971); Butler et al.
10,753	27.8		<1.1		6.8	(1972)
6,500	8		3.2		3.8	
1,867	4		1.3		2.9	
758	<1.1		<0.15		<0.2	
433	<20		13.9		12.4	
800	<20		7.6		23.8	
267	20		11.4		9.5	
181	25.5		7.9		6.4	
2.3	0.04		0.13		0.08	

(Cont'd)

Table 8 (Continued)

Species	Biological fluid	Absolute concentrations (mg/100 ml)					
		IgA	IgM	IgG			
				G_{2ab}	G_2	G_{2c}	G_1 (or T)
Bovine— *Cont'd*	Colostrum	440	490		190		7,500
	Colostrum	714	800		350		6,700
	Colostrum	–	–		–		–
	Milk	5	4		6		35
	Milk	< 20	< 10		< 10		50
	Serum						
	Pre-partum	10	–		–		1,070
	Post-partum	6	–		–		1,290
	Lacteal secretions						
	Pre-partum	183	–		–		3,160
	Post-partum	23	–		–		1,380
	Saliva						
	Pre-partum	30	–		–		5
	Post-partum	17	–		–		3
	Tears						
	Pre-partum	388	–		–		54
	Post-partum	375	–		–		49
Sheep	Serum	25	120		2,100		
	Colostrum	200	410		6,000		
	Colostrum	–	–	–			–
	Milk	6	3		30		
	Saliva	20	Traces		10		
	Saliva	–	–	–			–
Goat	Serum	32	160		2,200		
	Colostrum	170	380		5,800		
	Milk	6	3		25		
	Milk	–	–	–			–
	Saliva	20	Traces		10		
	Saliva	–	–	–			–
	Lacrimal secretions	–	–	–			–
	Bile	–	–	–			–
Pig	Serum	180	110		2,150		
	Serum	237	292		2,433		
	Serum (20 days old)	59	120		1,282		
	Intestinal secretions	374	10		70		
	Saliva (20–60 days old)	–	–		–		
	Urine (20 days old)	0.063	–		0.3		
	Colostrum	1,070	320		5,870		
	Colostrum	966	319		6,180		
	Colostrum	–	–		–		
	Milk (24 hr)	376	179		1,183		
	Milk (48 hr)	272	181		816		
	Milk (3–7 days)	341	117		191		
	Milk (6 days)	–	–		–		
	Milk (8–35 days)	304	89		137		
	Milk (29 days)	–	–		–		
Horse	Serum	200	180		1,800		
	Colostrum	900	400		8,000		
	Colostrum	–	–	–			–

| | | Secretion-serum concentration ratios ($\times 10^3$) | | | | |
| | | | IgG | | | |
IgA	IgM	G_{2ab}	G_2	G_{2c}	G_1 (or T)	Reference
14,667	1,960		241		7,143	
9,154	–		–		–	
5,000	1,491		65		3,432	
167	16		7.6		33.3	
<256	–		–		–	
–	–		–		–	
–	–		–		–	
18,300	–		–		2,953	
3,833	–		–		107	
3,000	–		–		46	
2,833	–		–		23	
38,800	–		–		504	
62,500	–		–		380	
–	–			–		Pahud and Mach (1970);
8,000	3,417			2,857		Vaerman (1970)
29,846	1,404		123		1,500	
240	25			14.3		
800	42			4.8		
800	<0.7		0.5		0.3	
–	–			–		Pahud and Mach (1970);
5,313	2,375			2,636		Vaerman (1970)
188	18.8			11.4		
7,280	196		0.6		73	
625	31.3			4.5		
375	0.1		<0.2		0.1	
3,750	2.2		<2.7		6.0	
187	45		<2.7		2.8	
–	–		–			Porter (1969); Porter and
–	–		–			Allen (1969); Vaerman
						(1970); Curtis and
–	–		–			Bourne (1971); Bourne
						et al. (1971)
1,578	34.2		28.8			
175	6.8		0.42			
1.1	–		0.23			
5,944	2,909		2,609			
4,076	1,092		2,540			
4,710	1,036		8,363			
1,586	613		486			
1,148	620		335			
1,439	401		78.5			
2,030	572		151			
1,283	305		56			
2,079	331		45			
–	–			–		Vaerman et al. (1971);
4,500	2,222			4,444		Pahud and Mach
7,115	4,504	6,963		205	1,854	(1972)

(Cont'd)

148   J. P. VAERMAN

Table 8 (Continued)

Species	Biological fluid	IgA	IgM	IgG			
				G_{2ab}	G_2	G_{2c}	G_1 (or T)
Horse—	Milk	80	4		35		
Cont'd	Milk	—	—	—		—	—
	Saliva	120	1.5		15		
	Saliva	—	—	—		—	—
	Lacrimal secretions	200	3		12		
	Nasal secretions	160	Traces		8		
	Seminal fluid	8	Traces		4		
Rabbit	Serum	18	—		—		
	Serum	34.5	—		2,430		
	Serum	1.2	15		950		
	Serum	1.0	52		3,200		
	Colostrum	364	—		—		
	Colostrum	450	10		240		
	Intestinal fluid	12	1.5		7.5		
	Intestinal perfusate	13.4	2.8		8.5		
Mouse	Serum (60–150 days old)	20–360	40–250	80–500			90–240
C3H	Serum (30–50 days old)	70–370	50–210	70–220			130–590
XVII	Serum (100–300 days old)	9–66	84–391	820–3500			31–150
C3H	Serum (100 days old)	170–279	535–582	—			78–119
C57bl/C3H	Serum (180 days old)	53	433	1,290			142
	Colostrum	—	—	—			—
Rat	Colostrum	—	—	—			—
	Bile	—	—	—			—
Hamster	Serum	>10	—		—		—
	Colostrum	40	—		—		—
Guinea pig	Serum	7.2	43		836		236
	Urine	0.14	0.16		1.9		0.95
	Bile	0.50	0.07		0.2		<0.1
	Saliva	0.48	0.10		0.6		<0.1
	Tears	14.8	0.9		1.0		<0.6
	Milk	75.8	11.0		49.5		13.8
Hedgehog	Saliva	—	—		—		—
	Bile	—	—		—		—
Chicken	Bile	—	—		—		

Secretion–serum concentration ratios ($\times 10^3$) — the columns G_{2ab}, G_2, G_{2c} and G_1 (or T) are IgG subclasses.

IgA	IgM	G_{2ab}	G_2	G_{2c}	G_1 (or T)	Reference
400	22.2			19.4		
321	29	21		1.3	11	
600	8.33			8.33		
75	<3	0.5		0.3	0.35	
1,000	16.7			6.7		
800	22.2			4.4		
40	11.1			2.2		
—	—			—		Cebra and Robbins (1966); O-Daly and Cebra (1968); Clough et al. (1971); Eddie et al. (1971)
—	—			—		
—	—			—		
—	—			—		
20,222	—			—		
375,000	667			253		
12,000	29			2.3		
13,400	54			2.7		
—	—	—			—	Barth et al. (1965); Fahey et al. (1965); Asofsky and Hylton (1968); Bazin and Malet (1969); Bazin and Doria (190); Bazin et al. (1971)
—	—	—			—	
—	—	—			—	
—	—	—			—	
—	—	—			—	
>1,000	—	—			—	
32,000	—	—			—	Bistany and Tomasi (1970); Stechschulte and Austen (1970)
1,000	—	50			50	
—	—		—		—	Bienenstock (1970); Haakenstad and Coe (1971)
<4,000	—		—		—	
—	—		—		—	Vaerman and Heremans (1972)
23.4	6.8		2.6		6.6	
83.7	3.0		0.27		<0.7	
98.5	5.33		0.65		<0.9	
3,036	47.5		1.08		<5.4	
10,514	256		48		46	
8.25	<1.5		0.38		0.43	Vaerman and Heremans (1971)
39.2	<9.6		4.4		4.6	
>10,000	<1,000			<20		Lebacq-Verheyden et al. (unpublished results)

few days of lactation, IgA becomes the predominant immunoglobulin, while IgG_{ab} and IgT fall to concentrations well below their serum level. IgG_c is not found in higher concentrations in colostrum than in serum, which suggests that some selection against it is made by the mammary gland (Vaerman et al., 1971).

e. Rabbit IgA

Neonatal thymectomy slightly (75%) reduces the concentration of rabbit serum IgA, but not of IgG, and induces a markedly depressed IgA-antibody response to arsanyl-azo-BSA, with moderately reduced IgM- and normal IgG-antibody responses (Clough, Mims, and Strober, 1971).

f. Mouse IgA

It is clear that mouse serum IgA levels vary widely according to age, strain, and immune status. Germ-free mice are known to have no or only very little IgA in their sera and secretions (Crabbé et al., 1968; Asofsky and Hylton, 1968; Crabbé et al., 1970a), although this has been denied (Benveniste, Lespinats, and Salomon, 1971; Benveniste et al., 1971). Conventional newborn mice are devoid of serum IgA. Detectable levels are reached between four and six weeks, and adult levels after from three to four months (Fahey and Barth, 1965).

Thymectomized mice have normal or elevated serum IgA (Humphrey, Parrott, and East, 1964; Fahey, Barth, and Law, 1965; Bazin and Duplan, 1966). In contrast, mice which are homozygous for the "nude" mutant gene and have a congenital insufficiency of the thymus have extremely low levels of serum IgA, reduced concentrations of IgG_{2a} and, to a smaller extent, of IgG_1, and normal concentrations of IgM (Salomon and Bazin, 1972).

B. Synthesis, Catabolism, and Secretion

1. Human IgA

The biological half-life of human serum IgA is 5–6 days. Forty per cent of the total exchangeable pool is intravascular. Synthesis of IgA, like that of IgG, amounts to 24–30 mg/kg/day, excluding IgA synthesized for exportation into secretions, which may be quite elevated. The fractional catabolic rate of IgA is independent of its serum concentration (Waldmann and Strober, 1969). Whether the molecular size of IgA (monomer versus polymer) and its subclass have any influence on the catabolism of IgA is not known.

One could classify the sites of synthesis of IgA into two groups: one comprising the bone marrow, the spleen, and those lymph nodes that do not drain mucosal or glandular areas; and another consisting of those sites which are closely associated with mucosal and exocrine glands. The latter group is represented chiefly by the digestive tract. It is a common statement that the former group contains only a minor population of IgA-producing cells, as compared to IgG- and IgM-producing cells. The reverse applies to the latter group, where the vast majority of immunocytes produce IgA. Another common opinion is that the number of IgA cells present in a given glandular mucosa is more or less proportional to the IgA concentration in the exocrine secretion of that gland, although this may not necessarily apply to the mammary gland.

However, Hijmans et al. (1971), in their studies on the bone marrow by immunofluorescence, found a striking similarity between the percentage of cells containing IgA, IgG, and IgM (37, 51, and 12%, respectively) and the ratios of the synthetic rates of immunoglobulins (40, 50, and 10%, respectively). They concluded that the synthetic rates of the three immunoglobulins per cell were equal, and deduced that the bone marrow was the major source of serum IgA in the human.

It is impossible to compare the respective masses belonging to each of these two groups of IgA-producing cells. The importance of the IgA plasma cell mass of the intestinal mucosa (Crabbé et al., 1965), together with the findings of Hijmans et al. (1971), suggest that human mucosae destine the major portion of their IgA for exportation into secretions. Thoracic duct lymph, in the human, does not contain a higher proportion of IgA than does serum (Cruchaud, Laperrouza, and Mégevand, 1968; Ballieux, personal communication; Vaerman, unpublished results). This implies that in the human, in contrast to the dog and the mouse (see below), the intestinal mucosa does not contribute a significant amount of IgA to the circulating pool of this immunoglobulin.

That the major part of IgA present in exocrine secretions is locally produced has been inferred from several lines of evidence, which have been reviewed (Heremans and Vaerman, 1971).

In the human transfer of serum IgA into secretions might occur on a very small scale (South et al., 1966; Butler, Rossen, and Waldmann, 1967; Strober, Blaese, and Waldmann, 1970; Dive, 1970) and would concern only the minor 7 S fraction of IgA found in secretions (Strober et al., 1970).

The exact mechanism by which the IgA synthesized in subepithelial plasma cells gains access to secretions, as well as the roles of the SC and J-chain in this mechanism, remain largely unknown. Several hypotheses have been put forward, based on immunohistochemical data (Heremans and Crabbé, 1967; Tourville and Tomasi, 1969; Tourville et al., 1969).

A unifying hypothesis has been proposed (Heremans and Vaerman, 1971), in which active transfer into secretion through epithelial surfaces is restricted to IgA dimers, which are synthesized primarily in subepithelial IgA cells, whereas IgA monomers would not be actively transferred, and can only reach secretions by passive diffusion. The high concentrations of IgA monomer in human serum would result from a large production of IgA by extramucosal sources, e.g., the bone marrow, and would be favored by its lack of transfer to secretions. That mucosal cells make a large proportion of polymers has been suggested on the basis of analyses of the molecular size of IgA in the venous return of *in vitro* perfusions of intestinal segments. In such perfusates the IgA synthesized *in vitro* was predominantly polymeric (80%), whereas in the intestinal lumen the amount of labeled IgA polymer was approximately equal to that of the monomer (Bull et al., 1971). It should be noted that, in such experiments lymphatic connections were disrupted, and that this may influence pressure gradients of interstitial fluid. It would be of interest to know the molecular size distribution of IgA present in human mesenteric lymph.

2. Dog IgA

In the dog the IgA plasma cells of the intestinal mucosa (Vaerman and Heremans, 1970b) have been shown to contribute about 70–80% of the IgA found in mesenteric lymph, whose concentration in IgA was higher than that of serum. From these data and deductions on catabolism of IgG in dogs and humans and of IgA in humans, it was inferred that the intestinal mucosa was the major source of serum IgA in the dog (Vaerman and Heremans, 1970b; Vaerman, 1970). In a three-week-old puppy, numerous IgA cells were already observed in the intestinal mucosa, particularly in the vicinity of Peyer's patches (Vaerman and Heremans, 1969a).

In contrast, studies on proteins from biliary, salivary, and intestinal secretions of dogs having received biosynthetically labeled plasma proteins by the intravenous route revealed that, in addition to local synthesis and passive diffusion, there occurred a selective transfer of IgA into secretions, particularly into hepatic bile, and to a smaller extent also into salivary and intestinal secretions (Dive, 1970). Confirmation of the latter data would add support to the unifying hypothesis proposed by Heremans and Vaerman (1971).

3. Cat IgA

Immunohistochemical studies revealed that the cat intestinal mucosa was, as expected, predominantly populated with IgA-synthesizing plasma cells, in contrast to spleen and lymph nodes (Vaerman, 1970).

4. IgA in Ruminants

Immunofluorescence studies have disclosed that IgA-synthesizing cells predominate in the lamina propria of the bovine intestinal mucosa, as well as in bovine mammary and salivary glands. SC was located in epithelial cells (Yurchak, Butler, and Tomasi, 1971).

In vitro incorporation of labeled amino acids, by tissue cultures, into bovine immunoglobulins revealed that IgA was the principal immunoglobulin synthesized by the duodenum, ileum, colon, lungs, nasal mucosa, oral pharynx, and parotid, lacrymal, and thymus glands. Spleen and lymph nodes labeled mainly IgG and IgM. The uterus, vagina, and mammary glands synthesized all classes of immunoglobulins. In calves the same results were found except that the lungs, ileum, and thymus did not synthesize immunoglobulins. Mammary gland cultures strongly labeled the SC (Butler et al., 1971; Hurlimann and Darling, 1971).

Similarly, sheep and goats have a majority of IgA-synthesizing cells in their intestinal mucosae (Vaerman, 1970; Lee and Lascelles, 1970; Curtain and Anderson, 1971). Local IgA antibody synthesis and

secretion by the mammary gland infused with antigen was demonstrated (Lascelles and McDowell, 1970). Parasitism of sheep abomasum
and intestine induces the appearance of vast populations of IgG_1 cells
in the mucosae of these organs, in numbers equal to or larger than
those of IgA cells (Curtain and Anderson, 1971).

5. *Pig IgA*

Synthesis of IgA in pigs has been demonstrated by im-
munofluorescence in spleen and lymph nodes as well as in the majority
of the immunocytes of the intestinal lamina propria (Vaerman, 1970;
Porter and Allen, 1970; Allen and Porter, 1970; Atkins et al., 1971).
The latter authors found an accumulation of IgA cells in the vicinity of
Peyer's patches, as has been observed for dogs and mice. A few IgA
cells were also found in the mammary gland (Porter, Noakes, and
Allen, 1970). Salivary glands of pigs synthesize IgA (Hurlimann and
Darling, 1971).

Half-lives of porcine immunoglobulins were estimated by following the decline of the concentration of IgA in the serum of piglets after
ingestion of colostrum. This was justified by the previous demonstration that protein absorption from the intestine in suckling piglets is
virtually stopped after the first 24–36 hr of life (Lecce and Morgan,
1962; Bourne, 1969c), and that piglets are born practically devoid of
serum immunoglobulins (Karlsson, 1966b; Kim et al., 1966). The
half-lives of IgM, IgA, and IgG found by this method were estimated
to be, respectively, 4.5 days, 3.5 days, and 14.2 days in the study of
Curtis and Bourne (1971), and 1.3 days, 3.5 days, and 7.5 days in that
of Porter and Hill (1970). These discrepancies could be explained by
considering that the decrease in concentration in serum after colostrum
ingestion is a function not only of catabolism, but also of hemodilution,
caused by the expansion of intra- and extravascular spaces in relation
to growth.

Colostral IgA antibodies against *Escherichia coli* have been stated
to be (Bourne, Honour, and Pickup, 1971) or not to be (Porter,
1969b) absorbed by the piglet. Amazingly, the latter authors agreed on
intestinal absorption of unspecific IgA by the piglet.

6. *Horse IgA*

The sites of biosynthesis of equine IgA were assigned by immunofluorescence to the intestinal mucosa, spleen, and lymph nodes

(Vaerman et al., 1971), and also, by radioimmunoelectrophoresis, to the salivary glands (Hurlimann and Darling, 1971).

7. Rabbit IgA

Rabbit IgA is synthesized in the spleen and lymph nodes (Cebra, Colberg, and Dray, 1966) and in the interstitial plasma cells of intestinal, mammary, salivary, and bronchial glands (Crandall et al., 1967; Cohen and Kern, 1969; Cebra, 1969; O'Daly and Cebra, 1968; Lawton et al., 1970b).

The mechanism of transfer of IgA from interstitial spaces to secretions was studied in the intestinal mucosa (O'Daly, Craig, and Cebra, 1971). Granules staining for α-chains, light chains, and SC were observed in the cytoplasm of epithelial cells of the crypts of Lieberkühn, but not in the enterocytes covering the villi. These granules increased in number toward the apex of the crypt cells, where they coalesced. It could be demonstrated that they moved from the basal part of the cell to its apex, and not the reverse. It was suggested that entry of IgA in these granules at the basal part was facilitated by a membrane receptor for IgA which could be SC.

It was recently found that Peyer's patches constitute a source of cells which can proliferate and differentiate into IgA-producing plasma cells. Cells from Peyer's patches were far more effective than were cells from blood or lymph nodes (Craig and Cebra, 1971).

8. Mouse IgA

The half-life of mouse serum IgA is reported to range from 0.7 to 1.3 days (Fahey and Sell, 1965) and from 10 to 13 hr (Bazin and Malet, 1969). The former values may be overestimates resulting from whole body counting. The catabolism of mouse IgA is not affected by low or high concentrations of immunoglobulins of any class, or by the germ-free status, or by X-irradiation, but it is increased by hydrocortisone (Levy and Waldmann, 1970).

A marked and selective drop of serum IgA level occurs after whole-body X-irradiation (Bazin and Micklem, 1967; Bazin and Doria, 1970). This drop is not seen when the gut is shielded (Bazin, Maldague, and Heremans, 1970), or in mice carrying IgA-producing tumors, provided the tumor is shielded, or in germ-free mice whose serum IgA level had been elevated artificially by transfusion (Bazin,

Levi, and Heremans, 1971b). The numbers of IgA plasma cells in the gut (Crabbé et al., 1968) and the rate of biosynthesis of IgA by gut slices were moderately affected (2/3) by irradiation, and this would not explain the fall in serum IgA (Bazin et al., 1971c). However, irradiation produced lesions in the intestinal epithelium and obstructions of lymphatic vessels, causing a rechannelling of the locally produced IgA which is entirely lost into the intestinal lumen, instead of being partly drained off into the circulating pool (Bazin et al., 1971c). In conclusion in mice the intestinal mucosa seems to be a major source of serum IgA.

In growing conventional animals and in "conventionalized" adult germ-free animals, significant numbers of IgA cells first appear after 10–15 days in the intestinal mucosa and mesenteric lymph nodes. The few IgA cells present in intestinal mucosa of adult germ-free mice are often located close to the mucosal edge of Peyer's patches (Crabbé et al., 1970b). Mice homozygous for the nude gene have only small numbers of IgA cells in their intestine (Bazin, personal communication).

In addition to the spleen, lymph nodes, and intestinal mucosa, another site of biosynthesis of mouse IgA may be found in the mammary gland (Asofsky and Hylton, 1968).

Intracellular IgA produced by plasma cell tumors appears to be essentially monomeric, regardless of the degree of polymerization found in serum IgA (Abel and Grey, 1968; Parkhouse, 1971). Two types of α-chains may be found intracellularly: one with and another without attached carbohydrate (Schubert, 1970).

9. Rat IgA

By immunofluorescence, cells producing rat IgA were found in small numbers in the spleen and lymph nodes, and in very large numbers in the intestinal mucosa (Nash et al., 1969).

10. Hamster IgA

The immunohistochemical localization of cells producing IgA in the hamster was the same as in the rat (Dolezel and Bienenstock, 1970). In addition, IgA was the only immunoglobulin detected in scant isolated plasma cells in the lamina propria of the normal bronchi (Fernald, Clyde, and Bienenstock, 1972).

11. Guinea Pig IgA

The intestinal mucosa was the major site where IgA-producing cells were found by immunofluorescence, besides a few foci in the spleen and lymph nodes (Vaerman and Heremans, 1972). The salivary gland may be involved in IgA synthesis (Hurlimann and Darling, 1971).

12. Hedgehog IgA

Similar immunohistochemical findings were obtained as for the rat (Vaerman and Heremans, 1971).

13. Chicken IgA

In this species, very large numbers of IgA-containing cells were detected by immunofluorescence in the intestinal mucosa, as compared to the spleen (Lebacq-Verheyden et al., 1972).

C. Complement Fixation. Opsonization

The lack of complement fixation, in the classical hemolytic reaction, by human IgA immunoglobulins, modified by interaction with antigen, or by physical and chemical means, has been well documented (Frommhagen and Fudenberg, 1962; Heremans, Vaerman, and Vaerman, 1963; Rawson and Abelson, 1964; Ishizaka et al., 1965, 1967; Vaerman, and Heremans, 1968; Audran and Steinbuch, 1966).

In addition, it was shown that neither C1 nor C1a was fixed onto red cell-IgA antibody complexes (Ishizaka et al., 1966).

A single report by Adinolfi et al. (1966b) mentions that colostral IgA antibodies against certain $E.coli$ strains interacted with lysozyme and complement. The precise mechanism of this reaction is far from understood.

It has now been found (Spiegelberg, unpublished) that both IgA_1 and IgA_2 myeloma proteins, as well as IgG_1, IgG_2, and IgG_3, but not IgG_4, IgM, or IgD, were able to convert a C3-proactivator into a C3-activator, with the ensuing splitting of C3 and consumption of the following components of complement C5–C9. This bypass reaction is obviously initiated by the $(Fab')_2$, fragment which is common to all immunoglobulins (Reid, 1971; Sandberg et al., 1970; Sandberg, Oliveira, and Osler, 1971).

Purified colostral IgA antibodies, in contrast to IgM and IgG, to blood group substance A, do not render A-cells adherent to monocytes and neutrophils *in vitro*, nor do they promote the phagocytosis of the erythrocyte-antibody complex by neutrophils and macrophages. The significance of this work is enhanced by the fact that purified antibodies were used, so as to avoid competition for receptor sites on the phagocytic cells by nonantibody immunoglobulins (Zipursky, Brown, and Bienenstock, submitted).

In contrast, Kaplan, Dalmasso, and Woodson (1972) found a high, complement-dependent, opsonizing activity in purified colostral IgA having anti-blood-group-B activity. More experimental data are obviously required before any generalization is permissible.

Few data are available in this respect for animal IgA. Porcine colostral IgA antibodies against *E. coli* were reported to be even more effective than IgG and IgM antibodies in their ability to promote phagocytosis and intracellular killing by peritoneal cells of normal mice (Wernet et al., 1971). On the other hand, direct bactericidal action of the same IgA antibodies was negligible (Knop et al., submitted).

In the rabbit, it was reported that intestinal and colostral IgA antibodies against *Salmonella* were very poorly bactericidal, and that no potentiation of this activity occurred after addition of lysozyme (Eddie, Schulkind, and Robbins, 1971). Furthermore, IgA antibodies were able to inhibit the bactericidal effect of IgM and IgG antibodies, if IgA was added to *Salmonella* suspension before antibodies and complement. The same IgA antibodies were very poor opsonins, as judged by an *in vivo* intravenous clearance test in specific pathogen-free mice. This contrasts with the high opsonic activity reported for rabbit colostral IgA antibody against *E. coli* by Wernet et al. (1971).

In mice, lack of complement fixation by IgA anti-SIII pneumococcal polysaccharide antibodies has been reported (Kearney and Halliday, 1970).

D. Precipitation, Agglutination, Valence, Affinity

1. *Human IgA*

Whether human IgA antibodies precipitate with soluble antigens is not clear. Ishizaka et al. (1965) obtained a positive interface ring test between blood group substance A and an IgA fraction containing serum anti-A antibody activity. However, relatively more antibody was required, and precipitation required more time, than with IgM and IgG antibodies. In contrast, an IgA myeloma protein was able to precipitate DNP-protein conjugates (Andersen, McAninch, and Patterson, 1971). Only the polymeric fraction of this IgA was able to precipitate, and reduction and alkylation abolished its activity. However, care must be exercised in interpreting precipitin reactions between proteins and DNP conjugates, since ionic strength, pH, and degree of conjugation of the hydrophobic DNP hapten may strongly influence such reactions (Terry et al., 1970; Potter, 1971).

Agglutinations of particulate antigens such as red cells, bacteria, antigen-coated latex particles and viruses, by IgA antibodies, have been commonly reported. On a weight basis, IgA polymers in serum have a higher agglutinating potency than monomers (Ishizaka et al., 1965).

The valence of IgA antibodies must be at least two, because of the structure of the molecule. However, whether dimers and n-polymers have valences of 4 and $2n$, respectively, has not been verified for human IgA. Terry et al. (1970) reported a valence of 2 for an IgA myeloma protein of unspecified molecular size with DNP-binding activity. The association constant was not given.

2. Dog IgA

Agglutination of *E. coli* has been obtained with purified preparations of colostral and fecal IgA (Reynolds and Johnson, 1970a).

3. Rabbit IgA

Streptococcal cell walls were strongly agglutinated by purified rabbit colostral IgA antibodies induced by intramammary injections of group A streptococci. Such antibodies did not precipitate with the streptotoccal group A carbohydrate, but were able to inhibit the precipitation of IgG antibodies with the same antigen. Colostral IgA antibodies had a valence of 4 (per mol wt of 370,000), as estimated by equilibrium dialysis. The association constant in this case was about 6–7×10^4 1 mole^{-1}, as compared for 6.5×10^3 1 mole^{-1} for the colostral IgG antibodies (Taubman and Genco, 1971).

4. Mouse IgA

In mice, several IgA myeloma proteins have been described with antihapten (DNP) antibody activity (Eisen et al., 1970). The monomeric 7 S forms of two of these proteins have relatively high affinity constants, i.e., 3×10^5 1 mole^{-1} for MOPC-460 (Jaffe et al., 1969), and 1.7–2×10^7 1 mole^{-1} for MOPC-315 (Eisen, Simms, and Potter, 1968). These affinity constants were, however, about tenfold larger if a bifunctional hapten was used (Green, Dourmashkin, and Parkhouse, 1971). These monomeric IgA proteins, in contrast to the polymers, did not precipitate with DNP-protein conjugates, despite their divalent nature (Jaffe et al., 1969; Green et al., 1971; Rockey, Montgomery, and Dorrington, 1971). Other anti-DNP IgA myeloma proteins, detected by precipitation with DNP-protein conjugates, had very low affinity constants. They were able to precipitate with the DNP-conjugates only because they were themselves polymeric molecules and the antigen (DNP-conjugates) was highly multivalent. The complexes formed with multivalent antigens were more stable than those formed with univalent DNP-haptens. In addition, several IgA myeloma proteins were also shown to precipitate with various bacterial polysaccharide antigens, having phosphorylcholine as their immunodominant group (Potter, 1971; Cohn, Notani, and Rice, 1969; Potter and Lieberman, 1970).

Acknowledgments

This work was financially supported by Grant no. 1192 from the Fonds de la Recherche Scientifique Médicale, Brussels, Grant no. 10-013 from the Fonds de la Recherche Fondamentale Collective, Brussels, and Grant no. 66-425 from the Ford Foundation.

The author is much indebted to all those who contributed to this review by sending information and/or preprints. The assistance of Prof. J. F. Heremans, Department of Experimental Medicine, University of Louvain in Brussels, who critically reviewed this article, is gratefully acknowledged.

Our thanks are also due to Miss C. de Poortere for promptly and expertly typing this manuscript.

Literature Cited

Aalund, O. 1968. Heterogeneity of ruminant immunoglobulins. Thesis. Munksgaard, Copenhagen.

Aalund, O., J. W. Osebold, and F. A. Murphy. 1965. Isolation and characterization of ovine gamma globulins. Arch. Biochem. Biophys. 109: 142–149.

Abel, C. A. 1971. The CNBr fragments of the heavy chains of a γA1 myeloma protein. Fed. Proc. 30:467 (Abstr.).

Abel, C. A., and H. M. Grey. 1967. Carboxy-terminal amino acids of γA and γM heavy chains. Science 156: 1609–1610.

Abel, C. A., and H. M. Grey. 1968. Studies on the structure of mouse γA myeloma proteins. Biochemistry 7: 2682–2688.

Abel, C. A., and H. M. Grey. 1969. Structural differences between human γA1 and γA2 myeloma proteins. Fed. Proc. 28:495 (Abstr.).

Abel, C. A., and H. M. Grey. 1971. Structural differences in the hinge region of human gamma A myeloma proteins of different subclasses. Nature 233: 29–31.

Acharya, U. S. V., M. D. Poulik, and M. Goodman. 1968. Phylogeny of human immunoglobulins IgG, IgA and IgM. Fed. Proc. 27: 490 (Abstr.).

Acharya, U. S. V., and S. S. Rao. 1966. Studies on horse antibodies. I. Development of antibody in different fractions of serum during immunization of horse with diphtheria toxoid. Indian J. Biochem. 3: 33–37.

Adinolfi, M., A. A. Glynn, M. Lindsay, and C. M. Milne. 1966a. Serological properties of γA-antibodies to *Escherichia coli* present in human colostrum. Immunology 10: 517–526.

Adinolfi, M., P. L. Mollison, M. J. Polley, and J. M. Rose. 1966b. γ_A-blood group antibodies. J. Exp. Med. 123: 951–967.

Allen, W. D., and P. Porter. 1970. The demonstration of immunoglobulins in porcine intestinal tissue by immunofluorescence with observations on the effect of fixation. Immunology 18: 799–806.

Ammann, A. J., and R. Hong. 1971a. Selective IgA deficiency: presentation of 30 cases and a review of the literature. Medicine 50: 223–236.

Ammann, A. J., and R. Hong. 1971b. Autoimmune phenomena in ataxia telangiectasia. J. Pediat. 78: 821–826.

Ammann, A. J., and R. Hong. 1971c. Unique antibody to basement membrane in patients with selective IgA deficiency and coeliac disease. Lancet i: 1264–1266.

Ammann, A. J., and E. R. Stiehm. 1966. Immune globulins levels in colostrum, breast milk and serum from formula and breast-fed newborns. Proc. Soc. Exp. Biol. Med. 122: 1098–1100.

Andersen, B. R., J. R. McAninch, and R. Patterson. 1971. The incidence of precipitating activity in monoclonal proteins. Clin. Exp. Immunol. 8: 263–269.

Anderson, T. O., R. H. Zschocke, and G. L. Bach. 1970. Studies on IgA. II. Isolation of IgA from small volumes of human serum by immunoadsorption. J. Immunol. 105: 146–153.

Apicella, M. A., and J. C. Allen. 1970. Antigenic specificity of γA polymers. J. Immunol. 104:455–462.

Arnason, B. G., C. de Vaux St-Cyr, and E. H. Relyveld. 1964. Role of the thymus in immune reactions in rats. IV. Immunoglobulins and antibody formation. Int. Arch. Allergy 25: 206–224.

Arnason, B. G., C. de Vaux St-Cyr, and J. B. Shaffner. 1964a. A comparison of immunoglobulins and antibody production in the normal and thymectomized mouse. J. Immunol. 93: 915–925.

Arnason, B. G., J. C. Salomon, and P. Grabar. 1964b. Anticorps antifoie et immunoglobulines sériques chez les souris axéniques; étude comparative après nécrose hépatique aiguë provoquée par le tétrachlorure de carbone (CCl_4). Compt. Rend. Acad. Sci., Paris 259:4882–4885.

Aschkenasy, A., C. de Vaux St-Cyr, and J. Courcon. 1967. Effets de la thymectomie tardive sur la production des protéines sériques et des anticorps antisérumalbumine bovine chez des rats carencés en protéines et restaurés après cette carence. Compt. Rend. Soc. Biol. 161: 264–268.

Ashimura, H., and J. Koyama. 1967. Formation of guinea pig 19 S antiovalbumin antibody by various lymphoid tissues. J. Biochem. 61: 478–484.

Askonas, B. A., and J. L. Fahey. 1962. Enzymatically produced subunits of proteins formed by plasma cells in mice. II. β-2a-myeloma protein and Bence-Jones protein. J. Exp. Med. 115: 641–653.

Asofsky, R., and M. B. Hylton. 1968. Secretory IgA synthesis in germfree and conventionally reared mice. Fed. Proc. 27: 617 (Abstr.).

Atkins, A. M., G. C. Schofield, and T. Reeders. 1971. Studies on the structure and distribution of immunoglobulin A-containing cells in the gut of the pig. J. Anat. 109: 385–395.

Audibert, F., and G. Sandor. 1968. Nature de la fraction antitoxine des immunsérums de cheval. Compt. Rend. Acad. Sci., Paris 267: 457–458.

Audran, R., and M. Steinbuch. 1966. Etude de l'activité anticomplémentaire des protéines sériques humaines: action "in vitro" de la globuline γA. Pathol. Biol. 14: 838–840.

Axelsson, H., B. G. Johansson, and L. Rymo. 1966. Isolation of immunoglobulin A (IgA) from human colostrum. Acta Chem. Scand. 20: 2339–2348.

Ballieux, R. E. 1963. Structuuranalyse en classificatie van β2a-paraproteinen. Thesis. **Schotanus en Jens, Utrecht.**

Ballieux, R. E., J. W. Imhof, and G. H. Niehaus. 1961. Identification of so-called atypical macroglobulinaemia as an atypical form of β2A-paraproteinaemia: a new immunological entity? Nature 189: 768–770.

Ballieux, R. E., J. W. Stoop, and B. J. M. Zegers. 1968. Comparative studies on polymer-type serum and exocrine IgA. Scand. J. Haemat. 5: 179–190.

Banowitz, J., and K. Ishizaka. 1967. Detection of five components having antibody activity in rat antisera. Proc. Soc. Exp. Biol. Med. 125: 78–82.

Bauer, K. 1970a. Die Antigenen Determinanten der α-und μ-Ketten menschlicher Immunglobuline. Naturwissenschaften 57: 90.

Bauer, K. 1970b. An immunological time scale for primate evolution consistent with fossil evidence. Humangenetik 10: 344–350.

Baumstark, J. S. 1968. Comparative studies on the fractionation of human and swine serum proteins by anion-exchange chromatography and gel filtration. Arch. Biochem. Biophys. 125: 837–849.

Bazin, H. 1966. Les immunoglobulines de la souris. I. Obtention des immunsérums spécifiques leur correspondant. Ann. Inst. Pasteur 111: 544–550.

Bazin, H. 1967a. Les immunoglobulines de la souris. II. Etude des anticorps synthétisés dans les différentes classes d'immunoglobulines en réponse à l'injection de deux antigènes protéiques solubles. Ann. Inst. Pasteur 112: 162–172.

Bazin, H. 1967b. Les immunoglobulines de la souris. Nouv. Rev. Franç. Hématol. 7: 507–526.

Bazin, H., F. Daburon, J. P. Vaerman, and J. F. Heremans. 1971a. Serum concentrations of three immunoglobulin classes in pigs after exposure to a γ-ray dose of 1600 rads. Int. J. Radiat. Biol. 20: 93–95.

Bazin, H., C. Deckers, A. Beckers, and J. F. Heremans. 1972. Transplantable immunoglobulin-secreting tumors in rats. I. General features of LOU/Wsl strain rat immunocytomas and their monoclonal proteins. Int. J. Cancer. 10:568–580, 1972.

Bazin, H., and G. Doria. 1970. The metabolism of different immunoglobulin classes in irradiated mice. III. Effects of supralethal doses of X-rays. Int. J. Radiat. Biol. 17: 359–365.

Bazin, H., and J. F. Duplan. 1966. Modifications du taux des immunoglobulines chez des souris thymectomisées á l'âge adulte et irradiées. Rev. Franç. et Clin. Biol. 11: 987–1000.

Bazin, H., G. Levi, and J. F. Heremans. 1971b. The metabolism of different immunoglobulin classes in irradiated mice. IV. Fate of circulating IgA of tumour or transfusion origin. Immunology 20: 563–570.

Bazin, H., P. Maldague, and J. F. Heremans. 1970. The metabolism of different immunoglobulin classes in irradiated mice. II. Role of the gut. Immunology 18: 361–368.

Bazin, H., P. Maldague, E. Schonne, P. A. Crabbé, H. Baudon, and J. F. Heremans. 1971c. The metabolism of different immunoglobulin classes in irradiated mice. V. Contribution of the gut to serum IgA levels in normal and irradiated mice. Immunology 20: 571–595.

Bazin, H., and F. Malet. 1969. The metabolism of different immunoglobulin classes in irradiated mice. I. Catabolism. Immunology 17: 345–365.

Bazin, H., and H. S. Micklem. 1967. Concentration of immunoglobulins in lethally X-irradiated mice. Nature 215: 742–744.

Benacerraf, B., Z. Ovary, K. Bloch, and E. C. Franklin. 1963. Properties of guinea pig 7 S antibodies. I. Electrophoretic separation of two types of guinea pig 7 S antibodies. J. Exp. Med. 117: 937–949.

Benedict, A. A., R. T. Hersch, and C. Larson. 1963. The temporal synthesis of chicken antibodies. The effect of salt on the precipitin reaction. J. Immunol. 91: 795–802.

Benveniste, J., G. Lespinats, C. Adam, and J. C. Salomon. 1971. Immunoglobulins in intact, immunized, and contaminated axenic mice: Study of serum IgA. J. Immunol. 107:1647–1655.

Benveniste, J., G. Lespinats, and J. C. Salomon. 1971. Serum and secretory IgA in axenic and holoxenic mice. J. Immunol. 107:1656–1662.

Bernier, G. M., K. Tominaga, C. W. Easley, and F. W. Putnam. 1965. Structural studies of the immunoglobulins. II. Antigenic and chemical properties of γA myeloma globulins. Biochemistry 4: 2072–2081.

Bienenstock, J. 1970. Immunoglobulins of the hamster. II. Characterization of the γA and other immunoglobulins in serum and secretions. J. Immunol. 104: 1228–1235.

Bienenstock, J., and K. J. Bloch. 1970. Immunoglobulins of the hamster. I. Antibody activity in four immunoglobulin classes. J. Immunol. 104: 1220–1227.

Bienenstock, J., and H. Strauss. 1970. Evidence for synthesis of human colostral γA as 11 S dimer. J. Immunol. 105: 274–277.

Bienenstock, J., and T. B. Tomasi. 1968. Secretory γA in normal urine. J. Clin. Invest. 47: 1162–1171.

Binaghi, R. A., and E. Sarandon de Merlo. 1966. Characterization of rat IgA and its non-identity with the anaphylactic antibody. Int. Arch. Allergy 30: 589–596.

Bistany, T. S., and T. B. Tomasi. 1970. Serum and secretory immunoglobulins of the rat. Immunochemistry 7: 453–460.

Blanc, B. 1964. Les protéines du lactosérum. Leurs relations avec l'immunité et le métabolisme du fer. Thesis. Editions Médecine et Hygiène, Geneva.

Bloch, K. J., H. C. Morse, and K. F. Austen. 1968. Biologic properties of rat antibodies. I. Antigen-binding by four classes of anti-DNP antibodies. J. Immunol. 101: 650–657.

Bloch, K. J., Z. Ovary, F. M. Kourilsky, and B. Benacerraf. 1963. Properties of guinea pig 7 S antibodies. VI. Transmission of antibodies from maternal to fetal circulation. Proc. Soc. Exp. Biol. Med. 114: 79–82.

Bloch, K. J., and R. J. M. Wilson. 1968. Homocytotropic antibody response in the rat infected with the nematode, *Nippostrongylus brasiliensis*. III. Characteristics of the antibody. J. Immunol. 100: 629–636.

Bloth, B., and S.-E. Svehag. 1971. Further studies on the ultrastructure of dimeric IgA of human origin. J. Exp. Med. 133: 1035–1042.

Bourne, F. J. 1969a. IgA immunoglobulin from porcine milk. Biochim. Biophys. Acta 181: 485–487.

Bourne, F. J. 1969b. IgA immunoglobulin from porcine serum. Biochem. Biophys. Res. Commun. 36: 138–145.

Bourne, F. J. 1969c. Antibody transfer and colostral whey proteins in the pig. Vet. Rec. 84: 607–608.

Bourne, F. J., J. Pickup. and J. W. Honour. 1971. Intestinal immunoglobulins in the pig. Biochim. Biophys. Acta 229: 18–25.

Bourne, F. J., J. W. Honour, and J. Pickup. 1971. Natural antibodies to *Escherichia coli* in the pig. Immunology 20: 433–436.

Brandtzaeg, P. 1970a. Human secretory immunoglobulins. Dissertation. Universitetsforlaget, Oslo.

Brandtzaeg, P. 1970b. Unfolding of human secretory immunoglobulin A. Immunochemistry 7: 127–130.

Brandtzaeg, P. 1971a. Human secretory immunoglobulins. V. Occurence of secretory piece in human serum. J. Immunol. 106: 318–323.

Brandtzaeg, P. 1971b. Human secretory immunoglobulins. VI. Association of free secretory piece with serum IgA *in vitro*. Immunology 21:323–332.

Brandtzaeg, P., I. Fjellanger, and S. T. Gjeruldsen. 1968. Immunoglobulin M: Local synthesis and selective secretion in patients with immunoglobulin A deficiency. Science 160: 789–791.

Brown, W. R., R. W. Newcomb, and K. Ishizaka. 1970. Proteolytic degradation of exocrine and serum immunoglobulins. J. Clin. Invest. 49: 1374–1380.

Brummerstedt-Hansen, E. 1967. The serum proteins of the pig. An immunoelectrophoretic study. Dissertation. Munksgaard, Copenhagen.

Bull, D. M., J. Bienenstock, and T. B. Tomasi. 1971. Studies on human intestinal immunoglobulin A. Gastroenterology 60: 370–380.

Burtin, P., L. Hartmann, J. Heremans, J. J. Scheidegger, F. Westendorp-Boerma, R. Wieme, C. Wunderly, R. Fauvert, and P. Grabar. 1957. Etudes immunochimiques et immuno-électrophorétiques des macroglobulinémies. Rev. Franç. Etudes Clin. Biol. 2: 5–177.

Butler, J. E. 1971. Physicochemical and immunochemical studies on bovine IgA and glycoprotein-a. Biochim. Biophys. Acta 251:435–449.

Butler, J. E., M. L. Groves, and E. J. Coulson. 1970. The identification of secretory immunoglobulin in the cow that is antigenically related to glycoprotein-A. Fed. Proc. 29:642 (Abstr.).

Butler, J. E., C. A. Kiddy, C. S. Pierce, and C. A. Rock. 1972. Quantitative changes associated with calving in the levels of bovine immunoglobulins in selected body fluids. I. Changes in the levels of IgA, IgG 1 and total protein. Can. J. Comp. Med. 36:234–242.

Butler, J. E., and C. F. Maxwell. 1972. Preparation of bovine immunoglobulins and free secretory component and their specific antisera. J. Dairy Sci. 55:151–164.

Butler, J. E., C. F. Maxwell, M. B. Hylton, C. A. Kiddy, E. J. Coulson, and R. Asofsky. 1971. Synthesis of immunoglobulins by various tissues of the cow. Fed. Proc. 30: 243 (Abstr.).

Butler, W. T., R. D. Rossen, and T. A. Waldmann. 1967. The mechanism of appearance of immunoglobulin A in the nasal secretions in man. J. Clin. Invest. 46: 1883–1893.

Carbonara, A. O., and J. F. Heremans. 1963. Subunits of normal and pathological γ 1A-globulins (β 2a-globulins). Arch. Biochem. Biophys. 102: 137–143.

Cebra, J. J. 1969. Immunoglobulins and immunocytes. Bacteriol. Rev. 33: 159–171.

Cebra, J. J., J. E. Colberg, and S. Dray. 1966. Rabbit lymphoid cells differentiated with respect to α-, γ- and μ-heavy polypeptide chains and to allotypic markers Aa1 and Aa2. J. Exp. Med. 123: 547–558.

Cebra, J., and J. B. Robbins. 1966. γ A-immunoglobulin from rabbit colostrum. J. Immunol. 97: 12–24.

Cebra, J. J., and P. A. Small. 1967. Polypeptide chain structure of rabbit immunoglobulins. III. Secretory γ A-immunoglobulins from colostrum. Biochemistry 6: 503–512.

Cederblad, G., B. G. Johansson, and L. Rymo. 1966. Reduction and proteolytic degradation of immunoglobulin A from human colostrum. Acta Chem. Scand. 20: 2349–2357.

Chordi, A., and I. G. Kagan. 1964. Analysis of normal sheep serum by immunoelectrophoresis. J. Immunol. 93: 439–445.

Clamp, J. R., and F. W. Putnam. 1967. Glycopeptides of immunoglobulins. Investigations on IgA myeloma globulins. Biochem. J. 103: 225–229.

Clausen, J., and J. Heremans. 1960. An immunologic and chemical study of the similarities between mouse and human serum proteins. J. Immunol. 84: 128–134.

Clough, J. D., L. H. Mims, and W. Strober. 1971. Deficient IgA antibody responses to arsanilic acid bovine serum albumin (BSA) in neonatally thymectomized rabbits. J. Immunol. 106: 1624–1629.

Cohen, H. J., and M. Kern. 1969. Synthesis and secretion of γ-globulin by lymph node cells. VI. Characteristics of the structure of immunoglobulin A and its pattern of secretion by appendix cell suspensions. Biochim. Biophys. Acta 188: 255–264.

Cohen, S. 1963. Properties of the peptide chains of normal and pathological human γ-globulins. Biochem. J. 89: 334–341.

Cohn, M., G. Notani, and S. A. Rice. 1969. Characterization of the antibody to the C-carbohydrate produced by a transplantable mouse plasmocytoma. Immunochemistry 6: 111–123.

Conway, T. P., S. Dray, and E. A. Lichter. 1969. Identification and genetic control of three rabbit γA immunoglobulin allotypes. J. Immunol. 102: 544–554.

Counitchansky, Y., G. Berthillier, and R. Got. 1970. Mise en évidence et caractérisation des complexes formés entre les immunoglobulines A (IgA) du colostrum humain et la trypsine ou la chymotrypsine. Clin. Chim. Acta 30: 83–92.

Crabbé, P. A. 1967. Signification du tissu lymphoide des muqueuses digestives. Thesis. Arscia, Brussels.

Crabbé, P. A., H. Bazin, H. Eyssen, and J. F. Heremans. 1968. The normal microbial flora as a major stimulus for proliferation of plasma cells synthesizing IgA in the gut. The germ-free intestinal tract. Int. Arch. Allergy 34: 362–375.

Crabbé, P. A., A. O. Carbonara, and J. F. Heremans. 1965. The normal human intestinal mucosa as a major source of plasma cells containing γA-immunoglobulin. Lab. Invest. 14:235–248.

Crabbé, P. A., D. R. Nash, H. Bazin, H. Eyssen, and J. F. Heremans. 1970a. Studies on the immunoglobulins of the mouse intestinal secretions. Progr. Immunobiol. Stand. 4: 308–311.

Crabbé, P. A., D. R. Nash, H. Bazin, H. Eyssen, and J. F. Heremans. 1970b. Immunohistochemical observations on lymphoid tissues from conventional and germ-free mice. Lab. Invest. 22: 448–457.

Craig, S. W., and J. J. Cebra. 1971. Peyer's patches: an enriched source of precursors for IgA-producing immunocytes in the rabbit. J. Exp. Med. 134: 188–200.

Crandall, R. B., J. J. Cebra, and C. A. Crandall. 1967. The relative proportions of IgG-, IgA- and IgM-containing cells in rabbit tissues during experimental trichinosis. Immunology 12: 147–158.

Cruchaud, A., C. Laperrouza, and R. Mégevand. 1968. Agammaglobulinaemia in monozygous twins: therapeutic prospects. Birth Defects Original Article Series IV: 315–327.

Cummings, N. A., and E. C. Franklin. 1965. Atypical γ1A-globulin with the electrophoretic properties of an α2-globulin occurring in multiple myeloma. J. Lab. Clin. Med. 65: 8–17.

Curtain, C. C., and N. Anderson. 1971. Immunocytochemical localization of the ovine immunoglobulins IgA, IgG1, IgG1$_A$ and IgG2: Effect of gastro-intestinal parasitism in the sheep. Clin. Exp. Immunol. 8: 151–162.

Curtis, J., and F. J. Bourne. 1971. Immunoglobulin quantitation in sow serum, colostrum and milk, and the serum of young pigs. Biochim. Biophys. Acta 236: 319–332.

Dawson, G., and J. R. Clamp. 1968. Investigations on the oligosaccharide units of an A myeloma protein. Biochem. J. 107: 341–352.

Delhanty, J. F., and J. B. Solomon. 1966. The nature of antibodies to goat erythrocytes in the developing chicken. Immunology 11: 103–113.

Deutsch, H. F. 1963. Molecular transformations of a γ1A-globulin of human serum. J. Mol. Biol. 7: 662–671.

Deutsch, H. F., and Suzuki, T. 1971. A crystalline γG1 human monoclonal protein with an extensive H chain deletion. Ann. N.Y. Acad. Sci. 190:472–486.

Diener, E., R. Wistar, and E. H. M. Ealey. 1967. Phylogenetic studies on the immune response. II. The immune response of the Australian echidna *Tachyglossus aculeatus*. Immunology 13: 329–337.

Dive, C. 1970. Les protéines de la bile. Leur composition et leur origine. Thesis. Arscia, Brussels.

Dolezel, J., and J. Bienenstock. 1970. Immunoglobulins of the hamster. 3. Immunofluorescent localization of γA, γ1 and γ2 in various tissues. Can. J. Microbiol. 16: 727–731.

Dorrington, K. J., E. Mihaesco, and M. Seligmann. 1970. The molecular size of three α-chain disease proteins. Biochim. Biophys. Acta 221: 647–649.

Dorrington, K. J., and J. H. Rockey. 1968. Studies on the conformation of purified human and canine γA-globulins and equine γT-globulin by optical rotatory dispersion. J. Biol. Chem. 243: 6511–6519.

Dorrington, K. J., and J. H. Rockey. 1970. Differences in the molecular size of the heavy chains from gamma A1 and gamma A2 globulins. Biochim. Biophys. Acta 200: 584–586.

Dourmashkin, R. R., G. Virella, and R. M. E. Parkhouse. 1971. Electron microscopy of human and mouse myeloma serum IgA. J. Mol. Biol. 56: 207–208.

Dreesman, G., C. Larson, R. N. Pinckard, R. M. Groyon, and A. A. Benedict 1965. Antibody activity in different chicken globulins. Proc. Soc. Exp. Biol. Med. 118: 292–296.

Eddie, D. S., M. L. Schulkind, and J. B. Robbins, 1971. The isolation and biologic activities of purified secretory IgA and IgG anti-*Salmonella typhimurium* "O" antibodies from rabbit intestinal fluid and colostrum. J. Immunol. 106: 181–190.

Eisen, H. N., M. C. Michaelides, B. J. Underdown, E. P. Schulenburg, and E. S. Simms. 1970. Myeloma proteins with antihapten antibody activity. Fed. Proc. 29: 78–84.

Eisen, H. N., E. S. Simms, and M. Potter. 1968. Mouse myeloma proteins with antihapten antibody activity. The protein produced by plasma cell tumor MOPC-315. Biochemistry 7: 4126–4134.

Fahey, J. L. 1961a. Immunochemical studies of twenty mouse myeloma proteins: evidence for two groups of proteins similar to gamma and beta-2A globulins in man. J. Exp. Med. 114: 385–398.

Fahey, J. L. 1961b. Physicochemical characterization of mouse myeloma proteins: demonstration of heterogeneity for each myeloma globulin. J. Exp. Med. 114:399–413.

Fahey, J. L. 1962. Heterogeneity of γ-globulins. Adv. Immunol. 2: 41–109.

Fahey, J. L. 1963a. Heterogeneity of myeloma proteins. J. Clin. Invest. 42: 111–123.

Fahey, J. L. 1963b. Studies of γ-and β2A-globulins. Comparison of immunochemical properties of S and F (papain) fragments of myeloma proteins from inbred mice. J. Immunol. 90: 576–583.

Fahey, J. L., and W. F. Barth. 1965. The immunoglobulins of mice. 4. Serum immunoglobulin changes following birth. Proc. Soc. Exp. Biol. Med. 118: 596–600.

Fahey, J. L., W. F. Barth, and L. W. Law. 1965. Normal immunoglobulins and antibody response in neonatally thymectomized mice. J. Nat. Cancer Inst. 35: 663–678.

Fahey, J. L., and S. Sell. 1965. The immunoglobulins of mice. V. The metabolic (catabolic) properties of five immunoglobulin classes. J. Exp. Med. 122: 41–58.

Fahey, J. L., J. Wunderlich, and R. Mishell. 1964. The immunoglobulins of mice. I. Four major classes of immunoglobulins: 7S γ_2-, 7S γ_1-, $\gamma_{1.1}$ (β_{2A})- and 18S γ_{1M}- globulins. J. Exp. Med. 120:223–242.

Faulkner, W., and L. Borella. 1970. Measurement of IgA levels in human cord serum by a new radioimmunoassay. J. Immunol. 105: 786–790.

Faust, C. H., and R. P. Tengerdy. 1970. Physicochemical properties of a purified IgG antibody. Immunochemistry 7: 744–746.

Feinstein, A. 1963. Character and allotypy of an immune globulin in rabbit colostrum. Nature 199: 1197–1199.

Feinstein, A., and M. J. Hobart. 1969. Structural relationship and complement fixing activity of sheep and other ruminant immunoglobulin G subclasses. Nature 223: 950–952.

Feinstein, D., and E. C. Franklin. 1966. Two antigenically distinguishable subclasses of human A myeloma proteins differing in their heavy chains. Nature 212: 1496–1498.

Felsenfeld, O., W. Burrows, G. Kasai, W. E. Greer, and Z. Jiřička. 1968a. The cellular immune response of nonhuman primates to crude type 2 cholera toxin. J. Infect. Dis. 118: 491–499.

Felsenfeld, O., A. D. Felsenfeld, W. E. Greer, and C. W. Hill. 1966. Relationship of some vibrio antibodies to serum immune globulins in man and in *Cercopithecus aethiops*. J. Infect. Dis. 116: 329–334.

Felsenfeld, O., W. E. Greer, and A. D. Felsenfeld. 1967. Cholera toxin neutralization and some cellular sites of immune globulin formation in *Cercopithecus aethiops*. Nature 213: 1249–1251.

Felsenfeld, O., W. E. Greer, and Z. Jiřička. 1968. Early immunoglobulin formation and hemagglutinating and bactericidal titers in *Erythrocebus patas* after oral administration of a weakly pathogenic Shigella strain. Lab. Invest. 19: 146–152.

Felsenfeld, O., W. E. Greer, B. Kirtley, and Z. Jiřička. 1968b. Cholera studies in non-human primates. Part 8. Comparison of methods for the enumeration of immunologically active cells and early immune globulin, precipitin, vibriocidin and antitoxin formation. Trans. R. Soc. Trop. Med. Hyg. 62: 278–284.

Fernald, G. W., W. A. Clyde, and J. Bienenstock. 1972. Immunoglobulin-containing cells in lungs of hamsters infected with *Mycoplasma pneumoniae*. J. Immunol. 108: 1400–1408.

Filkins, M. E., and D. D. Gillette. 1966. Initial dietary influences on antibody absorption in newborn puppies. Proc. Soc. Exp. Biol. Med. 122: 686–688.

Franěk, F., and J. Zikán. 1964. Limited cleavage of disulphide bonds of pig gamma globulin by S-sulphonation. Collect. Czech. Chem. Comm. 29: 1401–1412.

Frangione, B., F. Prelli, C. Mihaesco, C. Wolfenstein, E. Mihaesco, and E. C. Franklin. 1971. Structural studies of immunoglobulin G, M and A heavy chains. Ann. N.Y. Acad. Sci. 190:71–82.

Franklin, E. C. 1962. Two types of γ_{1A}-globulins in sera from normals and patients with multiple myeloma. Nature 195: 392–394.

Frommhagen, L. H., and H. Fudenberg. 1962. The role of aggregated γ-globulins in the anticomplementary activity of human and animal sera. J. Immunol. 89: 336–343.

Genco, R. J., L. Yecies, and F. Karush. 1969. The immunoglobulins of equine colostrum and parotid fluid. J. Immunol. 103: 437–444.

Gillette, D. D., and M. Filkins. 1966. Factors affecting antibody transfer in the newborn puppy. Amer. J. Physiol. 210: 419–422.

Green, N. M., R. R. Dourmashkin, and R. M. E. Parkhouse. 1971. Electron microscopy of complexes between IgA (MOPC 315) and a bifunctional hapten. J. Mol. Biol. 56: 203–206.

Grey, H. M 1963. Production of mercaptoethanol sensitive, slowly sedimenting antibody in the duck. Proc. Soc. Exp. Biol. Med. 113: 963–967.

Grey, H. M. 1969a. Phylogeny of immunoglobulins. Adv. Immunol. 10: 51–104.

Grey, H. M. 1969b. Presence of L-L interchain disulfide bonds in reconstituted gamma G molecules. J. Immunol. 102: 848–851.

Grey, H. M., C. A. Abel, W. J. Yount, and H. G. Kunkel. 1968. A subclass of human γA-globulins (γA$_2$) which lacks the disulfide bond linking heavy and light chains. J. Exp. Med. 128: 1223–1236.

Grey, H. M., C. A. Abel, and B. Zimmerman. 1971. Structure of IgA proteins. Ann. N.Y. Acad. Sci. 190: 37–48.

Grey, H. M., A. Sher, and N. Shalitin. 1970. The subunit structure of mouse IgA. J. Immunol. 105: 75–84.

Haakenstad, A. O., and J. E. Coe. 1971. The immune response in the hamster. IV. Studies on IgA. J. Immunol. 106: 1026–1034.

Halpern, M. S., and M. E. Koshland. 1970. Novel subunit in secretory IgA. Nature 228: 1276–1278.

Hanson, L. Å., and P. Brandtzaeg. 1972. Secretory antibody systems. *In* E. R. Stiehm and V. A. Fulginiti (eds.), Immunologic Disorders in Infants and Children. W. B. Saunders, Philadelphia.

Hanson, L. Å., and B. G. Johansson. 1967. Studies on secretory IgA. Nobel Symposium 3:141–151.

Hashimoto, N., S. Chandor, W. Mandy, and M. Yokoyama. 1970. Atypical IgA with hidden light chain. Clin. Exp. Immunol. 6: 941–949.

Hathaway, A., and J. H. Peters. 1969. Secretory immune globulin of the guinea-pig. Fed. Proc. 28: 766 (Abstr.).

Havez, R., J. P. Muh, M. Bonte, and G. Biserte. 1967. Etude des γA-globulines du colostrum humain. Clin. Chim. Acta 15: 7–18.

Havez, R., M. Bonte, and Y. Moschetto. 1965. Etude des protéines du sérum de cobaye. Définition électrophorétique et immunoélectrophorétique. Bull. Soc. Chim. Biol. 47: 223–238.

Havez, R., F. Gerrin, J. P. Muh, and G. Biserte. 1966. Caractérisation et isolement des immunoglobulines A de la muqueuse gastrique. Compt. Rend. Soc. Biol. 160: 571–576.

Heimburger, N., K. Heide, H. Haupt, and H. E. Schultze. 1964. Bausteinanalysen von Humanserenproteinen. Clin. Chim. Acta 10: 293–307.

Heimer, R., L. G. Clark, and P. H. Maurer. 1969. Immunoglobulins of sheep. Arch. Biochem. Biophys. 131: 9–17.

Heimer, R., D. W. Jones, and P. H. Maurer. 1969. The immunoglobulins of sheep colostrum. Biochemistry 8: 3937–3944.

Helms, C. M., and P. Z. Allen. 1971. A comparative immunological examination of some immunoglobulins of several equine species. Comp. Biochem. Physiol. 38B: 429–449.

Heremans, J. F. 1960. Les globulines sériques du système gamma. Leur nature et leur pathologie. Thesis. Arscia, Brussels, Masson, Paris.

Heremans, J. F. 1968. Immunoglobulin formation and function in different tissues. Current Topics in Microbiology 45: 131–203.

Heremans, J. F., and P. A. Crabbé. 1967. Immunohistochemical studies on exocrine IgA. Nobel Symposium 3: 130–139.

Heremans, J. F., M. T. Heremans, and H. E. Schultze. 1959. Isolation and description of a few properties of the β_{2a}-globulin of human serum. Clin. Chim. Acta 4: 96–102.

Heremans, J. F., and J. P. Vaerman. 1971. Biological significance of IgA antibodies in serum and secretions. First Int. Congr. Immunol. 695–710.

Heremans, J. F., J. P. Vaerman, and C. Vaerman. 1963. Studies on the immune globulins of human serum. II. A study of the distribution of anti-Brucella and anti-Diphtheria antibody activities among γ_{ss}-, γ_{1M}- and γ_{1A}-globulin fractions. J. Immunol. 91: 11–17.

Hijmans, W., H. R. Schuit, and E. Hulsing-Hesseling. 1971. An immunofluorescence study on intracellular immunoglobulins in human bone marrow cells. Ann. N.Y. Acad. Sci. 177: 290–305.

Hill, W. C., and J. J. Cebra. 1965. Horse anti-SI immunoglobulins. I. Properties of γM antibody. Biochemistry 4: 2575–2584.

Hong, R., B. Pollara, and R. A. Good. 1966. A model for colostral IgA. Proc. Nat. Acad. Sci. U.S.A. 56: 602–607.

Hudson, R. J., P. J. Bandy, and W. D. Kitts. 1970. Immunochemical quantitation of ovine immunoglobulins. Amer. J. Vet. Res. 31: 1231–1236.

Humphrey, J. H., D. M. V. Parrott, and J. East. 1964. Studies on globulin and antibody production in mice thymectomized at birth. Immunology 7: 419–428.

Hurlimann, J., and H. Darling. 1971. *In vitro* synthesis of immunoglobulin A by salivary glands from animals of different species. Immunology 21: 101–111.

Hurlimann, J., M. Waldesbühl, and C. Zuber. 1969. Human salivary immunoglobulin A. Some immunological and physicochemical characteristics. Biochim. Biophys. Acta 181: 393–403.

Hurvitz, A. I., J. D. Capra, J. M. Kehoe, and R. W. Leader. 1971. Isolation and characterization of four homogeneous canine immunoglobulins. Fed. Proc. 30: 399 (Abstr.).

Hurvitz, A. I., J. M. Kehoe, and J. D. Capra. 1971. Characterization of three homogeneous canine immunoglobulins. J. Immunol. 107: 648–654.

Ishizaka, K., T. Ishizaka, E. H. Lee, and H. Fudenberg. 1965. Immunochemical properties of human γA isohemagglutinin. I. Comparisons with γG- and γM-globulin antibodies. J. Immunol. 95: 197–208.

Ishizaka, K., T. Ishizaka, T. Tada, and R. W. Newcomb. 1971. Site of synthesis and function of gamma-E, pp. 71–80. *In* The Secretory Immunologic System, 1969. U.S. Government Printing Office, Washington, D.C.

Ishizaka, K., and R. W. Newcomb. 1970. Presence of γE in nasal washings and sputum from asthmatic patients. J. Allergy 46: 197–204.

Ishizaka., T., K. Ishizaka, T. Borsos, and H. Rapp. 1966. C'1 fixation by human isoagglutinins: Fixation of C'1 by γG and γM but not γA antibody. J. Immunol. 97:716–726.

Ishizaka, T., K. Ishizaka, S. Salmon, and H. Fudenberg. 1967. Biologic activities of aggregated γ-globulin. VIII. Aggregated immunoglobulins of different classes. J. Immunol. 99:82–91.

Iványi, J., V. Valentová, and J. Černy. 1966. The dose of antigen required for the suppression of the IgM and IgG antibody response in chickens. I. The kinetics and characterization of serum antibodies. Folia Biol. 12: 157–167.

Jacks, T. M., and P. J. Glantz. 1970. *Escherichia coli* agglutinins in cow serum, colostrum and the nursing calf. Can. J. Comp. Med. 34: 213–217.

Jaffe, B. M., H. N. Eisen, E. S. Simms, and M. Potter. 1969. Myeloma proteins with anti-hapten antibody activity: ϵ-2,4-dinitrophenyl lysine binding by the protein produced by mouse plasmacytoma MOPC-460. J. Immunol. 103: 872–874.

Jerry, L. M. 1971. Thesis. The Rockefeller University, New York.

Jerry, L. M., H. G. Kunkel, and H. M. Grey. 1970. Absence of disulfide bonds linking the heavy and light chains: A property of a genetic variant of γA2 globulins. Proc. Nat. Acad. Sci. U.S.A. 65: 557–563.

Johnson, J. S., and J. H. Vaughan. 1967. Canine immunoglobulins. I. Evidence for six immunoglobulin classes. J. Immunol. 98: 923–934.

Jonas, W. E. 1969. Immunoelectrophoretic analysis of sheep serum using guinea-pig antisera to particulate antigens treated with sheep antiserum. Res. Vet. Sci. 10: 397–404.

Jones, V. E., and B. M. Ogilvie. 1967. Reaginic antibodies and immunity to *Nippostrongylus brasiliensis* in the rat. II. Some properties of the antibodies and antigens. Immunology 12: 583–597.

Jordan, S. M., and E. H. Morgan. 1969. The serum and milk whey proteins of the Echidna. Comp. Biochem. Physiol. 29: 383–391.

Kaminski, M. 1965. Etude du sérum de canard. V. Analyse immunoélectrophorétique. Bull. Soc. Chim. Biol. 47: 611–619.

Kaplan, A. P., L. E. Hood, W. D. Terry, and H. Metzger. 1971. Amino terminal sequences of human immunoglobulin heavy chains. Immunochemistry 8:801–811.

Kaplan, M. E., A. P. Dalmasso, and M. Woodson. 1972. Complement-dependent opsonization of incompatible erythrocytes by human secretory IgA. J. Immunol. 108: 275–278.

Karlsson, B. W. 1966a. Immunoelectrophoretic studies on relationships between proteins of porcine colostrum, milk and blood serum. Acta Pathol. Microbiol. Scand. 67: 83–101.

Karlsson, B. W. 1966b. Immunochemical studies on changes in blood serum proteins in piglets after colostrum ingestion and during neonatal and juvenile development. Acta. Pathol. Microbiol. Scand. 67: 237–256.

Karlsson, B. W. 1966c. Milk composition and its influence on the blood serum proteins of the young during suckling. Immunochemical, enzymatic and electron microscopic studies on swine. Dissertation. Studentlitteratur, Lund, Sweden.

Kearney, R., and W. J. Halliday. 1970. Immunity and paralysis in mice. Serological and biological properties of two distinct antibodies to type III pneumococcal polysaccharide. Immunology 19: 551–560.

Keclik, M., R. H. Wolf, O. Felsenfeld, and H. F. Smetana. 1970. Immunoglobulins and antibodies in gallbladder bile. Amer. J. Gastroenterol. 54: 19–29.

Kim, Y. B., S. G. Bradley, and D. W. Watson. 1966. Ontogeny of the immune response. I. Development of immunoglobulins in germ-free and conventional colostrum deprived piglets. J. Immunol. 97: 52–63.

Klinman, N. R., J. H. Rockey, G. Frauenberger, and F. Karush. 1966. Equine antihapten antibody. III. The comparative properties of γ G- and γ A-antibodies. J. Immunol. 96: 587–595.

Knop, J., H. Breu, P. Wernet, and D. Rowley. Submitted. The relative antibacterial efficiency of IgM, IgG and IgA from pig colostrum.

Kobayashi, K. 1971. Studies on human secretory IgA: comparative studies of the IgA-bound secretory piece and the free secretory piece protein. Immunochemistry 8: 785–800.

Köhler, H., A. Shimizu, C. Paul, V. Moore, and F. W. Putnam. 1970. Three variable-gene pools common to IgM, IgG and IgA immunoglobulins. Nature 227: 1318–1320.

Kono, R., Y. Akao, A. Sasagawa, and Y. Nomura. 1969. Studies on the local immunity of intestinal tract of chickens after oral administration of Newcastle disease virus. Jap. J. Med. Sci. Biol. 22: 235–252.

Kunkel, H. G., and R. A. Prendergast. 1966. Subgroups of γA immune globulins. Proc. Soc. Exp. Biol. Med. 122: 910–913.

Kunkel, H. G., W. K. Smith, F. G. Joslin, J. B. Natvig, and S. D. Litwin. 1969. Genetic marker of the γA2 subgroup of γA immunoglobulins. Nature 223: 1247–1248.

Lamm, M. E., B. Lisowska-Bernstein, and V. Nussenzweig. 1967. Comparison of guinea-pig γ₁ and γ₂ immunoglobulins by peptide mapping. Biochemistry 6: 2819–2828.

Larsen, B., and O. Tönder. 1967. Serum proteins in the hedgehog. Acta Physiol. Scand. 69: 262–269.

Lascelles, A. K., and G. H. McDowell. 1970. Secretion of IgA in the sheep following local antigenic stimulation. Immunology 19: 613–620.

Laurell, C. B., and J. F. Heremans. 1961. Comparison between electrophoretic patterns and hexose content of different immunological types of M-components. Acta Med. Scand. (Suppl.) 367: 101–109.

Lavergne, M., M. Raynaud, and S. Iscaki. 1966. Fixation du complément et induction de la réaction d'anaphylaxie cutanée passive (PCA) par les γG-antitoxines de cheval. Ann. Inst. Pasteur 110: 155–160.

Lawton, A. R. 1971. Proteolytic fragments of rabbit colostral IgA, pp. 55–69. *In* The Secretory Immunologic System, 1969. U.S. Government Printing Office, Washington, D.C.

Lawton, A. R., R. Asofsky, and R. G. Mage. 1970a. Synthesis of the secretory IgA in the rabbit. III. Interaction of colostral IgA fragment with T chain. J. Immunol. 104: 397–408.

Lawton, A. R., R. Asofsky, and R. G. Mage. 1970b. Synthesis of the secretory IgA in the rabbit. II. Production of alpha, light and T chains by *in vitro* cultures of mammary tissue. J. Immunol. 104: 388–396.

Lawton, A. R., and R. G. Mage. 1969. The synthesis of secretory IgA in the rabbit. I. Evidence for synthesis as an 11S dimer. J. Immunol. 102: 693–697.

Lebacq-Verheyden, A. M., J. P. Vaerman, and J. F. Heremans. 1972. A possible homologue of mammalian IgA in chicken serum and secretions. Immunology 21: 165–175.

Lebacq-Verheyden, A. M., J. P. Vaerman, and J. F. Heremans. 1972. Immunohistologic distribution of the chicken immunoglobulins. J. Immunol. 109: 652–654.

Lecce, J. G., and D. A. Morgan. 1962. Effects of dietary regimen on cessation of intestinal absorption of large molecules (closure) in the neonatal pig and lamb. J. Nutr. 78: 263–268.

Lee, C. S., and A. K. Lascelles. 1970. Antibody-producing cells in antigenically stimulated mammary glands and in the gastro-intestinal tract of sheep. Austr. J. Exp. Biol. Med. Sci. 48: 525–535.

Leslie, G. A., and L. W. Clem. 1969. Phylogeny of immunoglobulin structure and function. III. Immunoglobulins of the chicken. J. Exp. Med. 130: 1337–1352.

Leslie, G. A., H. R. Wilson, and L. W. Clem. 1971. Studies on the secretory immunologic system of fowl. I. Presence of immunoglobulins in chicken secretions. J. Immunol. 106: 1441–1446.

Levy, A. L., and T. A. Waldmann. 1970. The effect of hydrocortisone on immunoglobulin metabolism. J. Clin. Invest. 49: 1679–1684.

Lichter, E. A., T. P. Conway, A. Gilman-Sachs, and S. Dray. 1970. Presence of allotypic specificities of the three loci, *a, b* and *f,* on individual molecules of rabbit colostral γA immunoglobulin. J. Immunol. 105: 70–74.

Lieberman, P., J. Ricks, L. W. Chakrin, J. R. Wardell, and R. Patterson. 1970. Immunoglobulins in respiratory secretions obtained from the canine tracheal pouch. Proc. Soc. Exp. Biol. Med. 135: 713–716.

Lieberman, R., J. F. Mushinski, and M. Potter. 1968. Two-chain immunoglobulin A molecules: Abnormal or normal intermediates in synthesis. Science 159: 1355–1357.

Ligouzat, B., and M. Kaminski. 1965. Etudes du sérum de canard. VII. Fractionnement par chromatographie et filtration sur gel. Bull. Soc. Chim. Biol. 47: 1043–1051.

Mach, J. P. 1970. *In vitro* combination of human and bovine free secretory component with IgA of various species. Nature 228: 1278–1282.

Mach, J. P., and J. J. Pahud. 1969. Une IgA à coefficient de sédimentation 11 S dans les sécrétions externes de l'espèce bovine. Experientia 25: 1083–1084.

Mach, J. P., and J. J. Pahud. 1971. Secretory IgA, a major immunoglobulin in most bovine external secretions. J. Immunol. 106: 552–563.

Mach, J. P., J. J. Pahud, and H. Isliker. 1969. IgA with "secretory piece" in bovine colostrum and saliva. Nature 223: 952–955.

Mannik, M. 1967. Binding of albumin to γA-myeloma proteins and Waldenström macroglobulins by disulfide bonds. J. Immunol. 99: 899–906.

Mansa, B. 1965. Hypo-7S-γ-globulinaemia in mature cattle. Acta Pathol. Microbiol. Scand. 63: 153–158.

Marchalonis, J. J., and G. M. Edelman. 1968. Phylogenetic origins of antibody structure. III. Antibodies in the primary immune response of the sea lamprey, *Petromyzon marinus.* J. Exp. Med. 127: 891–914.

Masson, P. L., and J. F. Heremans. 1966. Molecular size of gamma-A-immunoglobulin from bronchial secretions. Biochim. Biophys. Acta 120: 172–173.

Masuda, T., K. Kuribayashi, and M. Hanaoka. 1969. A new allotypic antigen of rabbit colostral γA immunoglobulin. J. Immunol. 102: 1156–1162.

Mattheus, W., and G. Korn. 1967. Die neutralisierende Antikörper in Schwein nach experimenteller Infektion mit Schweinepestvirus. Zentralbl. Bakteriol. Parasitol. Infektionskr. Hyg. 204: 173–180.

Mattheus, W., G. Korn, and J. Jakubik. 1970. Die Heterogeneität der Serum-γ-Globuline des Schweines nach der Infektion mit hochvirulentem Schweinepestvirus. Zentralbl. Vet. Med. B, 17: 677–685.

McDowell, G. H., and A. K. Lascelles. 1969. Local production of antibody by ovine mammary glands infused with Salmonella flagellar antigens. Austr. J. Exp. Biol. Med. Sci. 47: 669–678.

Mestecky, J., R. Kulhavy, and F. W. Kraus. 1971a. Method of serum IgA isolation. J. Immunol. 107: 605–607.

Mestecky, J., R. Kulhavy, and F. W. Kraus. 1971b. J-chain: class distribution and site of attachment to human immunoglobulins. Fed. Proc. 30: 468 (Abstr.).

Mestecky, J., R. Kulhavy, and F. W. Kraus. 1972a. Subunit structure of secretory IgA. J. Immunol. 108: 738–747.

Mestecky, J., J. Zikán, and W. T. Butler. 1971. IgM and secretory IgA: presence of a common polypeptide chain different from light chains. Science 171: 1163–1165.

Mestecky, J., J. Zikán, W. T. Butler, and R. Kulhavy. 1972b. Studies on human secretory immunoglobulin A — III. J chain. Immunochemistry 9: 883.

Metzger, J. J., and M. Fougereau. 1968. Caractérisations biochimiques des immunoglobulins γG et γM porcines. Rôle de la dose d'antigène pour l'immunisation des porcs adultes et en cours de gestation. Rech. Vét. 1: 37–61.

Mihaesco, E., M. Seligmann, and B. Frangione. 1971. Heavy-light chain disulphide bridge common to γA1 and a genetic variant of γA2 immunoglobulins. Nature 232: 220–221.

Mohr, U., and W. Dontenwill. 1964. Organ- und Blutveränderungen beim KG-13-Plasmocytom des Goldhamsters. Z. Krebsforsch. 66: 29–40.

Monte, V., and C. E. Arbesman. 1969. Immunoglobulins of rhesus monkey. Fed. Proc. 28: 820 (Abstr.).

Montgomery, P. C., A. C. Bello, and J. H. Rockey. 1970. N-terminal sequences of equine and human immunoglobulin heavy chains. Biochim. Biophys. Acta 200: 258–266.

Montgomery, P. C., K. J. Dorrington, and J. H. Rockey. 1969. Equine antihapten antibody. The molecular weights of the subunits of equine immunoglobulins. Biochemistry 8: 1247–1258.

Montreuil, J., A. Chosson, R. Havez, and S. Mullet. 1960. Isolement de β_{2A}-globulines du lait de femme. Compt. Rend. Soc. Biol. 154: 732–736.

Morein, B. 1970. Immunity against Parainfluenza-3 virus in cattle. IgA in nasal secretions. Int. Arch. Allergy 39: 403–414.

Morris, I. G. 1967. The transmission of bovine anti-*Brucella abortus* agglutinins across the gut of suckling rats. Immunology 13: 49–61.

Morrison, S. L., and M. E. Koshland. 1972. Characterization of the J chain from polymeric immunoglobulins. Proc. Nalt. Acad. Sci. U.S.A. 69: 124–128.

Muh, J. P. 1966. Particularités de structure des gamma A-globulines du colostrum humain. Thesis. Lille, France.

Mul, N. A. J., and R. E. Ballieux. 1968. Immunologic specificity of the antibody fragments of G- and A-immunoglobulins. Immunochemistry 5: 399–401.

Munn, E. A., A. Feinstein, and A. J. Munro. 1971. Electron microscope examination of free IgA molecules and of their complexes with antigen. Nature 231: 527–529.

Murphy, F. A., O. Aalund, J. W. Osebold, and E. J. Carroll. 1964. Gamma globulins of bovine lacteal secretions. Arch. Biochem. Biophys. 108: 230–239.

Murphy, F. A., J. W. Osebold, and O. Aalund. 1965. Physical heterogeneity of bovine γ-globulins: characterization of γM and γG globulins. Arch. Biochem. Biophys. 112: 126–136.

Mushinski, F. 1971. γA half molecules: Defective heavy chain mutants in mouse myeloma proteins. J. Immunol. 106: 41–50.

Nansen, P., and K. Nielsen. 1966. Metabolism of bovine immunoglobulin. I. Metabolism of bovine IgG in cattle with chronic pyogenic infections. Can. J. Comp. Med. 30: 327–331.

Nash, D. R., C. Deckers, and J. F. Heremans. 1970. Identification and characterization of three spontaneous myeloma proteins in Wistar rats. Fed. Proc. 29: 704 (Abstr.).

Nash, D. R., and J. P. Mach. 1971. Immunoglobulin classes in aquatic mammals. Characterization by serological cross-reactivity, molecular size and binding of human free secretory component. J. Immunol. 107: 1424–1430.

Nash, D. R., J. P. Vaerman, H. Bazin, and J. F. Heremans. 1969. Identification of IgA in rat serum and secretions. J. Immunol. 103: 145–148.

Nash, D. R., J. P. Vaerman, H. Bazin, and J. F. Heremans. 1970. Comparative molecular size of mouse IgA in different body fluids. Int. Arch. Allergy 37: 167–174.

Newcomb, R. W., D. Normansell, and D. Stanworth. 1968. A structural study of human exocrine IgA globulin. J. Immunol. 101: 905–914.

Niedermeier, W., M. Tomana, and J. Mestecky. 1972. The carbohydrate composition of J chain from human serum and secretory IgA. Biochim. Biophys. Acta 257: 527–530.

O'Daly, J. A., and J. J. Cebra. 1968. Structure and cellular localization of secretory IgA. Protides Biol. Fluids 16: 205–219.

O'Daly, J. A., and J. J. Cebra. 1971a. Rabbit secretory IgA. I. Isolation of secretory component after selective dissociation of the immunoglobulin. J. Immunol. 107: 436–448.

O'Daly, J. A., and J. J. Cebra. 1971b. Rabbit secretory IgA. II. Free secretory component from colostrum and its specific association with IgA. J. Immunol. 107: 449–455.

O'Daly, J. A., and J. J. Cebra. 1971c. Chemical and physicochemical studies of the component polypeptide chains of rabbit secretory immunoglobulin A. Biochemistry 10: 3843–3850.

O'Daly, J. A., S. W. Craig, and J. J. Cebra. 1971. Localization of b markers, α-chain and SC of the SIgA in epithelial cells lining Lieberkühn crypts. J. Immunol. 106: 286–288.

Oettgen, H. F., R. A. Binaghi, and B. Benacerraf. 1965. Hexose content of guinea-pig γ_1 and γ_2 immunoglobulins. Proc. Soc. Exp. Biol. Med. 118: 336–342.

Okoshi, S., I. Tomoda, and S. Makimura. 1967. Analysis of normal dog serum by immunoelectrophoresis. Jap. J. Vet. Sci. 29: 233–244.

Okoshi, S., I. Tomoda, and S. Makimura. 1968. Analysis of normal cat serum by immunoelectrophoresis. Jap. J. Vet. Sci. 29: 337–345.

Olson, G. B., and B. S. Wostmann. 1964. Electrophoretic and immunoelectrophoretic studies of the serum of germfree and conventional guinea-pigs. Proc. Soc. Exp. Biol. Med. 116: 914–918.

Onoue, K., Y. Yagi, and D. Pressman. 1964. Multiplicity of antibody proteins in rabbit anti-p-azobenzenearsonate antisera. J. Immunol. 92: 173–184.

Onoue, K., Y. Yagi, and D. Pressman. 1966. Isolation of rabbit IgA antihapten antibody and demonstration of skin-sensitizing activity in homologous skin. J. Exp. Med. 123: 173–190.

Orlans, E. 1968. Fowl antibody. X. The purification and properties of an antibody to the 2,4-dinitrophenyl group. Immunology 14: 61–67.

Orlans, E., and A. Feinstein. 1971. Detection of alpha, kappa and lambda chains in mammalian immunoglobulins using fowl antisera to human IgA. Nature 233: 45–47.

Osterland, C. K., and H. Chaplin. 1966. Atypical antigenic properties of a γA myeloma protein. J. Immunol. 96: 842–848.

Outteridge, P. M., D. D. S. MacKenzie, and A. K. Lascelles. 1968. The distribution of specific antibody among the immunoglobulins in whey from the locally immunized gland. Arch. Biochem. Biophys. 126: 105–110.

Pahud, J. J., and J. P. Mach. 1970. Identification of secretory IgA, free secretory piece and serum IgA in the ovine and caprine species. Immunochemistry 7: 679–686.

Pahud, J. J., and J. P. Mach. 1972. Equine secretory IgA and secretory component. Int. Arch. Allergy 42: 175–186.

Pan, I. C., A. M. Kaplan, R. L. Morter, and M. J. Freeman. 1968. Spectrum of ovine immunoglobulins. Proc. Soc. Exp. Biol. Med. 129: 867–870.

Parkhouse, R. M. E. 1971. Immunoglobulin A biosynthesis. Intracellular accumulation of 7 S subunits. F.E.B.S. Lett. 16: 71–73.

Parkhouse, R. M. E., G. Virella, and R. R. Dourmashkin. 1971. Structural characterization of a human monoclonal IgA protein. Clin. Exp. Immunol. 8: 581–591.

Patterson, R., M. Roberts, and J. J. Pruzansky. 1968. Types of canine serum immunoglobulins. J. Immunol. 101: 687–694.

Patterson, R., I. M. Suszko, and J. J. Pruzansky. 1965. Some antigenic characteristics and immunologic reactions of horse spleen ferritin. Proc. Soc. Exp. Biol. Med. 118: 307–311.

Penhale, W. J., and G. Christie. 1969. Quantitative studies on bovine immunoglobulins. I. Adult plasma and colostrum levels. Res. Vet. Sci. 10: 493–501.

Picard, J., J. Heremans, and G. Vandebroek. 1962a. Serum proteins found in primates. I. Proteins of man, macaccus irus and lemur mongoz. Vox Sang. 7: 190–213.

Picard, J., J. Heremans, and G. Vandebroek. 1962b. Serum proteins found in primates. II. Serum proteins of some other primates species. Vox Sang. 7: 425–448.

Picard, J., G. Vandebroek, J. Heremans, and G. Defossé. 1967. Les protéines sériques du hérisson. Bull. Soc. Chim. Biol. 49: 779–789.

Plaut, A. G., and T. B. Tomasi. 1970. Immunoglobulin M: pentameric Fc_μ fragment released by trypsin at higher temperatures. Proc. Nat. Acad. Sci. U.S.A. 65: 318–322.

Porter, D. D., and F. J. Dixon. 1966. Electrophoretic and immunoelectrophoretic characterization of normal mink serum proteins. Amer. J. Vet. Res. 27: 335–338.

Porter, P. 1969a. Transfer of immunoglobulins IgG, IgA and IgM to lacteal secretions in the parturient sow and their absorption by the neonatal piglet. Biochim. Biophys. Acta 181: 381–392.

Porter, P. 1969b. Porcine colostral IgA and IgM antibodies to *Escherichia coli* and their intestinal absorption by the neonatal piglet. Immunology 17: 617–626.

Porter, P. In press. The porcine secretory IgA antibody system. Acta Vet. Brno. (Suppl.) 2.

Porter, P., and W. D. Allen. 1969. Immunoglobulin IgA in the urine of conventional and colostrum-deprived hypogammaglobulinaemic pigs. Immunology 17: 789–800.

Porter, P., and W. D. Allen. 1970. Intestinal IgA in the pig. Experientia 26: 90–92.

Porter, P., and I. R. Hill. 1970. Serological changes in immunoglobulins IgG, IgA and IgM and *Escherichia coli* antibodies in the young pig. Immunology 18: 565–573.

Porter, P., and R. Kenworthy. 1970. Effects of *Escherichia coli* on germ-free and gnotobiotic pigs. II. Serum proteins and antibodies. J. Comp. Pathol. 80: 233–241.

Porter, P., and D. E. Noakes. 1970. Immunoglobulin IgA in bovine serum and external secretions. Biochim. Biophys. Acta 214: 107–116.

Porter, P., D. E. Noakes, and W. D. Allen. 1970. Secretory IgA and antibodies to *Escherichia coli* in porcine colostrum and milk and their significance in the alimentary tract of the young pig. Immunology 18: 245–257.

Potter, M. 1971. Myeloma proteins (M-components) with antibody-like activity. New Engl. J. Med. 284: 831–838.

Potter, M., and R. Lieberman. 1970. Common individual antigenic determinants in five of eight BALB/c IgA myeloma proteins that bind phosphoryl choline. J. Exp. Med. 132: 737–751.

Prahl, J. W., C. A. Abel, and H. M. Grey. 1971. The carboxyl-terminal structure of the α-chain of human IgA myeloma proteins. Biochemistry 10: 1808–1812.

Rádl, J., F. Klein, P. van den Bergh, A. M. de Bruyn, and W. Hijmans. 1971. Binding of secretory piece to polymeric IgA and IgM paraproteins *in vitro*. Immunology 20: 843–852.

Rask-Nielsen, R., J. F. Heremans, H. E. Christensen, and R. Djurtoft. 1961. Beta-2A (= Beta-3-II = Gamma-1A) mouse leukemia with "flame cells" in leukemic infiltrations and degenerative lesions in muscles. Proc. Soc. Exp. Biol. Med. 107: 632–636.

Rawson, A. J., and N. M. Abelson. 1964. Studies on blood group antibodies. VI. The blood group isoantibody activity of γ_{1A}-globulin. J. Immunol. 93: 192–198.

Raynaud, M., S. Iscaki, and R. Mangalo. 1965. Séparation chromatographique des γ G et γ A antitoxines antidiphtériques de cheval. Ann. Inst. Pasteur 109: 525–551.

Reid, K. B. M. 1971. Complement fixation by the F(ab')$_2$-fragment of pepsin-treated rabbit antibody. Immunology 20: 649–658.

Rejnek, J., J. Kostka, and O. Kotýnek. 1966. Electrophoretic behaviour of H- and L-chains of human serum and colostrum gamma-globulin. Nature 209: 926–928.

Rejnek, J., J. Kostka, and J. Trávníček. 1966. Studies on the immunoglobulin spectrum of porcine serum and colostrum. Folia Microbiol. 11: 173–178.

Reynolds, H. Y., D. C. Dale, S. M. Wolff, and J.S. Johnson. 1971. Serum immunoglobulin levels in grey collies. Proc. Soc. Exp. Biol. Med. 136: 574–577.

Reynolds, H. Y., and J. S. Johnson. 1970a. Canine immunoglobulins. IV. Copro-immunoglobulins. J. Immunol. 104: 888–895.

Reynolds, H. Y., and J. S. Johnson. 1970b. Canine immunoglobulins. III. Distribution of immunoglobulins in colostrum and isolation of secretory IgA and 7 S γ_1. J. Immunol. 104: 1000–1008.

Reynolds, H. Y., and J. S. Johnson. 1970c. Quantitation of canine immunoglobulins. J. Immunol. 105: 698–703.

Reynolds, H. Y., and J. S. Johnson. 1971. Structural units of canine serum and secretory immunoglobulin A. Biochemistry 10: 2821–2827.

Rice, C. E., J. Tailyour, and D. Cochrane. 1966. Ultracentrifugal studies of sera from cattle vaccinated or naturally infected with *Brucella abortus*. Can. J. Comp. Med. 30: 270–278.

Richardson, A. K., and P. C. Kelleher. 1970. The 11-S sow colostral immunoglobulin.

Isolation and physicochemical properties. Biochim. Biophys. Acta 214: 117–124.

Ricks, J., M. Roberts, and R. Patterson. 1970. Canine secretory immunoglobulins: Identification of secretory component. J. Immunol. 105: 1327–1333.

Rockey, J. H. 1967. Equine antihapten antibody. The subunits and fragments of anti-β-lactoside antibody. J. Exp. Med. 125: 249–275.

Rockey, J. H., N. R. Klinman, and F. Karush. 1964. Equine antihapten antibody. I. 7S β_{2A} and 10 S γ_1-globulin components of purified anti-β-lactoside antibody. J. Exp. Med. 120: 589–609.

Rockey, J. H., P. C. Montgomery, and K. J. Dorrington. 1971. Induced optical activity (circular dichroism) of antibody-hapten complexes. Fed. Proc. 30: 349 (Abstr.).

Rockey, J. H., and R. M. Schwartzmann. 1967. Skin sensitizing antibodies: a comparative study of canine and human PK and PCA antibodies and a canine myeloma protein. J. Immunol. 98: 1143–1151.

Rossen, R. D., R. H. Alford, W. T. Butler, and W. E. Vannier. 1966. The separation and characterization of proteins intrinsic to nasal secretion. J. Immunol. 97: 369–378.

Rothman, U.S.E. 1966. Passive transfer of a delayed skin reactivity to 2,4-dinitrochlorobenzene (DNCB) with the immunoglobulin A (IgA) fraction of serum and lymphoid cells. Acta Soc. Med. Uppsal. 71: 141–155.

Rouse, B. T., and D. G. Ingram. 1970. The total protein and immunoglobulin profile of equine colostrum and milk. Immunology 19: 901–907.

Rowlands, D. T. 1970. The immune response of adult opossums (*Didelphys virginiana*) to the bacteriophage f2. Immunology 18: 149–155.

Rowlands, D. T., and M. A. Dudley. 1968. The isolation of immunoglobulins of the adult opossum (*Didelphys virginiana*). J. Immunol. 100: 736–743.

Salomon, J. C., and H. Bazin. 1972. Low levels of some serum immunoglobulin classes in nude mice. Rev. Europ. et Clin. Biol. 17: 880–882.

Sandberg, A. L., B. Oliveira, and A. G. Osler. 1971. Two complement interaction sites in guinea pig immunoglobulins. J. Immunol. 106: 282–285.

Sandberg, A. L., A. G. Osler, H. S. Shin, and B. Oliveira. 1970. The biologic activities of guinea pig antibodies. II. Modes of complement interaction with $\gamma 1$ and $\gamma 2$ immunoglobulins. J. Immunol. 104: 329–334.

Sardesai, S. K., and S. S. Rao. 1968. Immunoglobulins in hyperimmune horse serum. Indian J. Biochem. 5: 46–49.

Schubert, D. 1970. Immunoglobulin biosynthesis. IV. Carbohydrate attachment to immunoglobulin subunits. J. Mol. Biol. 51: 287–301.

Schultze, H. E., and J. F. Heremans. 1966. *In* Molecular biology of human proteins. Volume 1. Elsevier, Amsterdam, London, New York.

Schwartzmann, R. M., R. E. Halliwell, and J. H. Rockey. 1970. Spontaneous anti-ragweed and induced anti-dinitrophenyl reaginic antibody of the atopic dog. Fed. Proc. 29: 575 (Abstr.).

Schwick, G., and H. E. Schultze. 1960. Immunoelectrophoretische Studien bei der Hyperimmunisierung von Pferden. I. Mitteilung. Protides Biol. Fluids 8: 162–165.

The Secretory Immunologic System. Proceedings of a Conference, Vero Beach, Florida, 1969. D. H. Dayton, P. A. Small, R. M. Chanock, H. E. Kaufman, and T. B. Tomasi (eds.), U.S. Government Printing Office, Washington, D.C., 1971.

Seki, T., E. Appella, and H. A. Itano. 1968. Chain models of 6.6 S and 3.9 S mouse myeloma γA immunoglobulin molecules. Proc. Nat. Acad. Sci. U.S.A. 61: 1071–1078.

Seligmann, M., E. Mihaesco, and B. Frangione. 1971. Studies on alpha chain disease. Ann. N.Y. Acad. Sci. 190: 487–500.

Seligmann, M., E. Mihaesco, D. Hurez, C. Mihaesco, J. L. Preud'homme, and J. C. Rambaud. 1969. Immunochemical studies in four cases of alpha chain disease. J. Clin. Invest. 48: 2374–2389.

Sell, S. 1967. Isolation and characterization of rabbit colostral IgA. Immunochemistry 4: 49–55.

Shim, B. S., Y. S. Kang, W. J. Kim, S. H. Cho, and D. B. Lee. 1969. Self-protective activity of colostral IgA against tryptic digestion. Nature 222: 787–788.

Shuster, J. 1971. Pepsin hydrolysis of IgA. Delineation of two populations of molecules. Immunochemistry 8: 405–411.

Silverstein, A. M., G. J. Thorbecke, K. L. Kraner, and R. J. Lukes. 1963. Fetal response to antigenic stimulus. III. γ-globulin production in normal and stimulated fetal lambs. J. Immunol. 91: 384–395.

Small, P. A., J. H. Curry, and R. H. Waldman. 1971. Characteristics of the secretory immunologic system, pp. 13–27. *In* The Secretory Immunologic System, 1969. U.S. Government Printing Office, Washington.

South, M. A., M. D. Cooper, F. A. Wollheim, R. Hong, and R. A. Good. 1966. The IgA system. I. Studies of the transport and immunochemistry of IgA in the saliva. J. Exp. Med. 123: 615–627.

Stechschulte, D. J., and K. F. Austen. 1970. Immunoglobulins of rat colostrum. J. Immunol. 104: 1052–1062.

Steinbuch, M., C. Reuge, and R. Audran. 1969. Digestion papaïnique de l'IgA humaine normale. Résultats physicochimiques. Compt. Rend. Acad. Sci. Paris. 268: 462–464.

Steiner, L. A., and R. R. Porter. 1967. The interchain disulfide bonds of a human pathological immunoglobulin. Biochemistry 6: 3957–3970.

Steward, M. W. 1971. Resistance of rabbit secretory IgA to proteolysis. Biochim. Biophys. Acta 236: 440–449.

Stoop, J. W., R. E. Ballieux, W. Hijmans, and B. J. M. Zegers. 1971. Alpha-chain disease with involvement of the respiratory tract in a Dutch child. Clin. Exper. Immunol. 9: 625–635.

Strober, W., R. M. Blaese, and T. A. Waldmann. 1970. The origin of salivary IgA. J. Lab. Clin. Med. 75: 856–862.

Sullivan, A. L., R. A. Prendergast, L. J. Antunes, A. M. Silverstein, and T. B. Tomasi. 1969. Characterization of the serum and secretory immune systems of the cow and sheep. J. Immunol. 103: 334–344.

Sullivan, A. L. and T. B. Tomasi. 1964. Studies on bovine serum and salivary γ-globulins. Clin. Res. 12: 452 (Abstr.).

Surján, J. 1969a. Studies on swine serum immunoglobulins. I. Protein fractions in swine serum. Acta Microbiol. Acad. Sci. Hung. 16: 107–112.

Surján, J. 1969b. Studies on swine serum immunoglobulins. II. Relationship between immunoglobulins and antibodies. Acta Microbiol. Acad. Sci. Hung. 16: 279–287.

Svehag, S.-E., and B. Bloth. 1970. Ultrastructure of secretory and high-polymer serum immunoglobulin A of human and rabbit origin. Science 168: 847–849.

Taubman, M. A., and R. J. Genco. 1971. The purification and characterization of rabbit secretory γA antibodies directed to group A streptococcus. Fed. Proc. 30: 528 (Abstr.).

Tenenhouse, H. S., and H. F. Deutsch. 1966. Some physical-chemical properties of chicken γ-globulins and their pepsin and papain digestion products. Immunochemistry 3: 11–20.

Terry, W. D., M. M. Boyd, J. S. Rea, and R. Stein. 1970. Human M-proteins with antibody activity for nitrophenyl ligands. J. Immunol. 104: 256–259.

Thompson, R. A. 1970. Secretory piece linked to IgM in individuals deficient in IgA. Nature 226: 946–948.

Thompson, R. A., and P. Asquith. 1970. Quantitation of exocrine IgA in human serum in health and disease. Clin. Exper. Immunol. 7: 491–500.

Thompson, R. A., P. Asquith, and W. T. Cooke. 1969. Secretory IgA in the serum. Lancet ii: 517–519.

Tomasi, T. B., and J. Bienenstock. 1968. Secretory immunoglobulins. Adv. Immunol. 9: 1–96.

Tomasi, T. B., and N. Calvanico. 1968. Human secretory IgA. Fed. Proc. 27: 617 (Abstr.).

Tomasi, T. B., E. M. Tan, A. Solomon, and R. A. Prendergast. 1965. Characteristics of an immune system common to certain external secretions. J. Exp. Med. 121: 101–124.

Tomasi, T. B., and S. D. Zigelbaum. 1963. The selective occurrence of γ 1A-globulin in certain body fluids. J. Clin. Invest. 42: 1552–1560.

Tormo, J., A. Chordi, A. Rodriguez-Burgos, and R. Diaz. 1967. Immunoelectrophoresis of normal pig serum. Vet. Rec. 81: 392–395.

Tourville, D. R., R. H. Adler, J. Bienenstock, and T. B. Tomasi. 1969. The human secretory immunoglobulin system. Immunohistological localization of γA, secretory "piece", and lactoferrin in normal human tissues. J. Exp. Med. 129: 411–429.

Tourville, D. R., and T. B. Tomasi. 1969. Selective transport of γA. Proc. Soc. Exp. Biol. Med. 132: 473–477.

Vaerman, J. P. 1970. Studies on IgA immunoglobulins in man and animals. Thesis. Sintal, Louvain.

Vaerman, J. P. 1971. A comparison between several mammalian IgAs, including the bovine. J. Dairy. Sci. 54: 1317 (Abstr.).

Vaerman, J. P., J. B. Arbuckle, and J. F. Heremans. 1970. Immunoglobulin A in the pig. II. Sow's colostral and milk IgA: Quantitative studies and molecular size estimation. Int. Arch. Allergy 39: 323–333.

Vaerman, J. P., H. H. Fudenberg, C. Vaerman, and W. J. Mandy. 1965. On the significance of the heterogeneity in molecular size of human serum γA-globulin. Immunochemistry 2: 263–272.

Vaerman, J. P., and J. F. Heremans. 1966. Subclasses of human immunoglobulin A based on differences in the alpha polypeptide chains. Science 153: 647–649.

Vaerman, J.P., and J. F. Heremans. 1968a. The immunoglobulins of the dog. I. Identification of canine immunoglobulins homologous to human IgA and IgM. Immunochemistry 5: 425–432.

Vaerman, J. P., and J. F. Heremans. 1968b. Effect of neuraminidase and acidification on complement fixing properties of human IgA and IgG. Int. Arch. Allergy 34: 49–52.

Vaerman, J. P., and J. F. Heremans. 1969a. Distribution of various immunoglobulin containing cells in canine lymphoid tissue. Immunology 17: 627–633.

Vaerman, J. P., and J. F. Heremans. 1969b. The immunoglobulins of the dog. II. The immunoglobulins of canine secretions. Immunochemistry 6: 779–786.

Vaerman, J. P., and J. F. Heremans. 1970a. Immunoglobulin A in the pig. I. Preliminary characterization of normal pig serum IgA. Int. Arch. Allergy 38: 561–572.

Vaerman, J. P., and J. F. Heremans. 1970b. Origin and molecular size of immunoglobulin-A in the mesenteric lymph of the dog. Immunology 18: 27–38.

Vaerman, J. P., and J. F. Heremans. 1971. IgA and other immunoglobulins from the European hedgehog. J. Immunol. 107: 201–211.

Vaerman, J. P., and J. F. Heremans. 1972. The IgA system of the guinea pig. J. Immunol. 108: 637–648.

Vaerman, J. P., J. F. Heremans, and C. B. Laurell. 1968. Distribution of α-chain subclasses in normal and pathological IgA-globulins. Immunology 14: 425–432.

Vaerman, J. P., J. F. Heremans, and G. Van Kerckhoven. 1969. Identification of IgA in several mammalian species. J. Immunol. 103: 1421–1423.

Vaerman, J. P., P. Querinjean, and J. F. Heremans. 1971. Studies on the IgA system of the horse. Immunology 21: 443–454.

Valentine, R. C., and N. M. Green. 1967. Electron microscopy of an antibody-hapten complex. J. Mol. Biol. 27: 615–617.

van Munster, P. J. J., G. B. A. Stoelinga, and S. Poels-Zanders. 1971. Isolation of free secretory component (S.C.) from human milk, determination of its molecular weight. Immunochemistry 8: 471–477.

Vyas, G. N., and H. H. Fudenberg. 1969. Am(1), the first genetic marker of human immunoglobulin A. Proc. Nat. Acad. Sci. U.S.A. 64: 1211–1216.

Waldman, R. H., J. P. Mach, M. M. Stella, and D. S. Rowe. 1970. Secretory IgA in human serum. J. Immunol. 105: 43–47.

Waldmann, T. A., and W. Strober. 1969. Metabolism of immunoglobulins. Progr. Allergy 13: 1–110.

Wang, A. C., and H. H. Fudenberg. 1970. Heterogeneity of carbohydrate content of human IgA myeloma proteins. J. Immunol. 105: 1286–1288.

Wang, A. C., J. W. Goodman, and H. H. Fudenberg. 1969. N-terminal residues of heavy chains of human IgA myeloma proteins. J. Immunol. 103: 1149–1151.

Wang, A. C., J. R. L. Pink, H. H. Fudenberg, and J. Ohms. 1970. A variable region subclass of heavy chains common to immunoglobulins G, A, and M and characterized by an unblocked amino-terminal residue. Proc. Nat. Acad. Sci. U.S.A. 66: 657–663.

Wang, A. C., J. Shuster, A. Epstein, and H. H. Fudenberg. 1968. Evolution of antigenic determinants of transferrin and other serum proteins in primates. Biochem. Genet. 1: 347–358.

Warner, N. L., and J. J. Marchalonis. 1972. Structural differences in mouse IgA myeloma proteins of different allotypes. J. Immunol. 109: 657–661.

Weinheimer, P. F., J. Mestecky, and R. T. Acton. 1971. Species distribution of J-chain. J. Immunol. 107: 1211–1212.

Weir, R. C., R. R. Porter, and D. Givol. 1966. Comparison of the C-terminal amino-acid sequence of two horse immunoglobulins IgG and IgG(T). Nature 212: 205–206.

Wernet, P., H. Breu, J. Knop, and D. Rowley. 1971. The antibacterial action of specific IgA and the transport of IgM, IgA and IgG from serum into the small intestine. J. Infect. Dis. 24: 223–226.

World Health Organization. 1964. Nomenclature for human immunoglobulins. Bull. Wld. Hlth. Org. 30: 447–450.

World Health Organization. 1966. Notation for human immunoglobulin subclasses. Bull. Wld. Hlth. Org. 35: 953.

Wicher, K., and C. E. Arbesman. 1971. Distribution of immunoglobulin containing cells in human and monkey organs. Fed. Proc. 30: 244 (Abstr.).

Wiedermann, G., W. Auerswald, and H. Denk. 1968. Gegen subzelluläre Leberzellfraktionen gerichtete Serumfaktoren bei Ratten. III Mitteilung: Nähere physikalische Charakterisierung. Z. Immun. Forsch. 136: 230–236.

Williams, C. A. 1954. Immunoelectrophoresis: A new method for the analysis of complex antigen and antibody mixtures. Application to human serum antigens and hyperimmune horse serum. Thesis. Rutgers University, New Brunswick, N.J.

Williams, R. C., J. D. Russel, and A. J. Kenyon. 1966. Anti-gamma-globulin factors and immunofluorescent studies in normal mink and mink with Aleutian disease. Amer. J. Vet. Res. 27: 1447–1454.

Wilson, I. D. 1971. Studies on the products of peptic digestion of IgA. Immunology 20: 327–339.

Wilson, I. D., and R. C. Williams. 1969. Two distinct groups of immunoglobulin A (IgA) revealed by peptic digestion. J. Clin. Invest. 48: 2409–2416.

Wolfenstein, C., Frangione, B. and Franklin, E. C. 1971. Structural studies of $\gamma A1$ immunoglobulin. Fed. Proc. 30: 467 (Abstr.).

Yakulis, V., N. Costea, and P. Heller. 1969. Cleavage of the Fc fragment of IgA. J. Immunol. 102: 488–491.

Yurchak, A. M., J. E. Butler, and T. B. Tomasi. 1971. Fluorescent localization of immunoglobulins in the tissues of the cow. J. Dairy Sci. 54: 1324 (Abstr.).

Zimmerman, B., and H. M. Grey. 1971. Non-covalent bonding of immunoglobulin poplypeptide chains. Fed. Proc. 30: 594 (Abstr.).

Zipursky, A., E. J. Brown, and J. Bienenstock. Submitted. The attachment and ingestion of anti-A sensitized erythrocytes by monocytes and neutrophils.

Author's address: Dr. J. P. Vaerman, Department of Experimental Medicine, University of Louvain, Avenue Chapelle-aux-Champs 4, B-1200, Brussels (Belgium).

Methods of Labeling Antibodies for Electron Microscopic Localization of Antigens

MANFRED WAGNER

Akademie der Wissenschaften der DDR, Forschungszentrum für Molekularbio-
logie und Medizin, Zentralinstitut für Mikrobiologie und Experimentelle Therapie,
Jena

Contents

I. Introduction 186
II. Immunoferritin Technique 187
   A. Principle 187
   B. Ferritin 187
   C. Preparation of Ferritin-Labeled Antibodies 189
      1. Immunoglobulin 189
      2. Coupling Agents 189
      3. Conjugation Procedures 191
   D. Purification of Conjugates 192
   E. Methods for the Assay of Ferritin-Labeled Antibodies 195
      1. Electrophoretic and Immunoelectrophoretic Analysis 195
      2. Labeling with Fluorescein Isothiocyanate 195
   F. Properties of Ferritin-Labeled Antibodies 195
      1. Immunological Activity 195
      2. Molecular Ratio of Antibody and Ferritin 196
   G. Treatment of Specimens and Staining Methods 197
      1. Staining Before Embedding 197
      2. Postembedding Staining 199
      3. Hybrid Antibody Method 200
      4. Specificity Controls 201
   H. Applications of Ferritin-Labeled Antibodies 201
      1. Tissue Antigens and Antibody Synthesis 201
      2. Microbial and Parasitic Antigens 204
III. Immunoenzyme Technique 208
   A. Principle 208
   B. Enzymes 209
   C. Coupling Reagents and Procedures 209
   D. Purification and Properties of Enzyme-Labeled Antibodies ... 217
   E. Tagging of Antigen Structures with Enzyme-Labeled Antibodies ... 218
      1. Staining Methods 218

        2. Cytochemical Reaction Procedures.. 221
        3. Specificity Controls.. 222
    F. Applications of Enzyme-Labeled Antibodies................................. 222
        1. Synthesis of Immunoglobulins.. 222
        2. Tissue Antigens... 224
        3. Microbial Antigens 226
IV. Iodinated and Heavy Metal-Conjugated Antibodies 228
    A. Iodine 228
    B. Mercury 229
    C. Ferrocene 229
    D. Uranium and Osmium 230
        1. Immunouranium Technique 230
        2. Immunouranium-Thiocarbohydrazide-Osmium Tetroxide Technique... 231
        3. Immunodiazothioether-Osmium Tetroxide (Immuno-DTO) Technique. 232
        4. Quantitation of the Immunouranium Technique.......................... 232
V. Evaluation of the Immune Electron Microscopic Labeling Methods............ 232
    Literature Cited 233
    Supplementary References 247

I. Introduction

The development of the immunofluorescence technique by Coons and co-workers led to a search for similar methods with immunological specificity in electron microscopy. It is true that in some instances antigenic structures can be demonstrated specifically by the adsorbed antibody with the negative-staining technique, e.g., isolated muscle fibers, flagellae, fimbriae, F-pili, or phages and other virus particles (Ritchie and Fernelius, 1968; Pepe et al., 1961). But the negative-staining technique is not applicable in the study of tissue sections and several other specimens. Therefore the antibody itself must be labeled with an electron-dense compound. This problem has been solved in the past 14 years in different manners. Several authors labeled antibodies with organic salts of heavy metals or introduced iodine into the antibody molecule. A fruitful approach was that of Singer (1959) who coupled the iron-rich protein ferritin on the antibody globulin. This is now called the immunoferritin technique. Recently Franz (1968) used another iron-containing compound, the ferrocene, for labeling antibodies. Possibly the most ingenious method was the use of stable enzymes which can be localized by the electron-dense reaction products of their substrates (Nakane and Pierce, 1966). The present review describes different methods of antibody labeling, discusses their advantages and limitations, and gives a survey of their applications.

II. Immunoferritin Technique

A. Principle

The immunoferritin technique was developed by Singer (1959). Ferritin is an iron-containing protein that is characterized by its high electron density. Conjugation of antibody and ferritin by low-molecular bifunctional reagents results in a bimolecular complex. This complex retains the immunological activity of the antibody, and it is visible in the electron microscope because of its dense iron core of ferritin. Thus the location of an antigen can be detected by the iron particle of the ferritin-antibody complex.

Detailed reviews on the immunoferritin technique have been given by Pierce et al. (1964), Andres et al. (1967), and Schäfer (1970), and short descriptions can be found in Singer (1963, 1964), Rifkind et al. (1964), Vogt et al. (1967) and Sternberger (1967).

Eskeland (1967) suggested the use of another big molecule, the hemocyanin, for antibody labeling.

B. Ferritin

Ferritin is composed of a protein shell with a diameter of about 100–120 Å, which envelops a core of ferric hydroxide micells of 55–60 Å in diameter. The molecular weight of ferritin is approximately 750,000. The iron content amounts to about 23%. This corresponds to 2000–3000 atoms of iron per molecule.

Ferritin can be obtained from many animal sources. In general, it is extracted from horse spleen by Granick's method (Granick, 1942) (Figure 1). This product also can be purchased commercially in good

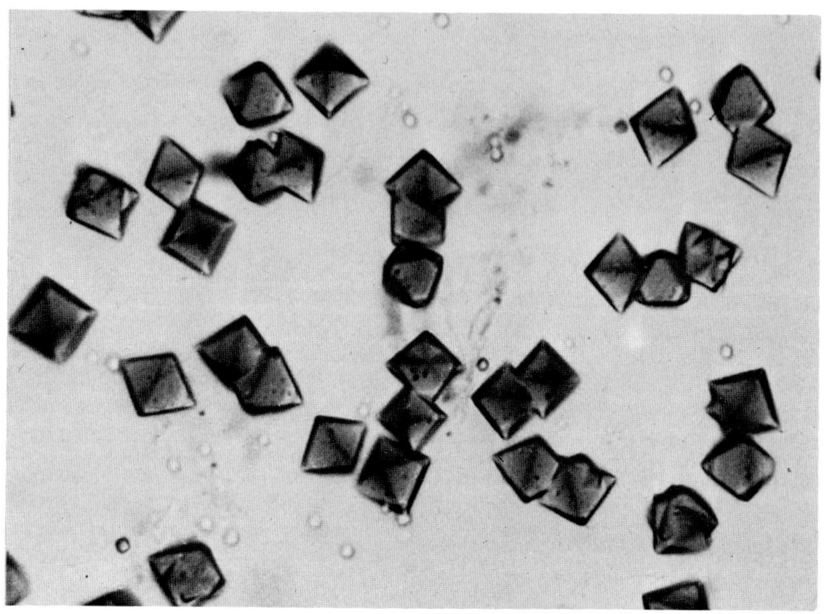

Fig. 1. Crystals of ferritin, extracted from horse spleen and purified by repeated recrystallization with cadmium sulphate. × 400.

quality from some suppliers. Crystallized ferritin is not a chemical entity but consists of a mixture of the colorless component apoferritin ($S_{20} = 17.6$; mol wt 465,000) and the heterogenous colored iron-containing ferritin. By using starch gel or polyacrylamide gel electrophoresis it is possible to separate the ferritin into at least three (in some cases four) fractions (Figure 2). As Kopp et al. (1963) have shown, the two minor fractions do not represent artifacts of electrophoresis or artificial stable or metastable dimers and polymers. They consist of ferritin molecules which seem to be serologically identical but differ in their sedimentation coefficients and possibly also in their iron contents. For the immunoferritin technique, their separation is not necessary. But in order to get very clear electron microscopic pictures, it is advisable to purify Granick's product further by recrystallization with cadmium sulfate, reprecipitation with ammonium sulfate, and ultracentrifugation. A convenient procedure, which avoids the crystallization with the cytotoxic cadmium salt, is described by Vogt et al. (1968).

Fig. 2. Disc electrophoresis of ferritin. The unstained gel column shows three brown zones of ferritin.

C. Preparation of Ferritin-Labeled Antibodies

1. Immunoglobulin

Of course, it is desirable to use the antibody in a somewhat purified state. In most cases the globulin fraction of high titer antisera is convenient. Further purification can be accomplished by chromatography on a DEAE-cellulose column or by immunoadsorption.

2. Coupling Agents

There are many bifunctional reagents of low molecular weight for the coupling of two protein molecules. Singer (1959) first employed

meta-xylylene diisocyanate (XC), but in the original method he had to
take precautions in order to avoid the inactivation of antibodies by this
reagent. He later suggested the use of toluene-2,4-diisocyanate (TC)
(Singer and Schick, 1961). Tawde and Sri Ram (1962) proposed
p,p'-difluoro-*m,m'*-dinitrodiphenylsulphone (FNPS) as coupling agent
(Figure 3). Another convenient reagent was found by Borek (1961) in
bis-diazotized-3,3'-dimethoxy benzidine, dianisidine (BDD). Gregory
and Williams (1967) have described tetrazotized benzidine as a suitable
reagent. Recently we have shown that glutaraldehyde is convenient for
coupling of antibody and ferritin (Wagner and Wagner, 1972).

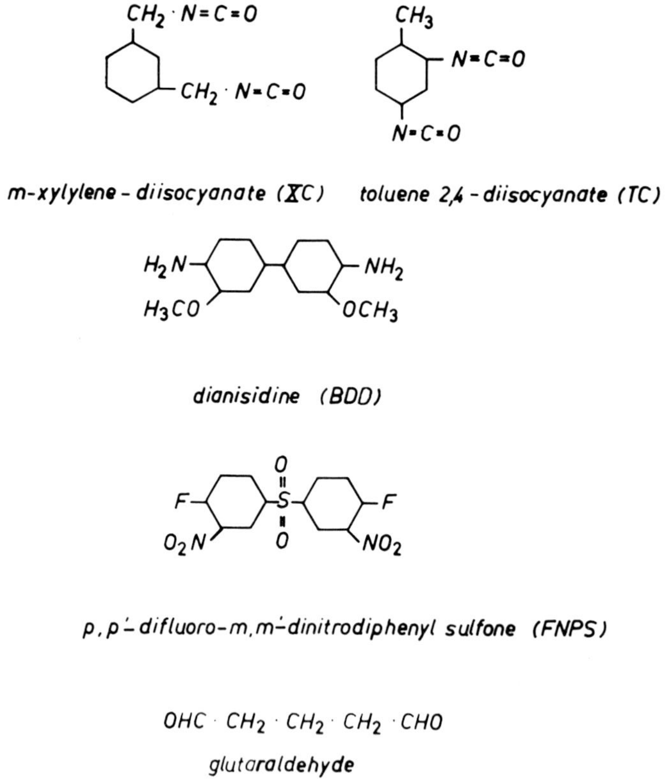

m-xylylene - diisocyanate (XC)   *toluene 2,4 - diisocyanate (TC)*

dianisidine (BDD)

p, p'- difluoro-m, m'-dinitrodiphenyl sulfone (FNPS)

$$OHC \cdot CH_2 \cdot CH_2 \cdot CH_2 \cdot CHO$$

glutaraldehyde

Fig. 3. Reagents for the coupling of ferritin to antibody globulin.

3. Conjugation Procedures

In the ferritin labeling of antibodies, one must remember that it is unreasonable to aspire to a very high coupling ratio, since, in several investigations, it was shown that as the degree of coupling increases, the antibody activity decreases. With both XC and TC as coupling reagents, ferritin and globulin are coupled in a two-step process. In the first stage the coupling agent is linked to ferritin by forming the ferritin-XC-mono-ureido and ferritin-TC-mono-ureido-substituted compound, respectively. The ferritin intermediate then is conjugated with an antibody through ureido linkage of the remaining unreacted isocyanate groups with ϵ-amino groups of the globulins. Andres et al. (1967) give the following modified procedures: XC: In an ice-bath, purified ferritin is mixed with 0.05 M phosphate buffer, pH 7.5, and 0.3 M borate buffer, pH 9.5, in volumes calculated to achieve a final concentration of 20–25 mg per milliliter of ferritin in 0.1 M borate buffer. XC is added to the mixture in the proportion of 0.1 ml per 100 mg of ferritin. The mixture is stirred vigorously in an ice-bath for 45 min and then centrifuged at 4°C and 1500g for 30 min. The clear brown supernatant is placed in an ice-bath for one hour to complete the reaction. Immunoglobulin is then added in the proportion of one part of globulin to four parts of ferritin by weight. Fresh borate buffer is added to maintain 0.1 molarity and pH 9.5, and the mixture is stirred gently for 48 hr at 4°C.

TC: Solid TC (stored under refrigeration) is melted at room temperature and added to a 2–2.5% solution of purified ferritin in 0.05 M phosphate buffer, pH 7.5, in the proportion of 0.1 ml per 100 mg of ferritin. The mixture is stirred in an ice-bath for 25 min and centrifuged at 4°C. The supernatant is then placed in an ice-bath for one hour. Next the immune globulin is added as above and the mixture is stirred for one hour at 37°C.

The reaction by means of BDD is a mild diazonium coupling which has relatively little effect on antibody activity. Borek (1961) proposed the following procedure: A solution of 160 mg of ferritin and 80 mg of rabbit globulin in 7 ml of 0.1 M citrate buffer, pH 5.0, was treated at 4°C with 1 ml aliquot of a solution of 6.7 mg of dianisidin and 3.8 mg of sodium nitrite in 10 ml of 0.017 N hydrochloric acid. The solution was stirred in the cold for two hours and then dialyzed overnight against 0.08 M borate, pH 9.4, and finally against neutral saline.

With FNPS as coupling agent the conjugation also proceeded in a one-step process. Sri Ram et al. (1963) described the following procedure as giving optimal conditions for the conjugation: To a mixture of 160 mg of rabbit globulin and 460 mg of ferritin, dissolved in sufficient cold 2% aqueous sodium carbonate to constitute a 4% protein solution, was added 1 ml of chilled acetone containing 5 mg of FNPS. After being stirred in the cold (2–4°C) for 24 hr, the reaction mixture was dialyzed exhaustively against normal saline and centrifuged to remove a small precipitate. In this procedure, the pH value and the FNPS concentration are critical, since at higher pH and FNPS concentration there is excessive precipitation.

Conjugation with glutaraldehyde can be performed at room temperature (Wagner and Wagner, 1972). To a solution of 30 mg of immunoglobulin G (or globulin) in 1 ml of 0.1 M phosphate buffer, pH 6.8 (within the range of pH 6.0 to pH 7.0 the value is not critical), 0.2 ml of a 10% sterile solution of cadmium-free ferritin is added. While the solution is gently stirred, 0.1 ml of a 0.5% aqueous solution of glutaraldehyde is added in drops. After two hours the reaction mixture is transferred into a dialysis bag and dialyzed overnight at 4°C against a large volume of PBS.

D. Purification of Conjugates

After termination of the coupling procedure, the reaction mixture contains the ferritin-antibody complex, unconjugated globulin, unconjugated ferritin, and residues of the bifunctional coupling reagent. The latter can be removed by dialysis against phosphate buffered saline (PBS, pH 7.2) or by gel filtration on Sephadex G-25 or G-50. The elimination of unconjugated antibody globulin is particularly necessary, since these antibodies compete with the conjugate at the antigen binding sites. Also, the elimination of free ferritin is favorable, since it could lead to unspecific precipitations and misinterpretations.

Many procedures have been developed for the elimination of globulin and ferritin.

Ultracentrifugation at $100,000 \times g$ or more for at least two hours separates by sedimentation the conjugate and the unconjugated ferritin, whereas most of the unconjugated globulins are retained in the supernatant and can be discarded. The procedure must be repeated at least twice. The pellet is resuspended in 0.05 M phosphate buffer at pH 7.2, but often the solubility is low.

A more complete removal of the uncoupled antibody globulin by centrifugation is achieved in a sucrose density gradient (Vogt and Kopp, 1964; Vogt et al. 1968; Binz, 1969; Birnbaum et al. 1970).

Unconjugated ferritin and globulin can be separated from the conjugate by continuous-flow paper electrophoresis (Borek and Silverstein, 1961), starch block electrophoresis, and preparative zone electrophoresis using polyvinyl powder (Pevikon C 870, Geon X427, etc.) as described by Charles (1966) and Vogt et al. (1968). The purified conjugate is eluted with successive aliquots of buffer and is transferred to dialyzing tubes to be concentrated by ultrafiltration, evaporation, or dialysis against certain polysaccharides (e.g., Aquacide) or polyvinylpyrrolidone.

Chromatographical procedures are more convenient. Amstey (1967) used chromatography on DEAE-cellulose columns for this purpose. As shown by immunodiffusion and ultracentrifugation, the procedure yields a pure conjugate.

By gel filtration on 4% agarose, which was prepared in spherical beads, we have separated raw ferritin-antibody conjugates into three distinct fractions (Figure 4): the pure antibody-ferritin complex, the unconjugated ferritin, and the unconjugated 7 S globulin (Wagner, 1967a). The raw mixture can be applied on the column as a very concentrated solution, and the eluted ferritin-labeled antibody fraction is then ready for use. Electrophoretically, all three peaks are homogeneous (Figure 5). Unfortunately, some commercially available 4% agarose gel bead preparations did not give the same good results (Vogt, personal communication; Binz, 1969).

Freezing of ferritin-labeled antibodies causes partial denaturation and should therefore be avoided.

The best way to conserve the purified conjugate is sterile filtration, e.g., with the Millipore sterile filter equipment (Millipore filter HA, 0.45 μ pore size). The sterilized solutions can be stored at 4°C for over a year.

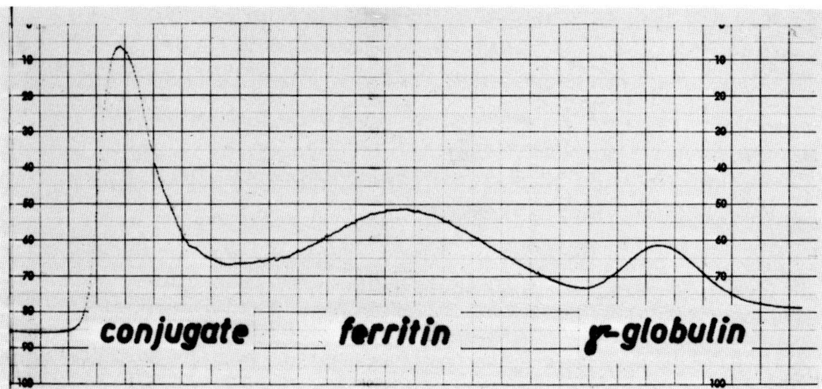

Fig. 4. Gel filtration pattern of raw ferritin-antibody conjugate fractionated on a column of 4% agarose beads.

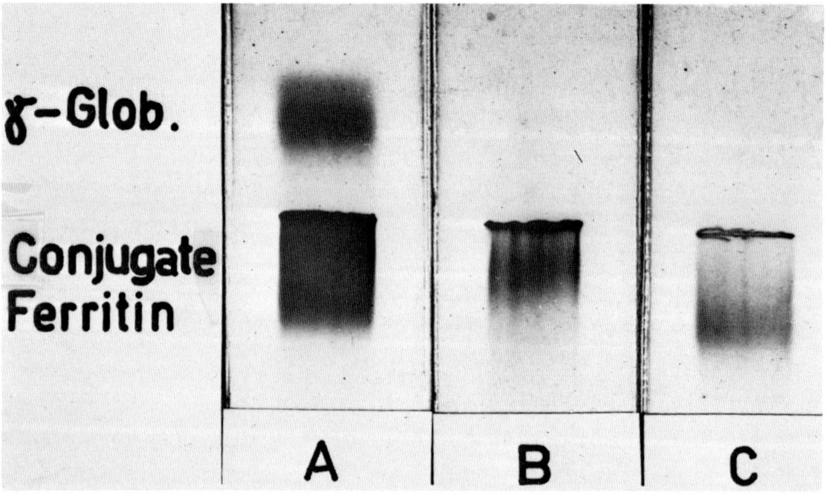

Fig. 5. Comparative agar electrophoresis patterns of fractions obtained by gel filtration of raw ferritin-antibody conjugate on 4% agarose beads. Electropherogram developed with amido black 10 B. *A*, Conjugate before gel filtration; *B*, purified conjugate (first fraction of Figure 4); *C*, unconjugated ferritin (second fraction of Figure 4).

E. Methods for the Assay of Ferritin-Labeled Antibodies

The success of immunoferritin experiments depends on many factors. Since the preparation of the electron microscopic specimens is very laborious and time-consuming, it is desirable for one to know about the purity and activity of the labeled antibodies before the staining procedure. Below are some recommended tests.

1. Electrophoretic and Immunoelectrophoretic Analysis

The coupling ratio can be estimated by simple electrophoretic analysis on paper strips or agar (Smith and Metzger, 1961). Ferritin-labeled globulin is faster than γ-globulin and slower than the ferritin in its electrophoretic mobility. The strips can be dyed with amido black 10B for protein or by the "prussian blue" reaction for iron, and the concentrations can be estimated densitometrically.

Immunoelectrophoretic analysis is much more sensitive than simple electrophoretic analysis for the detection of traces of unconjugated globulin. Also, in special cases one can ascertain whether the conjugated antibody is still reactive with its specific antigen.

2. Labeling with Fluorescein Isothiocyanate

For a rapid previous testing of the serological activity of ferritin-labeled antibodies, the complex can be further labeled by fluorescein isothiocyanate (see Wagner, 1967b). The doubly labeled antibody may then be tested on simple microscopic preparations of the same antigenic structure by fluorescent microscopy (Hsu et al., 1963; Dales et al., 1965). It is also possible to label the antibody first with fluorescein and then with ferritin.

F. Properties of Ferritin-Labeled Antibodies

1. Immunological Activity

Of course, the most essential prerequisite for the success of immunoferritin experiments is the conservation of the serological activity of the antibody after ferritin-labeling. This has been shown in many investigations. Nevertheless, generally there are significant decreases in the antibody titers. In most cases the ferritin-labeled antibodies have more or less lost their precipitating activity but further bind to the antigen structure. Vogt and Kopp (1964), using the tanned cell hemagglutination technique in very pure conjugates, could not show any significant antibody activity regardless of the conjugation reagent (XC, TC, or FNPS) used. Therefore, precipitation and agglutination tests are not always useful for the assay of ferritin-labeled antibodies. This may possibly be done by steric hindrance (masking) of one antigen binding site during coupling, which leads to the formation of functionally univalent antibody molecules.

These suggestions imply a contradiction to the results of Rifkind et al. (1960) and others, who hold that the conjugation with ferritin did not reduce the precipitating and hemagglutinating activity. But one must keep in mind that exact data on this problem can be obtained only if the conjugate is free from any traces of unreacted antibody globulin.

Some other biological phenomena, such as the virus neutralization (Amstey, 1967) and the nephritogenic potency of nephrotoxic globulin (Vogt et al., 1968), also show the loss of antibody activity after labeling.

However, Isliker et al. (1964) have shown that the univalent antibody fragments Fab can be labeled with ferritin and that they react with the homologous antigen structures. Such conjugates show a higher iron content, and in the electron micrographs a high percentage of ferritin particles forming "doublets" are seen.

Recently, Birnbaum et al. (1970), using radioactivity measurements after electrophoresis of the antigen-conjugate complex in polyacrylamide gel, have shown that the activity of a rabbit antibody against human serum albumin after conjugation with ferritin was not significantly reduced. The ferritin-labeled antibodies were found in soluble and insoluble complexes.

2. Molecular Ratio of Antibody and Ferritin

On the basis of the electrophoretic mobility of the conjugate, estimated by moving boundary electrophoresis, Borek and Silverstein (1961) postulated an equimolar ratio of ferritin to γ-globulin. By determination of the iron content in the conjugates, Sri Ram et al. (1963)

found the molecular ratio ranging from 1 : 1.1 to 1 : 1.3 for ferritin and γ-globulin.

More recently, Marinis et al. (1969) determined the molecular ratio in conjugates prepared from ^{125}I-labeled antibody globulin and ferritin free of apoferritin. All conjugates from which uncoupled γ-globulin was separated entirely showed exactly equimolecular ratios of ferritin and globulin.

The single localization of ferritin particles along linearly arranged antigen structures shows that generally the ferritin-antibody complex contains one ferritin molecule. Therefore, it seems established that the complex is a dimer composed of one ferritin molecule and one antibody molecule.

On the basis of these data, it should be possible to use pure conjugates for quantitative immunological investigations at the ultrastructural level by counting the ferritin particles in electron micrographs.

G. Treatment of Specimens and Staining Methods

1. Staining Before Embedding

Generally, the ferritin conjugate of a specific antiserum under consideration can be applied to living or fixed material which is then washed and embedded for electron microscopic examination. This is the direct method of immunoferritin staining technique.

Baxandall et al. (1962, 1963) proposed a two-layer or indirect technique corresponding to the indirect immunofluorescent technique. In the two-layer method, the specific antiserum is used in a free unconjugated state where it combines with its homologous antigen on the cell surface or in the cell. The removal of any excess of antiserum proteins is followed by a ferritin conjugate of an anti-γ-globulin serum prepared in a different animal species. Thus the antigen site is labeled indirectly by the ferritin anti-γ-globulin conjugate with the unmodified antibody as the intermediate.

As in the immunofluorescent technique, the two-layer method has several practical advantages. First, only one ferritin conjugate, the ferritin-labeled anti-IgG serum, is needed for all types of immunoferritin experiments with antisera from the same animal species. This not only saves time but also is economical with respect to specific antisera. The latter is especially important, since often there is not an abundant supply of specific antiserum against a particular cellular antigen and all labeling techniques are somewhat wasteful.

The antigenic structures amenable to study by the immunoferritin technique can be localized on the surface of single cells, on the surface of cells in tissues and organs, or within the cells. The first case provides no technical difficulties. Many cell surface antigens simply can be tagged with ferritin-labeled antibodies on living or fixed cells. After treatment, the cells are washed with saline, fixed in osmium tetroxide, and embedded as usual.

In tagging predominantly extracellular antigens in solid tissues, it is necessary to disintegrate the tissue somewhat. For example, following a brief fixation in phosphate buffered formalin, small blocks of tissue are finely minced with sharp razor blades and the tiny fragments are immersed in the conjugate solution. As an alternative, following brief formalin fixation, the tissue may be quickly frozen in a dry ice-alcohol bath and sectioned in a cryostat. Sections of 10–50 μ in thickness are then treated with the conjugate, washed, and treated further as usual.

The tagging of intracellular antigens is a difficult problem. Normally the intact cell is impenetrable for both labeled and unlabeled antibodies. Presectioning of the frozen specimen or dissecting and mincing allows only partial and irregular entry of the labeled antibody. The best way to tag intracellular antigens is the postembedding staining (see p. 199), but this method is not yet fully developed.

For the detection of intracellular virus antigens, some methods involving a slight disintegration of the cell membranes were developed. Oshiro et al. (1967) facilitated the penetration by treatment with dimethylsulfoxide (DMS) and freezing and thawing: monolayers of cells were washed in 0.1 M phosphate buffer (pH 7.2), fixed for 5 min at 4°C with 4% formalin in phosphate buffer, and treated for 30 min at room temperature with 10% DMS in buffer. The cells were then scraped from the glass into the DMS solution, pelleted by centrifugation at low speed, frozen for 3 min in a CO_2-ethanol bath, rapidly thawed, and suspended in ferritin-labeled antibody for one hour at room temperature. After being washed several times in 0.1% phosphate buffer containing 0.1% glucose, the cells were pelleted, fixed in 1% glutaraldehyde, washed again, postfixed in osmium tetroxide, dehydrated, and embedded as usual.

Another means of increasing the permeability of cell membranes is the treatment with digitonin (Levinthal et al. 1967a,b). In this method the cell monolayer is washed briefly with PBS (pH 7.4) and then allowed to react for one minute with 1.2×10^{-4} M digitonin in cacodylate, Millonig, or Sörensen's phosphate buffer, pH 7.4, followed immediately by one minute of treatment with 0.5% formaldehyde in similar buffers. After three ten-minute washes with PBS, the cells were scraped, decanted into small tubes, and centrifuged at $100 \times g$; the pellet volume was adjusted to 0.05 ml. Four volumes of diluted whole serum were added, and the cells were mixed and allowed to react with the serum for one to two hours at room temperature. After exhaustive washings with PBS, the cells were dispersed in four volumes of ferritin-labeled antiglobulin, allowed to react for one to two hours, and washed as above. The pellet, usually about 0.02–0.03 ml in volume, was postfixed undisturbed in 1–2% osmic acid for 30–45 min, dehydrated, and embedded. Ultrathin sections of conjugate-incubated materials remain unstained or are stained with uranyl acetate only. Lead salts are not used because of the possibility of mistaking fine lead precipitate for ferritin.

2. Postembedding Staining

Unfortunately, on the commonly used highly polar resins the ferritin-labeled antibody is strongly adsorbed nonspecifically. This difficulty is averted by the use of hydrophilic cross-linked polyampholytes (charged methacrylate polymers), but staining on sections of this material in routine work was not successful (Singer and McLean, 1963, 1964).

Molenaar et al. (1966) also observed heavy nonspecific adsorption of the labeled protein when it was added directly to the ultrathin sections. Trying several cleaning procedures, they succeeded by electrophoresis of the section, which was floated on a buffer solution.

No unspecific adsorption was observed when immunospecifically purified antibody conjugate was used (Striker et al., 1966). Unfortunately, the amount of ferritin particles as opposed to antigen-containing structures was sparse.

An interesting approach to postembedding staining was recently made by McLean and Singer (1970). Cells to be embedded were fixed in formaldehyde or other fixatives and dispersed in 0.5 ml of a 30% solution of bovine serum albumin (BSA) in 0.15 M NaCl. This mixture was then concentrated by placing it in a short glass tube. One end of the tube was attached to a collodion dialysis membrane and immersed in the dehydrating agent, Aquacide II (Calbiochem). When the BSA had attained the consistency of a gel, the membrane-covered end of the tube was cleaned and immersed in a solution of either 2% glutaraldehyde in PBS, pH 7.5, or 2% formaldehyde in the same buffer. These fixatives diffused through the gel and cross-linked the BSA in about three hours.

The cross-linked BSA was cut into narrow strips which were washed briefly with water, drained, and dried above silica gel. The strips were then cemented onto an epoxy resin block and sectioned. The sections were collected on water, and were then mounted on carbon-coated formvar or collodion grids which were first treated with a 4% solution of BSA in phosphate buffer. Staining with ferritin-labeled antibody was carried out by placing a drop of conjugate on the mounted section. After five minutes the grid was floated face down on a succession of phosphate buffer solutions and was washed with water and dried.

The method was illustrated by specific staining of hemoglobin inside the nucleated red cells of the pigeon and of the T4-phages inside infected *Escherichia coli* cells.

3. Hybrid Antibody Method

Hämmerling et al. (1968) developed a method of labeling which depends on the specific combination of ferritin with antiferritin antibody. The antiferritin antibody is hybridized with the antibody against the cell antigen (direct method) or with anti-IgG (indirect method) by Nisonoff's method. The latter method is based on the observation that antibody of dual specificity can be obtained by combining univalent fragments of pepsin-treated antibodies of different specificity. The hybridization technique is relatively laborious and time consuming, but it gives a sensitive and specific labeling and avoids some disadvantages of the chemical coupling of ferritin and antibody globulin. Comparative investigations of surface antigen structures treated according to the conventional indirect immunoferritin method and the indirect hybrid immunoferritin method, respectively, show dense aggregates of ferritin at variable distances from the cell surface in the former, and sparser distribution of the ferritin with more constant distances from the cell membrane in the latter (Aoki et al., 1969).

A special advantage of the hybrid method is the possibility of using other visual markers, such as plant viruses or bacteriophages (Hämmerling et al., 1969). This allows the demonstration of several different antigens simultaneously.

Néauport-Sautès et al. (1970) used this method to localize the histocompatibility antigens of the HLA system on the surface of human lymphocytes. The hybridized antibodies possessed activity against human immunoglobulin and against ferritin and turnip yellow mosaic-virus, respectively. Whereas a polyvalent HLA antiserum tagged about 20–25% of the surface of the lymphocytes, the antigenic zones demonstrated by a specific anti-HL A2 serum are much more restricted.

4. Specificity Controls

Criteria for the specificity of the staining reactions are similar to those for immunofluorescent techniques (see Wagner, 1967b): (a) Application of unlabeled homologous antibody prior to incubation with the ferritin-labeled antibody inhibits or at least reduces the tagging of the antigen structure (Blocking test). (b) Application of a labeled heterologous antibody does not tag the antigen. (c) Adsorption of the conjugate with the homologous antigens eliminates the tagging of the antigen structure.

H. Applications of Ferritin-Labeled Antibodies

1. Tissue Antigens and Antibody Synthesis

Using ferritin-labeled antibodies, Rifkind et al. (1962) revealed the localization of γ-globulin in a mouse plasma cell tumor (X5563). At a stage of the secretory process, when the remainder of the cytoplasm was essentially free of myeloma globulin, the content of cis-

ternae of the endoplasmic reticulum is labeled heavily with ferritin.
Later the accumulation of globulin results in distention of the endoplasmic reticulum, rupture of the distended vesicles, and extrusion of the
secretory globulin.

Baxandall and co-workers used the indirect immunoferritin technique to study ultrastructural events associated with stages of fertilization in sea urchin eggs (Baxandall, 1966a; Baxandall et al., 1962, 1963,
1964a, b). The data suggest that most of the antigenic sites detected in
the fertilized eggs were associated with sperm substances.

Ferritin-labeled antibodies to whole ascites tumor cells localize
primarily on the surface of the cell membrane and within pinocytic
vacuoles (Easton et al., 1962a). In the presence of complement, cytotoxic antibodies produce lysis of the tumor cells. The combination of
antibodies with cell membranes and the smooth membranes of the
endoplasmic reticulum indicate that antigens in these structures are
most important in the formation of cytotoxic antibodies (Easton et al.,
1962b).

The fine structure of skeletal muscle was studied by Douglas et al.
(1966) and by Samosudova et al. (1968).

After treatment with ferritin-labeled antihuman γ-globulin, sections from rheumatic hearts showed large amounts of ferritin in some
regions of the endocardium and subendocardium (Lannigan and Zaki,
1968). The ferritin was heavily concentrated in relation to collagen
fibrils, whereas the elastic tissues showed only occasional ferritin particles, and the cells of the endocardium were not tagged.

Human fibrin was localized by means of ferritin-labeled antifibrinogen in blood clots, in experimentally produced deposits within rat
muscle (Wyllie, 1964) and in human atherosclerotic lesions (e.g., the
deposits present between the elastica and the smooth muscle cells of
the aorta) (Haust et al., 1965).

Paul and Cohen (1963) demonstrated that amyloid fibrils from
human liver and spleen did not contain undenatured γ-globulin, as
was postulated in theories on the pathogenesis of amyloidosis.

The rabbit intestinal sucrase was demonstrated at the luminal
surface of the enterocytes (Gitzelmann et al., 1970). The staining was
pronounced after removal of the enteric surface coat by careful trypsinization.

Studies on mouse parietal yolk sac carcinoma, which secretes basement membrane-like material, showed that the basement membrane originates in the endoplasmic reticulum of the epithelial cell (Pierce et al., 1963). There is no antigenic relationship to collagen, reticulin, and the basement membranes of blood vessels.

In several studies the blood group antigens, as well as other surface antigens of erythrocytes, were demonstrated (Harris, 1964; Lee and Feldman, 1964; Suzuki, 1970; Haberman et al., 1967). On erythrocytes of newborns the AB0 blood group antigens are difficult to demonstrate, but on red cells of adults the antigens were readily located. Tagging with labeled anti-D antibodies resulted in a pattern of fairly evenly spaced sites of the Rh (D) antigen, which are about 100-fold rarer than those of antigen A (Lee and Feldman, 1964).

Davis et al. (1968) studied the localization of the Rh isoantigens and the antigens associated with idiopathic and drug-induced antibody hemolytic anemias. They found interesting differences in the periodicity of the antigenic sites as well as in the concentrations of the different antigens.

Autoantibodies belonging to the IgG were demonstrated on the erythrocytes of a patient with autoimmune hemolytic anemia (Tonietti et al., 1969).

On hemoglobin-free membranes and intact erythrocytes of group 0, antibody to purified virus receptor substance was bound in sites similar to those observed for isoantibodies (Howe et al., 1970). The authors discuss the relationship between the virus receptor substance-reactive sites to those containing blood group antigens.

By using the hemagglutination reaction with ferritin-labeled antibodies, Haferkamp et al. (1969) confirmed Heidelberger's lattice theory of the antigen-antibody reaction. After incubation with specific antibodies, unfixed erythrocytes assumed an irregular shape; the surfaces in contact together were enlarged and myriads of ferritin-labeled antibodies became bound between two cells, producing a stable agglutination. The failure of formalin-fixed red blood cells to agglutinate in the presence of a specific antiserum was a result of the inability of the antiserum to cause the shape of the cells to change, even though they were layered with a heavy coat of ferritin-labeled antibody (Schäfer et al., 1968). When fresh unfixed red cells were added to the formalin-fixed sensitized cells, agglutination was obtained (Haferkamp et al., 1969).

Kourilsky et al. (1970) demonstrated the antigens of the HLA system on human lymphocytes, myelocytes, reticulocytes, and several other nucleated cell types, but not on erythocytes. The antigens were situated on the cell membrane in irregular plaques.

In studies on glomerulonephritis, the immunoferritin technique has provided definitive information concerning the sites of reaction. With the use of ferritin-labeled antibodies against the infected nephrotoxic globulin, the toxic antibody was localized in the glomerular basement membrane and in the cytoplasm of the epithelial and endothelial cells (Andres et al., 1962a, b; Arhelger et al., 1963). In rabbits which died of anaphylactic shock, embolic precipitates of antigen-antibody complexes were present in the lumina of the capillaries (Andres et al., 1963). Similar studies were carried out using an *in vivo* tagging (Vogt et al., 1966, 1968). Ferritin-labeled nephrotoxic antibodies injected intravenously localized almost exclusively at the endothelial site of the glomerular basement membrane. There was no evidence of specific reaction with constituents of glomerular cells. Quantitative studies with highly purified conjugates showed that at least 40 basement membrane-fixed antibody molecules from the rabbit per 3,000 $m\mu^2$ of filtration surface were needed to cause immediate nephritis.

Masugi (1969) investigated the interaction between the immune complexes and the local vascular components and described the mechanism of the beginning and progression of nephrotoxic nephritis.

Studies on the pathogenesis of severe acute human glomerulonephritis have shown the localization of human γ-globulin and β_{1c} (C'3) in foreign material present in capillary lumens, between proliferating cells, in subendothelial and certain subepithelial deposits, in Bowman's space, and in the walls of some arterioles. Products of the nephritogenic group A streptococcus type 12 have been demonstrated in all these areas except the subepithelial deposits (Seegal et al., 1965; Andres et al., 1966).

2. *Microbial and Parasitic Antigens*

Bacteria.—Preliminary immunoferritin studies on bacteria to demonstrate the activity and specificity of the ferritin-labeled antibodies were performed by several workers (Smith et al., 1960; Spendlove and Singer, 1961; Metzger and Smith, 1962; Hsu et al., 1963; Rifkind et al., 1964; Mergenhagen et al., 1966). As shown in Figure 6, in mixtures of different bacteria, only cells of the homologous species were tagged by the ferritin-labeled antibodies (Wagner, unpublished results). Tagging of *Spirillum serpens* resulted in the location of ferritin particles on the outermost layer of the cell surface (Figure 7). Neighboring cells were bound ("agglutinated") by clusters of ferritin particles (Wagner, unpublished results).

The somatic antigens of *Salmonella typhimurium* and *Escherichia coli* O113 were demonstrated in considerable quantities on the cell surface (Shands, 1965). High magnification pictures show that the antigen appears to be structurally a fibril, which can extend from the surface up to 150 mμ.

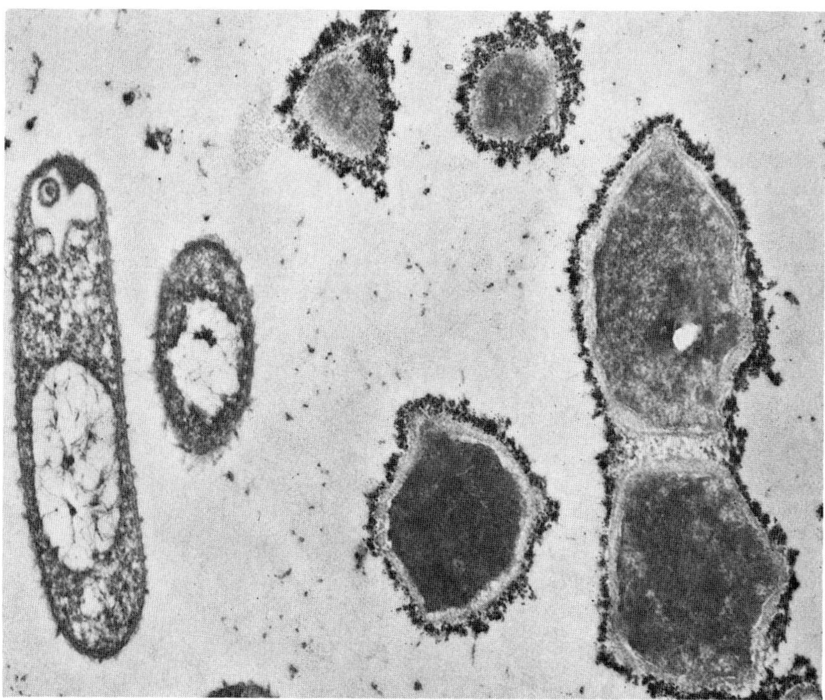

Fig. 6. Mixture of *Streptococcus pyogenes (right)* and *Escherichia coli (left)*, treated with ferritin-labeled antibody against group A-streptococci. Ferritin is localized only on the surface of streptococci. × 34,000.

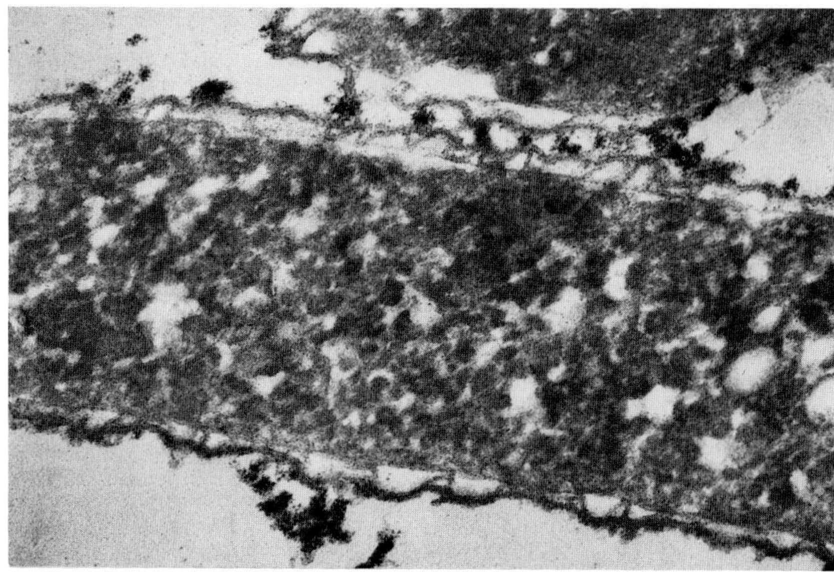

Fig. 7. *Spirillum serpens,* treated with ferritin-labeled specific antibody. Two cells are "agglutinated" by several clusters of labelled antibodies. × 79,000.

The Vi-antigen and the O-antigen of virulent strains of *Pasteurella* (*Francisella*) *tularensis* are located along the entire thickness of the capsule-like coat and on the surface, respectively (Katz et al., 1970a, b). In an avirulent strain the O-antigen is located along the capsule.

Investigations by Walker and co-workers showed that in *Bacillus cereus* and *B. subtilis* ferritin-labeled antibody to the vegetative cell stained the cell wall of young vegetative and of sporulating cells, as well as the cortical membrane in partially disintegrated spores (Walker et al., 1966, 1967b; Thomson et al., 1966). Ferritin-labeled spore antibody stained only the exosporium in *B. cereus* and the spore coat in *B. subtilis.*

Similar specificity of labeled cell wall and spore antisera was shown in three clostridial species, *Cl. bifermentans, Cl. sordelli,* and *Cl. sporogenes* (Walker et al., 1967a).

Duda and Slack (1969) used ferritin-labeled antitoxin to locate *Clostridium botulinum* toxin in bacteria and spores. Following injection of labeled β-toxin of *Cl. botulinum* into mice, the electron microscopic examination of the intercostal muscles revealed the presence of the toxin in the synaptic clefts of the postsynaptic apparatus (Zacks et al., 1962).

With ferritin-labeled antibody the M-protein of *Streptococcus pyogenes* was demonstrated on the surface of M-positive cells (Swanson et al., 1969; Wagner and Wagner, 1973). The M-protein is bound to threadlike structures, which originate from the outer cell wall layer. On the cell surface it forms a flocculent envelope (Figure 8). After trypsinization the threadlike structures are removed but reappear when the cells are incubated in fresh broth.

An unusual application of ferritin-labeled antibody is described by Knöll and Tresselt (1965). These authors have shown that Sarcina tagged with ferritin-labeled antibodies were moved in a powerful magnetic field to the pole piece.

Parasites including free-living protozoa. — The variable antigens of *Trypanosoma brucei,* from which each relapse population in the blood has a different character from its predecessor, are located in the surface coat including the filiform appendages ("plasmanemes") (Vickerman and Luckins, 1969).

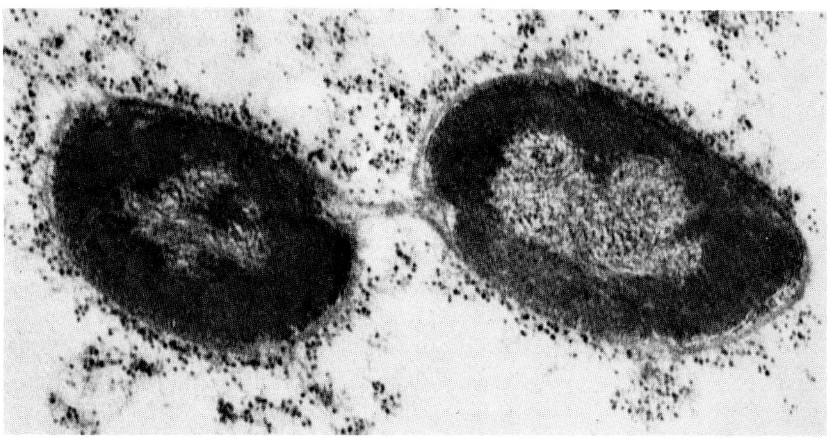

Fig. 8. Streptococcus pyogenes, type 19, treated with ferritin-labeled antibodies against the homologous M-protein. The ferritin particles are localized along filaments extending from the cell wall. The cells are connected by a small funiculus formed by the cell wall. ×98,000.

Matsubayashi et al. (1966) localized parasite-derived antigens in the limiting membrane of the vacuole surrounding Toxoplasma organisms in peritoneal exudate cells from mice.

The immobilization antigens of *Paramecium aurelia* were demonstrated on the pellicle and cilia (Mott, 1963). After transformation from one antigenic type to another, the new antigen appeared initially on the pellicle and subsequently on the cilia (Mott, 1965).

Despommier et al. (1967) investigated antigenic sites on the larva of *Trichinella spiralis*.

Rickettsia.— Immunoferritin studies on *Coxiella burneti* phases I and II confirm previous data indicating that the phase antigens are localized on the cell surface (Avakyan et al., 1970; Crăcea et al., 1970). Phase I antigen seems to be located more peripherally than phase II antigen.

Viruses.— In a great number of investigations the immunoferritin technique has been successfully used to localize viral antigens in infected cells. This allows for the continuation of the immunofluorescent studies on virus development at the electron microscopic level. These papers are summarized in Table 1. An excellent review on virologic applications of ferritin-labeled antibodies was given by Howe et al. (1969). Micheel (1971) resumed studies on tumor virus antigens.

III. Immunoenzyme Technique

A. Principle

The immunoenzyme technique was developed independently by Nakane, Pierce, and co-workers (Nakane and Pierce, 1966a, b; Sri Ram et al., 1966) for electron microscopy, and by Avrameas and Uriel (1966) for immunodiffusion in gel studies. The principle of this technique is the coupling of the antibody to a relatively stable enzyme, for which there exists a cytochemical detection method at the ultrastructural level. Since the enzyme produces an increasingly larger number of product molecules with increasingly greater concentrations of substrate and increasingly greater reaction times, the immunocytochemical reaction can be greatly intensified. A detailed review of the immunoenzyme technique was given by Avrameas (1970).

B. Enzymes

Nakane et al. (1966) and Sri Ram et al. (1966) first conjugated acid phosphatase from wheat germ. Now, the most frequently employed enzyme is the peroxidase from horseradish (Nakane and Pierce, 1966). This enzyme is preferred because its molecule is smaller than that of phosphatase and it is less abundant in mammalian tissues, except in erythrocytes. Other convenient enzymes are the glucose oxidase from *Aspergillus niger,* the tyrosinase from mushroom, the alkaline phosphatase from *E. coli* and the acid phosphatase from potato (Avrameas, 1969a, 1970). In general, the use of the purest available enzyme preparation is recommended.

C. Coupling Reagents and Procedures

Antibody and enzyme can be conjugated by the same bifunctional reagents as those used in the immunoferritin technique. Acid phosphatase and horseradish peroxidase were conjugated to antibody by the use of FNPS or 1-ethyl-3-(3-dimethylamino propyl) carbodiimide (Nakane and Pierce, 1966).

In the coupling of peroxidase, optimal yields were obtained with the following method: 0.25 ml of 0.5% FNPS in acetone was added to 50 mg of horseradish peroxidase and 50 mg of γ-globulin dissolved in 2 ml of 0.5 M cold carbonate buffer at pH 10. The mixture was agitated gently for six hours at 4°C and was dialyzed against PBS.

Avrameas (1969a) proposed glutaraldehyde as a very effective and suitable reagent for producing enzyme-antibody globulin complexes with enzymatic and immunologic specificity. The following example of the procedure involves the coupling of anti-rabbit γ-globulin with peroxidase: 12 mg of peroxidase (RZ3) are dissolved in 1 ml of

Table 1. Application of ferritin-labeled antibodies (FAb) in virologic studies

Virus group and species	Host cells	Structures binding FAb	Reference
		RNA containing animal viruses	
Picorna viruses			
Poliomyelitis virus	Primary and continuous cultures of human and monkey cells	Viral antigen on fibrils, vesicles, and smooth endoplasmic reticulum; full and empty virus particles in cytoplasm aligned on fibrils, emerging at the cell membrane and extracellular	Levinthal et al., 1969
Mengo virus	L-cells	Viral antigen in cytoplasm and on the nucleus membrane; virus particles on cytoplasmic vesicles and emerging from the cell membrane (Figure 9)	Wagner and Veckenstedt, 1970
Foot-and-mouth-disease virus	Primary swine kidney cells	Virus crystals and unknown structures in the cytoplasm	Breese, 1969, 1970
Reovirus	L-cells	Virus crystals and virus particles; viral antigen on mitotic-spindle tubules, but not on the characteristic kinky filaments	Dales et al., 1965
Arbo viruses			
Colorado tick fever virus	BHK-21, KB-cells	Virus particles; intranuclear and intracytoplasmic fibres	Oshiro and Emmons, 1968

Chikungunya virus	VERO cells	Spheric and rod-shaped virus particles and giant forms; cell membrane beneath virus precursors	Higashi et al., 1967
Influenza virus	Chorio-allantoic membrane	Extracellular virus particles; dense aggregates (soluble antigen) in the nucleus, except the nucleoli; dispersed antigen in the cytoplasm; circumscribed sites of the cell surface and free and budding virions	Rifkind et al., 1960; Morgan et al., 1961b,c, 1962; Morgan et al., 1961a
		As infection proceeded, viral antigen progressively accumulated at the cell surface, while host cell antigen diminished in amount	Duc-Nguyen et al., 1966
	Primary monkey kidney cells	Extracellular virus particles, but not the elongated tubular structures in the infected cell	Archetti et al., 1970
Paramyxo viruses			
Parainfluenza virus type 2	HeLa cells, human amnion cells	Perinuclear aggregates of viral ribonucleoprotein; pleomorph virus particles inclusive abortive forms	Howe et al., 1970
Parainfluenza virus type 3	Calf kidney cells	Virus particles of the cell membrane and sites	Reczko and Bögel, 1963
Mumps virus	Chick embryo fibroblasts	Large masses of cytoplasmic nucleoproteins; modified cell membrane and virus particles	Duc-Nguyen and Rosenblum, 1967
Rubella virus	BHK-21, BS-C-1 cells	Virus particles in various stages of budding and sites of the cell membrane	Oshiro et al., 1969

(Cont'd)

Table 1 (Continued)

Virus group and species	Host cells	Structures binding FAb	Reference
		RNA containing animal viruses *(Continued)*	
Rinderpest virus	Lymphocytes, reticular cells, mucosal epithelial cells, calf kidney cells	Filaments with a tubular structure in cytoplasmic inclusions	Tajima et al., 1967
Rabies virus	BHK 21, C-13 cells	Virus particles in the cytoplasm and filaments and spheric particles on the cell surface	Atanasiu et al., 1963
RNA tumor viruses			
Rous sarcoma virus	Rat sarcoma cells	Diffuse sites at the periphery of the cytoplasm	Lindberg and Biberfeld, 1967
Mouse mammary tumor virus	Tumor specimens from RIII and C57BL mice	Only B particles of virus, not the intracytoplasmic A particles; oncogenic MTV and the far less oncogenic nodule-inducing virus are antigenically related	Tanaka and Moore, 1967
Graffi virus	Graffi leukemia cells	Extracellular virus particles and circumscribed sites of the cell surface	Micheel and Bierwolf, 1969
Gross leukemia virus	Leukemia cells	G(gross)- and H-2 cell surface antigens in circumscribed areas of the cell membrane, not on free or budding virions	Aoki et al., 1970

DNA containing animal viruses

Adenoviruses			
Adenovirus type 12	Hamster and human amnion cells	T-antigen on bundles of fibers in the nuclei of infected cells and in the cytoplasm of neoplastic cells	Kalnins et al., 1966, 1967
	Human amnion cells (AV-3)	Viral antigen in the virus coat, in complexes consisting of electron dense and light areas and in patches of amorphous material	Stich et al., 1967
	Infected and transformed hamster, human, and monkey cells	Filaments of T-antigen in the cytoplasm and nucleus of infected and transformed cells; spots and rings of viral antigen in the nucleus	Levinthal et al., 1967a
Papova viruses			
Polyoma virus	Mouse embryo cells	Virus particles in nuclei and cytoplasm	Biberfeld and Ringerts, 1966
SV40	Transformed hamster cells	Aggregates of T-antigen in the nuclear matrix except the nucleoli	Oshiro et al., 1967a; Levinthal et al., 1967a
	BSC-1, MA-104 cells	Virus particles in the cytoplasm; nuclear virus and virus in tubules and vacuoles is unstained	Levinthal et al., 1967b; Oshiro et al., 1967b

(Cont'd)

Table 1 (Continued)

Virus group and species	Host cells	Structures binding FAb	Reference
		DNA containing animal viruses (Continued)	
Herpes viruses			
Herpes simplex virus	HeLa, FL-cells	Small aggregates in the nuclear matrix; large masses in the cytoplasm; structurally altered sites of the cell surface. Intracellular virus particles did not tag.	Nii et al., 1968
Epstein-Barr virus	BHK-21 cells, human lymphoid cells	Virus capsids; no cross-reaction with Herpes simplex virus.	Hampar et al., 1970
Pox viruses			
Vaccinia virus	HeLa cells	Mature virus particles and aggregates of viral antigen; immature virus particles did not tag.	Morgan et al., 1962a
Miscellaneous viruses			
African swine fever virus	Pig kidney cells	Virus particles	Breese et al., 1967

Vesicular stomatitis virus	L-cells, HeLa cells	Extracellular virus particles	Paucker et al., 1970
Serum hepatitis		Australia SH antigen	Almeida et al., 1969
Plant viruses			
Tobacco mosaic virus	Virus spray	Virus particles	Singer and Schick, 1961
	Cells of tomato leaves	Viral antigen in nucleus and cytoplasm; virus particles in cytoplasm	Shalla and Amici, 1967
Bacteriophages			
T2-phage	*E. coli* K12 spheroblasts	Phage particles in spheroblasts	Lee, 1960
		Demonstration of the interaction with IgG and IgM antibodies	Höglund, 1967

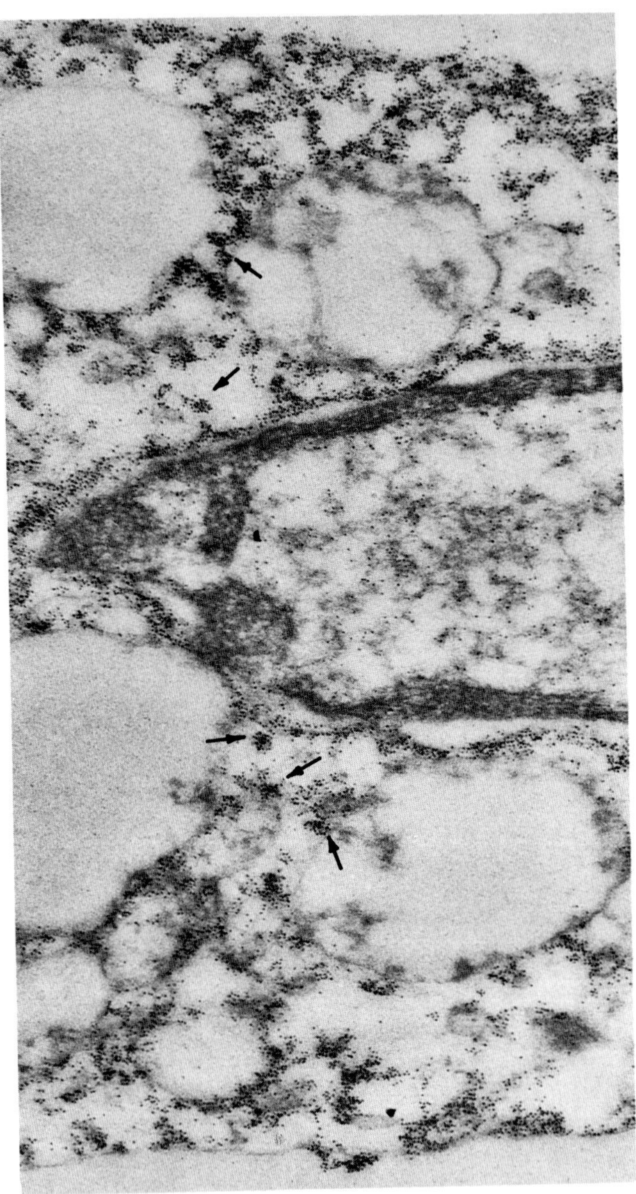

Fig. 9. Mengovirus-infected L-cell, eight hours after infection, treated with virus-specific antibody and ferritin-labeled antiglobulin. The surfaces of cytoplasmic vesicles and nucleus membrane are heavily coated with virus antigen. Aggregates of ferritin particles *(arrows)* indicate single virus particles (Wagner and Veckenstedt, 1970). × 58,000.

0.1 M phosphate buffer, pH 6.8, containing 5 mg of antibody. While the solution is stirred gently, 0.05 ml of a 1% aqueous solution of glutaraldehyde is added in drops. The reaction mixture is allowed to stand for two hours at room temperature and then dialyzed against a large volume of PBS at 4°C overnight. The precipitate is removed by centrifugation for 30 min at 4°C and 20,000 rev/min. This stock solution of peroxidase-labeled antibodies is kept at 4°C and can be used for at least three months without any appreciable loss in its catalytic and immunologic activities.

D. Purification and Properties of Enzyme-Labeled Antibodies

As in the immunoferritin technique, after termination of the coupling reaction, the reaction mixture contains labeled antibodies, unreacted globulin, and unreacted enzyme.

Nakane et al. (1966) have tried the purification of the acid phosphatase-labeled antibodies by gel filtration on Bio-Gel P-300. The unreacted peroxidase can be separated from labeled and unlabeled γ-globulin by precipitating the latter with 50% ammonium sulphate. The precipitate must be resuspended in PBS and dialyzed.

Avrameas (1969) generally avoided such purification procedures, but he used only pure antibody preparations isolated by immunoadsorption techniques. He found that immunodiffusion and immunoelectrophoresis of the raw conjugates show a picture of high heterogeneity. By gel filtration on Sephadex G-200, the IgG-enzyme complex can be eluted with the void volume of the column.

Zeromski (1970) reported that in brain sections the presence of unbound peroxidase in the conjugate resulted in severe unspecific reactions.

The activity of enzyme-labeled antibody can be proved by immunoelectrophoresis. The precipitation line formed by the reaction of labeled antibody and homologous antigen will be specifically stained by incubation with an appropriate enzyme substrate (Figure 10).

Similarly, with enzyme-labeled antigens, immunoelectrophoresis can be used to reveal antibodies in serological investigations.

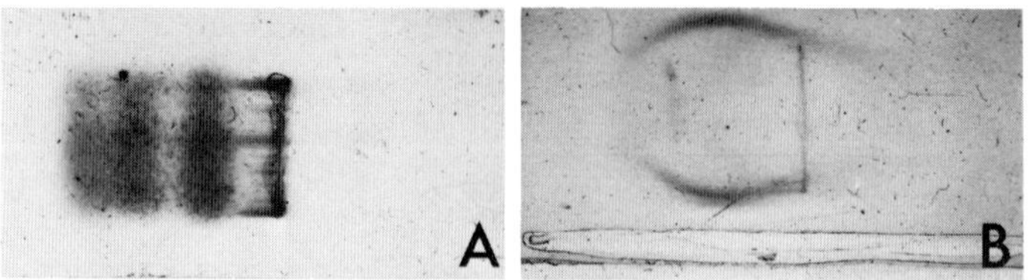

Fig. 10. A, Agar electrophoresis pattern of raw peroxidase-antibody conjugate. After staining with 3,3'-diaminobenzidine, the electropherogram shows several fractions with peroxidase activity. *B,* Immunoelectrophoresis pattern of peroxidase-labeled anti-rabbit IgG antibodies and rabbit serum (trough). The precipitation line was stained with 3,3'-diaminobenzidine.

E. Tagging of Antigen Structures with Enzyme-Labeled Antibodies

1. Staining Methods

Cell and tissue preparations are treated with the enzyme-labeled antibody following procedures similar to those described for the immunoferritin technique. Penetration of antibody into the cells may be difficult, and can be facilitated by prefixation or other convenient pretreatments. In general, the type of fixation is important for the quality of the antigen demonstration.

Recently, Kawarai and Nakane (1970) described a method for the localization of tissue antigens directly on ultrathin sections. Sections from methacrylate-embedded tissues were placed on coated grids, and parts of the embedding medium were removed with a water-saturated solution of xylene. Exhaustive washing of the grids is necessary to remove all traces of xylene. The sections are placed face down on a droplet of antiserum for 10–30 min, washed in several changes of PBS, placed on a droplet of peroxidase-labeled antiglobulin, and washed again in PBS. The incubation with the substrate must be carried out in a constant flow; otherwise there is heavy nonspecific precipitation. The developed grids are washed with distilled water in a syringe and dried.

This technique is still being developed, but such a procedure would eliminate the problem of penetration of antisera and conjugates through the tissue and cell membranes, and therefore it deserves great attention.

Enzyme-labeled antibodies may be used in the direct method or as labeled antiimmunoglobulin antibodies in the indirect (double-layer) method.

Autoradiography combined with the immunoenzyme technique has several advantages over a combination of autoradiography and immunofluorescence (Wicker and Avrameas, 1970). By contrast, the combination of the latter with the immunoenzyme technique may be used for simultaneous localization of different antigens, e.g., two different antibodies in one immunocompetent cell (Guillien et al., 1968).

Recently, some new techniques have been described, in which the enzyme is not coupled to the antibody by covalent linkages. Avrameas (1969b) called this procedure an indirect immunoenzyme technique, but since there is no similarity to the already known indirect immunofluorescent technique, this designation could be misleading and should be avoided.

Mixed antibody method for the demonstration of cell-bound immunoglobulin (Avrameas, 1969b).—For the localization of immunoglobulin of species A, an antiimmunoglobulin A of species B and an antienzyme of species A are necessary. The antiimmunoglobulin A binds to the cell-bound immunoglobulin and to the antienzyme. The free active site of the latter can then react with the enzyme added last, which now catalyzes the reaction for the histochemical detection.

Immunoglobulin-enzyme bridge method (Mason et al., 1969).— This technique is similar to the above-mentioned method for visualizing tissue antigens. The reaction is performed with the following components, given in order of their use:

(a) specific antiserum to the tissue antigen,
(b) antiserum against the immunoglobulin of the species for serum (a),
(c) specific antiserum against the enzyme label (peroxidase), prepared in the same species as serum (a), and
(d) enzyme label followed by the histochemical reaction.

Sternberger and Cuculis (1969) independently developed the same method and demonstrated its usefulness on the staining of syphilis spirochetes.

Hybrid antibody method (Avrameas 1969b).—The principle of this method is similar to that of the antiferritin hybrid antibody method of Hämmerling et al. (1968). The yield of hybrid (antienzyme, anti-immunoglobulin) antibody varies between 20% and 50%, but the capacity to detect antigens is less than that of enzyme-coupled antibodies.

Amplification antibody method (Avrameas, 1969b).—Since the enzyme has several numbers of antigenic determinants, an antienzyme antibody can be used to enhance the sensitivity of the immunoenzyme technique. These antibodies are linked to the immobilized enzyme by one of their active sites, and the free combining site can react with subsequently added enzyme which finally can be revealed by histochemical staining.

Tagging with soluble complexes of enzyme and antienzyme immunoglobulin (Sternberger et al., 1970).—In this method the antibody against the specific antigen to be detected also remains unlabeled and the enzyme (horseradish peroxidase) is bound to rabbit-antienzyme immunoglobulin as a soluble complex. The antigen then was identified by sequential application of:

(a) specific rabbit antiserum,
(b) sheep antiserum to rabbit IgG, added in sufficient excess to leave one combining site free after reaction with the rabbit antibody,
(c) specifically purified, soluble peroxidase-rabbit antiperoxidase complex (PAP),
(d) 3,3'-diaminobenzidine and H_2O_2, and
(e) osmium tetroxide.

High yields of PAP were obtained by precipitation of antibody from specific rabbit antiserum with horseradish peroxidase (PO) at equivalence, solubilization of the washed precipitate with excess PO at pH 2.3 (1°C), followed by immediate neutralization and separation of PAP from PO by half-saturation with ammonium sulfate. It is very interesting that the ratio of PO to anti-PO in PAP constantly was 3 : 2, irrespective of the preparation and source of antiserum. On electron micrographs, the PAP shows a pentagonal shape, with a diameter of about 205 Å, in which three corners are suspected to be PO and two antibody fragment Fc. Sensitivity and specificity of this method, as demonstrated by the staining of spirochetes, were about 100- to 1000-fold that of immunofluorescence.

2. Cytochemical Reaction Procedures

In general, the reaction of coupled enzyme with the appropriate substrate, i.e., the "staining reaction," immediately follows the tagging of the antigenic structure with labeled antibody and the washing away of the residues of antiserum and/or conjugate.

Specimens, treated with acid phosphatase-labeled antibodies, were stained in Gomori's medium for 30 min at 37°C, washed in acetate buffer for one hour, postfixed at 1.2% veronal-buffered glutaraldehyde for one hour, and washed in 0.25 M sucrose for one hour. The specimens then were transfered to 2% OsO_4 buffered with S-collidine, dehydrated, and embedded (Nakane and Pierce, 1967).

A convenient histochemical method for demonstrating peroxidase activity uses 3,3'-diaminobenzidine as an oxidizable substrate. The substrate is oxidized to an indamine polymer which then may be altered by oxidative cyclization to a phenazine polymer. This reaction product is brown and strongly osmiophilic. When reacted with osmium tetroxide, a distinct, amorphous, nondroplet reaction product is formed that is easily seen in both light and electron microscopes. The antibody-tagged and washed specimens were incubated at room temperature, for 10–30 min, in a solution of 75 mg of 3,3'-diaminobenzidine and 0.001% hydrogen peroxide in 100 ml of 0.05 M tris buffer, pH 7.6, washed in the same buffer, osmicated in 2% OsO_4 in distilled water, washed again, dehydrated, and embedded.

The possibility of producing stable reaction products of peroxidase substrates in different colors induced Nakane (1969) to develop a method for the simultaneous localization of multiple tissue antigens in the light microscope. Since the antibody can be eluted without removing the reaction product, the section can be incubated with another antibody and the histochemical procedure repeated with a different substrate. Convenient substrates are 3,3'-diaminobenzidine (free base), α-naphthol followed by pyronin staining, and 4-Cl-1-naphthol, which gives yellowish brown, reddish pink, and grayish blue reaction products, respectively.

Glucose oxidase activity was localized by incubating the preparation in the absence of light in 20 ml of 0.1 M phosphate buffer, pH 7.0, containing 150 mg of D-glucose, 10 mg of thiozyl blue, and 2 mg of phenazine methasulphate. The preparation then was washed for 3–5 min in phosphate buffer and rinsed with distilled water (Avrameas, 1969). A convenient substrate for tyrosinase is dihydroxyphenylalanine.

3. Specificity Controls

The specificity of the staining can be proved with the same control methods as are used in the immunoferritin technique (see page 201). Furthermore, the eventual presence of endogenous enzyme activity must be considered. For example, deposition of reaction product from 3,3′-diaminobenzidine substrate in intracristate spaces of mitochondria was carried out on the endogenous cytochrome oxidase activity of these organelles (Abelson et al., 1969). In erythrocytes an endogenous peroxidase activity is present.

F. Applications of Enzyme-Labeled Antibodies

Immunoenzyme techniques can be used to demonstrate antigens or antibodies at the electron microscopic level as well as at the light microscopic level. Since the light microscopic studies often are the first stage toward further electron microscopic investigations, they also are included in this review. Another field using enzyme-labeled antibodies is gel immunodiffusion studies (Avrameas and Uriel, 1966). Recently, Stanislawski (1970) employed labeling with peroxidase for the quantitative estimation of antigens or antibodies following electroimmunodiffusion. He stated that the sensitivity of this technique is about 5–20 times higher than the conventional method.

1. Synthesis of Immunoglobulins

In spleen cells of rabbits immunized against human IgG, synthesized antibodies were located by means of peroxidase-labeled IgG in the perinuclear cisternae and on the ribosomes (Bouteille and Avrameas, 1967).

In bone marrow cells from a myeloma patient, the intracellular site of immunoglobulin synthesis was revealed specifically with anti-body against the κ-type light chain (Suzuki and Takahashi, 1969). The unresponsiveness to labeled antibodies against light chain type λ and heavy chain classes α, γ, and μ was consistent with the observation that the patient secreted into serum and urine only free κ-type light chains.

In cells of a long-term culture line (R.P.M.I., No. 4666) from peripheral blood of a patient with chronic myelogenous leukemia which produced both monoclonal IgA of κ-type and free κ-type light chains, a different localization of light and heavy chains was observed (Suzuki et al., 1969). With antiserum, free polysomes were stained selectively in the cytoplasm, indicating that they are the dominant site of heavy chain accumulation. On the other hand, κ-type light chains were mainly localized in the endoplasmic reticulum and ribosomes lining the ergastoplasmic membranes and in the external layer of the nuclear membrane.

Several interesting investigations were performed using enzymes as antigen and tracing the ultrastructural distribution of the antien-zyme antibody by incubation with the same enzyme followed by the appropriate cytochemical reaction (Avrameas and Lespinat, 1967; Leduc et al., 1968, 1969; Scott et al., 1968; Straus, 1968, 1970a,b; Sordat et al., 1970).

The antibody synthesis starts from the perinuclear space of the hemocytoblasts, where it persists through differentiation into immature plasma cells. Later the antibody fills the cisternae of the endoplasmic reticulum and the lamellar portion of the Golgi apparatus. In late stages some cisternae are distended to large globules and form the so-called Russell bodies (Avrameas and Leduc, 1970). In popliteal lymph nodes from rabbits, antibody was found in three types of cells: large lymphocytes, typical plasma cells, and modified small lymphocytes, which tentatively were called "lymphoplasmacytes." These types of cells seem to be responsible for the immunologic memory, since it could be shown that after an additional antigenic stimulation a second cycle of antibody synthesis may start around the nucleus in the same cell, even before the previously synthesized antibody has been entirely secreted.

A paired-staining technique which combines direct immuno-enzyme and immunofluorescent methods was used to prove the specificity of the antibody production by single spleen cells of rabbits

(Guillien et al., 1970). The results confirm once more the general concept of the narrow specificity of the antibody production by immunocompetent cells.

2. Tissue Antigens

Swope et al. (1970) compared the peroxidase-labeled antibody technique on adjacent sections with a permanganate-Alcian Blue (AB)-aldehyd fuchsin (AF) procedure on the anterior pituitary gland of female rats. The AB + /AF + cells correspond to positive reaction with antiserum against the thyroid-stimulating hormone, whereas the AF + /AB − cells correspond to the follicle-stimulating hormone. Cells that reacted with antiserum against the luteinizing hormone do not react with either AB or AF.

Nakane (1970) localized six hormones of the anterior pituitary gland of male rats at both the light and electron microscopic levels. Growth hormone, adenocorticotropic hormone, prolactin, and thyrotropic hormone were found in separate cells, whereas the follicle-stimulating hormone and the luteinizing hormone frequently were localized in the same cell. On the same organ, also the direct staining of ultrathin sections was demonstrated (Kawarai and Nakane, 1970). The hormones were localized in secretion granules and in endoplasmic reticulum but not in nucleus or mitochondria.

Using immunoenzyme and immunofluorescent techniques, we have demonstrated tissue antigens in the brain and the corpora cardiaca of the cockroach (*Periplaneta americana*), which correspond to the PAF-positive neurosecretes (Eckert et al., 1971). In the brain, two secretory types of PAF-negative neurosecretory neurons could also be found. One type of these cells is situated in the pars intercerebralis, the other in the rostro-dorsal region of the protocerebrum (Figure 11).

Chymotrypsinogen was found by staining with peroxidase-labeled antibodies both in the zymogen granules of the apical portion of acinar cells of some pancreas acini and in the basal portion and surrounding the nuclei in other acini (Schiff et al., 1970). This indicated an asynchronous proenzyme production.

With peroxidase- or fluorescein-labeled antibodies against proinsulin, positive immunoreactions were obtained in the β-cells of islets of both fetal and adult bovine pancreas (Logothetopoulos et al., 1970).

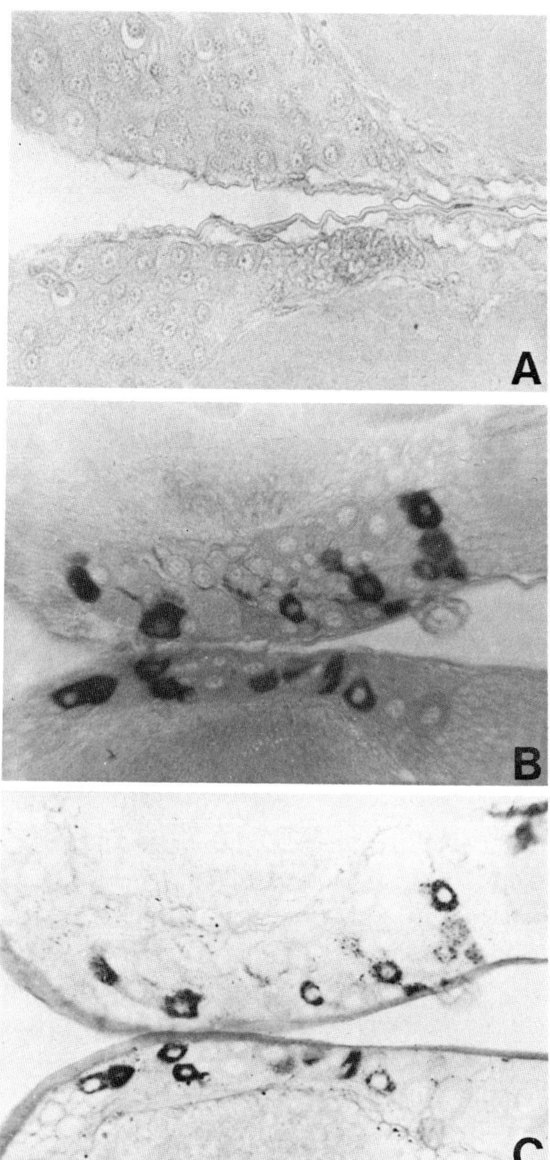

Fig. 11. Intercerebral part of the brain of the cockroach *(Periplaneta americana)* stained by the indirect immunoenzyme technique. *A,* Control section, treated with normal rabbit serum and peroxidase-labeled anti-rabbit IgG. *B,* Section treated with antiserum against the neuroendocrine retrocerebral complex (NRC) and peroxidase-labeled anti-rabbit IgG. The NRC positive cells are heavily stained. *C,* Same section as in *B.* Bound antibodies were eluted with HCl-glycine buffer, pH 2.2, and the section was poststained with paraldehyde fuchsin (PAF). The NRC positive cells are also PAF positive. × 375.

Antibodies to parietal cells, which are present in the sera of most patients with pernicious anemia, react with an antigen on the cell membrane, forming the microvilli of the gastric parietal cells (Hoedemaker and Ito, 1970). The labeled antibody stains parietal cells of some other mammals, too, but no other cell types (e.g., the pepsinogenic cells).

Bretton and Lespinats (1969) located surface antigens on suspended tumor cells from plasmocytomes of mouse strain BALB/c.

In sera of patients with sensory carcinomatous neuropathy, an antibody against neurons was demonstrated with peroxidase-labeled antihuman γ-globulin (Zeromski, 1970). Positive reactions were indicated by heavy brown deposits in nerve cells from different parts of unfixed guinea pig brain sections.

Using human antinuclear antibodies, Beck et al. (1965) demonstrated the nuclear structure of isolated rat liver cell nuclei. Their results confirm previous fluorescent antibody observations.

In studies on glomerulonephritis, the staining of the glomerular basement membrane by peroxidase-labeled antibodies was the same as that obtained with the fluorescein antibody method (Davey and Busch, 1970).

3. Microbial Antigens

Nakane et al. (1968) localized the leucine-binding protein of *E. coli* in the cell envelope.

The cellular localization of M-protein in *Streptococcus pyogenes* was investigated comparatively by both the indirect immunoperoxidase and the indirect immunoferritin technique (Wagner and Wagner, 1973). The M-protein forms threadlike structures, which originate from the middle lamella of the electron permeable outer cell wall layer. Whereas the fine structure of the M-protein on the cell surface is well demonstrated by the latter method, the M-protein structure within the cell wall can be localized only by the immunoperoxidase technique.

A specific but nonimmunologic reaction between Staphylococcus protein A and the Fc portion of certain γ-globulins (especially γG_1-myeloma protein) provided the basis for the ultrastructural localization of protein A in the outmost layer of the cell wall (Nickerson et al., 1970).

Mouse skeletal muscle poisoned with tetanus toxin and incubated with peroxidase-labeled tetanus antitoxin showed histochemical reaction products in the lumen of T-tubules, in the region between T-tubules and longitudinal components, and within terminal sacs of the sarcoplasmic reticulum (Zacks and Sheff, 1967). It is interesting that both the sites where tetanus toxin was localized are involved in the relaxation-contraction cycle.

Several authors investigated the localization of virus antigens in infected cell cultures. In studies on lymphocytic choriomeningitis virus-infected 3T3 cells, the extracellular virions were intensely stained (Abelson et al., 1969). Virus-specific antigens were demonstrated to be associated with large cytoplasmic ribosomal aggregates which had not been described previously.

In vaccinia virus-infected L-cells, the virus antigen was demonstrated in the cytoplasm of many cells six hours after infection (Siverd and Sharon, 1969). The nucleus and the cytoplasm were pale; only the inclusions were stained distinctly dark brown. After about 48 hr the entire cytoplasm became darker, and localization of the vaccinia antigen was not well defined.

The development and localization of antigens of the densonucleosis virus were investigated in the larvae of *Galleria mellonella* (Kurstak et al., 1969, 1970). In addition to a faint intracytoplasmic staining four hours after infection, which is suggestive of early proteins, an intense staining on the nuclear membrane was observed six to eight hours after infection. Later the nucleus was entirely filled with the antigen and the virus spread to the cytoplasm.

Wicker and Avrameas (1969) studied the localization of antigens of SV40, adenovirus 12, and rat K-virus in infected cell cultures by means of horseradish peroxidase, alkaline phosphatase, and glucose oxidase as antibody labels. Using histochemical procedures resulting in reaction products of different colors, they revealed the T-antigens and the structural antigens simultaneously. The T-antigen of SV40 was also localized at the ultrastructural level (Leduc et al., 1969). In monkey kidney cells, strain MA 104, it appeared first in the reticular network of the nucleus, though not in the nucleolus. Unfortunately, there was heavy nonspecific staining in the cytoplasm and on the cell surface in both control and infected cell cultures.

IV. Iodinated and Heavy Metal-Conjugated Antibodies

Several attempts have been made to render the antibody itself sufficiently electron scattering by means of iodination or the introduction of heavy metals. Considerations in choosing convenient heavy metals are the following:

1. The metal must be of as high a molecular weight as possible to be effective in electron scattering.
2. The metal must be introduced in sufficient quantity to increase visibily the electron opacity of the antibody.
3. The metal should be covalently linked directly or indirectly to the protein to eliminate the possibility of dissociation and subsequent binding to other tissue constituents.
4. Introduction of the metal into the antibody molecule must not diminish the reaction between antibody and antigen.
5. The metal should be stable in the electron beam.
6. The amount of metal needed to give adequate electron opacity to the final conjugated antibody must not result in the insolubility of the modified antibody.

Attempts to introduce metals into the antibody molecule were made with compounds of mercury, uranium, osmium, and iron. A review of some of these techniques was given by Sternberger (1967).

A. Iodine

Methods for the iodination of antibody were described by Mekler et al. (1964, 1967). For example, iodine-labeled antibodies retaining immunological specificity could be obtained if a 2% solution of γ-globulin in 1.5% solution of $NaHCO_3$, pH 8.4, at 0–2°C, were reacted with a 0.2 N solution of iodine in ethanol. Iodinated antibodies were employed to demonstrate the antigens of influenza virus (Mekler et al., 1964) and measles virus (Parfanovich et al., 1965). On *Leptospira canicola* the iodinated IgG and IgM molecules are visible as electron-dense particles along the cell surface (Osechinsky et al., 1969).

B. Mercury

Pepe (1961) used diazotized tetraacetoxy mercuriarsanilic acid as labeling agent. Since this compound is rather unstable in the electron beam, Pepe and Fink (1961) overlayed the stained sections with a carbon film to prevent volatilization. Unspecific staining, because of the binding of mercury to sulfhydryl groups in the tissue, was prevented by blocking with iodoacetic acid and formaldehyde.

Kulberg and Azadova (1963) described the coupling with *p*-aminophenylmercuryl acetate (PAFMA), which can be prepared simply from mercuric acetate and aniline. After treatment with an excess of monoiodoacetate (pH 7.5, 25°C, 2 hr), the globulin fraction was labeled according to the following procedure: 10 mg of $NaNO_2$ was added to 50 mg of PAFMA dissolved in 1 ml of 50% acetic acid, and the mixture was cooled to 0–2°C. After 30 min the pH of the diazotized PAFMA was raised to 4.5, and the globulin solution was added. During the conjugation process the pH was maintained at 8.5–9.0.

Antibodies labeled with PAFMA were used for tagging the antigens of Sendai virus (Zhdanov et al., 1962, 1965) and of virulent and avirulent strains of *Francisella tularensis* (Meshcheryakova et al., 1967).

Kendall (1965) described a further procedure for labeling with mercury. He applied a monofunctional thiol-specific mercurial (methylmercuric hydroxide) to antibody after a large proportion of the protein groups had been thiolated using N-acetylhomocysteinethiolactone. The labeled antibody globulin contained 3.2–3.5% of mercury by weight, or 25–27 mercury atoms per antibody molecule, and possessed 50% or more of the activity of the unmodified protein.

C. Ferrocene

The potential utility of ferrocene derivates as tracers of antibody globulin was first tested by Wagner and Wunderwald (1964). Ferrocenyl sulfochloride was coupled in the presence of acetone; the purified conjugate fraction showed a yellowish color. Unfortunately, the staining efficiency of this conjugate was very weak. Similar insufficient results were obtained with *p*-ferrocenyl phenylisothiocyanate (Franz, 1967a,b), which is also insoluble in water.

In order to improve the water solubility, Franz (1968) introduced a carbonyl group into the phenyl side chain. The preparation of 3-carboxy-4-ferrocenyl-phenylisothiocyanate (CFPI) proceeds over the steps 2-ferrocenyl-5-nitro-benzoic acid and 2-ferrocenyl-5-amino-benzoic acid, which is converted by means of thiophosgene to the CFPI, as seen in the following diagram:

CFPI can be conjugated to antibody globulin in alkaline-buffered aqueous solution similar to fluorescein isothiocyanate. The unreacted CFPI is removed by gel filtration on Sephadex G-50. Tagging of microbial cells with ferrocene-labeled antibodies resulted in a more or less dense homogeneous lining of the cell surface (Franz, 1968).

D. Uranium and Osmium

A series of investigations were carried out by Sternberger, Donati, Petrali, and co-workers using uranium and osmium for immunospecific labeling.

1. Immunouranium Technique

Uranium readily chelates with protein, but antibody activity is progressively destroyed. By complexing the antibody molecule with the specific antigen prior to exposure to uranyl acetate, Sternberger and co-workers protected the specific combining sites on the antibody. In a subsequent step, the antigen was separated from the antibody. Thus, an antibody was recovered which contained uranium in the nonspecific areas of the molecule, but possessed specific combining sites devoid of uranium and hence still capable of reacting with antigen.

Specific protection first was achieved by adsorption of anti-*Bordetella bronchiseptica* antibody on *B. bronchiseptica* cells (Sternberger et al., 1963). The washed agglutinates were exposed to uranium, and the antibody was recovered by brief alkali treatment.

To avoid the need for preparing uranium-labeled antibody for each antigen to be localized, these workers developed an indirect staining method. Antibodies against immunoglobulins were removed from serum by adsorption on antigen insolubilized by coupling with diazotized *p*-aminobenzyl cellulose (Sternberger et al., 1965, 1966a). The reaction of the purified uranium-labeled antibody with its antigen resulted in the precipitation of 50–85% of total protein and somewhat lower proportions of total uranium contents. By means of the indirect staining technique, vaccinia antigen was localized in infected HeLa cells (Donati et al., 1965).

In another study the flagella of *Bordetella bronchiseptica* was marked (Wilson et al., 1966). While specific contrast was conferred to antigen, the surrounding structures were indistinct, and focusing of the specimens was difficult. Furthermore, the sections were unstable in the electron beam and, hence, only low beam intensity could be used for visualization.

2. *Immunouranium-Thiocarbohydrazide-Osmium Tetroxide Technique*

In a bridging reaction, uranium of the labeled antibody is capable of chelation with one of the hydrazine groups and the thiocarbonyl group of thiocarbohydrazide ($NH_2 \cdot NH \cdot CS \cdot NH \cdot NH_2$), leaving its second hydrazine group free to react with osmium tetroxide. Exposure to moist osmium tetroxide vapor resulted in osmium black being deposited on the sites of uranium-labeled antibody. Thus, the contrast of the preparations was intensified and the stability in the electron beam was improved (Sternberger et al., 1966b).

Specimens embedded in methacrylate can be stained by this method after sectioning. In the case of sections of linear methacrylate, etching with benzene-saturated water proved satisfactory for making antigen accessible to antibody. With divinylbenzene cross-linked methacrylate sections, etching with a solution of 0.01% benzene and 1% ethanol in water was successful.

3. Immunodiazothioether-Osmium Tetroxide (Immuno-DTO) Technique

Since diazotized diazothioethers couple rapidly with aromatic amines, an excess of diazotized 4'-(3-aminobenzyl-thio)-diazo-2',5'-diethoxybenzanilide was reacted with immunospecifically protected antibody. Essentially pure, extensively coupled antibody was obtained (Sternberger et al., 1966a). The specific contrast of the osmicated antigen structure following exposition of the ultrathin sections to this diazothioether antibody exceeded by far the constrast resulting from the natural affinity of embedded tissue to osmium tetroxide. Donati et al. (1966) compared this technique with the nonintensified immunouranium technique in investigations on the antigen formation of vaccinia virus in HeLa cells. Unfortunately, the osmiumtetroxide-binding power of diazothioether antibodies is unstable even on storage in dry ice or liquid nitrogen.

4. Quantitation of the Immunouranium Technique

Since, by the immunouranium technique, staining of experimental and control probes can be performed on successive sections of the same tissue block, the staining intensity is useful in quantitative antigen determinations (Sternberger, 1969). By densitometry of electron micrography plates, the location of lysozyme in the lysosomes of monocytes, as well as in the granules of granulocytes, was confirmed. Quantitation confirmed also the visual impression that platelets contain fibrinogen in their granulomeres.

V. Evaluation of Immune Electron Microscopic Labeling Methods

The immunoferritin technique is not only the oldest of all labeling techniques for immune electron microscopy, but it is also the most elaborate one. It offers the highest sensitivity of all methods. Thus, it is possible to localize a single antigenic site on a cell surface by a single ferritin-labeled antibody molecule (e.g., the Rh(D) antigen on erythrocytes). Although the immunoferritin technique is the method of choice in the location of surface antigens, several difficulties must be overcome in tagging intracellular structures because of the large dimension of the conjugate. It is hoped that the further development of postembedding staining will overcome this difficulty. The new hybrid immunoferritin antibody method reduces the danger of unspecific staining and offers the possibility of localizing several different antigens simultaneously, using ferritin and other large marker molecules.

Advantages of the immunoenzyme techniques are the large amplification factor resulting from the catalyzing action of the enzyme on the substrate, the ease of preparation of the antibody conjugate, the permanence of the preparation, and the ability to study antigen localization at both the light and electron microscope levels. This permits close correlation of the cytological structures observed at the two levels. However, there are also some disadvantages. Because of the intense deposition of the reaction products, the resolution of the antigen sites at the electron microscopic level is not as high as in the immunoferritin technique. Several authors observed a considerable background staining. In some cases staining by endogenous enzyme activity can lead to misinterpretation.

It is difficult to assess the labeling techniques with heavy metals and by iodination, since so far most of them have been applied only in the laboratories in which they were developed. In the present author's opinion, in many of the reproduced micrographs, the contrast of the tagged antigenic structures with the background is not convincing. Nevertheless, these methods should be further developed, since they offer possibilities for double staining and for a better penetration of labeled antibodies into the cell.

Literature Cited

Abelson, H. T., G. H. Smith, H. A. Hoffman, and W. P. Rowe. 1969. Use of enzyme-labeled antibody for electron microscope localization of lymphocytic choriomeningitis virus antigens in infected cell cultures. J. Nat. Cancer Inst. 42: 497–515.

Almeida, J. D., A. J. Zuckerman, P. E. Taylor, and A. P. Waterson. 1969. Immune electron microscopy of the Australia-SH (serum hepatitis) antigen. Microbios 1: 117.

Amstey, M. S. 1967. Purification of ferritin-conjugated antibody by DEAE-cellulose chromatography. J. Lab. Clin. Med. 69: 997–1002.

Andres, G. A., L. Accinni, K. C. Hsu, J. B. Zabriskie, and B. C. Seegal. 1966. Electron microscopic studies of human glomerulonephritis with ferritin-conjugated antibody. Localization of antigen-antibody complexes in glomerular structures of patients with acute glomerulonephritis. J. Exp. Med. 123: 399–412.

Andres, G. A., K. C. Hsu, and B. C. Seegal. 1967. Immunoferritin technique for the identification of antigens by electron microscopy, pp. 527–570. *In* D. M. Weir, (ed.), Handbook of experimental immunology. Blackwell Scientific, Oxford.

Andres, G. A., C. Morgan, K. C. Hsu, R. A. Rifkind, and B. C. Seegal. 1962a. Use of ferritin-conjugated antibody to identify nephrotoxic sera in renal tissue by electron microscopy. Nature, London 194: 590–591.

Andres, G. A., C. Morgan, K. C. Hsu, R. A. Rifkind, and B. C. Seegal. 1962b. Electron microscopic studies of experimental nephritis with ferritin conjugated antibody. The basement membranes and cisternae of visceral epithelial cells in nephritic rat glomeruli. J. Exp. Med. 115: 929–936.

Andres, G. A., B. C. Seegal, K. C. Hsu, M. S. Rothenberg, and M. L. Chapeau. 1963. Electron microscopic studies of experimental nephritis with ferritin-conjugated antibody. Localization of antigen-antibody complexes in rabbit glomeruli following repeated injections of bovine serum albumin. J. Exp. Med. 117: 691–704.

Aoki, T., E. A. Boyse, L. J. Old, E. de Harven, U. Hämmerling, and H. A. Wood. 1970. G (gross) and H-2 cell surface antigens: Location on gross leukemia cells by electron microscopy with visually labeled antibody. Proc. Nat. Acad. Sci. U.S.A. 65: 569–576.

Aoki, T., U. Hämmerling, E. de Harven, E. A. Boyse, and L. J. Old. 1969. Antigenic structure of cell surfaces. An immunoferritin study of the occurrence and topography of H-2, θ, and TL alloantigens on mouse cells. J. Exp. Med. 130: 979–1001.

Archetti, I., E. Bereczky, F. Rosati-Valente, and D. Steve-Bocciarelli. 1970. Elongated structures present in cells infected with influenza viruses. Arch. ges. Virusforsch. 29: 275–286.

Arhelger, R. B., J. A. Gronvall, O. B. Carr, and J. G. Brunson. 1963. Electron microscopic localization of nephrotoxic serum in rabbit glomeruli with ferritin-conjugated antibody. Lab. Invest. 12: 33–37.

Atanasiu, P., G. Orth, J. Sisman, and C. Barreau. 1963. Identification immunologique de virion rabique en cultures cellulaires par les anticorps spécifiques conjugués à la ferritine. C. R. Acad. Sci., Ser. D, 257: 2204–2207.

Avakjan, A. A., S. M. Kulagin, R. I. Kudelina, S. A. Gulevskaja, and V. M. Kusnarev. 1970. Investigation of the antigen structure of *Rickettsia burneti*, phase I and II by the method of electron microscopic immunochemistry. [In Russian.] Zh. Mikrobiol. (1) 133–136.

Avrameas, S. 1969a. Coupling of enzymes to proteins with glutaraldehyde. Use of the conjugates for the detection of antigens and antibodies. Immunochemistry 6: 43–52.

Avrameas, S. 1969b. Indirect immunoenzyme techniques for the intracellular detection of antigens. Immunochemistry 6: 825–831.

Avrameas, S. 1970. Immunoenzyme techniques: Enzymes as markers for the localization of antigens and antibodies. Int. Rev. Cytol. 27: 349–385.

Avrmeas, S., and E. H. Leduc. 1970. Detection of simultaneous antibody synthesis in plasma cells and specialized lymphocytes in rabbit lymph nodes. J. Exp. Med. 131: 1137–1168.

Avrameas, S., and G. Lespinats. 1967. Enzymes couplées aux protéines: leur utilisation pour la détection des antigènes et des anticorps. C. R. Acad. Sci., Ser. D, 265: 1149–1152.

Avrameas, S., and J. Uriel. 1966. Méthode de marquage d'antigènes et d'anticorps avec des enzymes et son application en immunodiffusion. C. R. Acad. Sci., Ser. D, 262: 2543–2545.

Baxandall, J. 1966a. The surface reactions associated with fertilization of the sea urchin egg as studied by immunoelectron microscopy. J. Ultrastruct. Res. 16: 158–180.

Baxandall, J., P. Perlmann, and B. A. Afzelius. 1962. A two-layer technique for detecting surface antigens in the sea urchin egg with ferritin-conjugated antibody. J. Cell Biol. 14: 144–151.

Baxandall, J., P. Perlmann, and B. A. Afzelius. 1963. Immune electron microscopy using a two-layer method of ferritin labeling. J. Roy. Micr. Soc. 81: 155–158.

Baxandall, J., P. Perlmann, and B. A. Afzelius. 1964a. Immuno-electron microscope analysis of the surface layers of the unfertilized sea urchin egg. I. Effects of the antisera on the cell ultrastructure. J. Cell Biol. 23: 609–628.

Baxandall, J., P. Perlmann, and B. A. Afzelius. 1964b. Immuno-electron microscope analysis of the surface layers of the unfertilized sea urchin egg. II. Localization of surface antigens. J. Cell Biol. 23: 629–650.

Beck, J. S., G. B. Scott, H. N. Munro, S. Waddington, and D. MacSeveney. 1965. A new immuno-chemical technique for electron microscopic study of nuclear structure using human antinuclear antibodies. Exp. Cell Res. 39: 292–296.

Biberfeld, P., and N. Ringertz. 1966. The application of immune electron microscopy to the demonstration of polyoma virus antigen in cultured mouse embryo cells. J. Nat. Cancer Inst. 37: 451–465.

Binz, H. 1969. Konjugation von Ferritin mit Anti-Kaninchensaccharase Immunoglobulin G. Pathol. Microbiol. 34: 305–315.

Birnbaum, U., A. Vogt, and S. Marinis. 1970. Isolation and characterization of immunoferritin conjugates. II. Antibody binding capacity in vitro. Immunology, London 18: 443–448.

Borek, F. 1961. A new two-stage method for cross-linking proteins. Nature; London 191: 1293–1294.

Borek, F., and A. M. Silverstein. 1961. Characterization and purification of ferritin-antibody globulin conjugates. J. Immunol. 87: 555–561.

Bouteille, M., and S. Avrameas. 1967. Étude au microscope électronique de la formation d'anticorps à l'aide d'antigènes marqués à la péroxydase. C. R. Acad. Sci., Ser. D, 265: 2097–2099.

Breese, S. S. 1969. Reactions of intercellular crystals of foot-and-mouth disease virus with ferritin-tagged antibody. J. Gen. Virol. 4: 343–346.

Breese, S. S. 1970. An indirect ferritin-tagged antibody system for foot-and-mouth disease virus. J. Gen. Virol. 8: 153–155.

Breese, S. S., S. S. Stone, C. J. DeBoer, and W. R. Hess. 1967. Electron microscopy of the interaction of African swine fever virus with ferritin-conjugated antibody. Virology 31: 508–513.

Bretton, R., and G. Lespinats. 1969. Localisation ultrastructurale d'antigènes à la surface de cellules tumorales. C.R. Acad. Sci., Ser. D, 268: 3223–3225.

Charles, A. 1966. Purification of ferritin-labelled immunoglobulines. Experientia 22: 486–487.

Crăcea, E., R. Voilescu, G. Zarnea, M. Ionescu, and D. Bolez. 1970. Electron microscopic study of phase I and II C. burneti in the chick yolk sac by use of ferritin conjugated antibody. Z. Immun. Forsch. 140: 358–365.

Dales, S., P. J. Gomatos, and K. C. Hsu. 1965. The uptake and development of reovirus in strain L cells followed with labeled viral ribonucleic acid and ferritin-antibody conjugates. Virology 25: 193–211.

Davey, F. R., and G. J. Busch. 1970. Immunohistochemistry of glomerulonephritis using horseradish peroxidase and fluorescein-labeled antibody: A comparison of two technics. Amer. J. Clin. Pathol. 53: 531–536.

Davis. W. C., S. D. Douglas, L. D. Petz, and H. H. Fudenberg. 1968. Ferritin-antibody localization of erythrocyte antigenic sites in immunohemolytic anemias. J. Immunol. 101: 621–627.

Despommier, D. D., M. Kajima, and B. S. Wostmann. 1967. Ferritin-conjugated antibody studies on the larvae of Trichinella spiralis. J. Parasitol. 53: 618–624.

Donati, E. J., F. H. J. Figge, and L. A. Sternberger. 1965. Staining of vaccinia antigen by immunouranium technique. Exp. Mol. Pathol. 4: 126–129.

Donati, E. J., J. P. Petrali, and L. A. Sternberger. 1966. Formation of vaccinia antigen studied by immunouranium and immunodiazothioether-osmium tetroxide techniques. Exp. Mol. Pathol. Suppl. 3: 59–74.

Douglas, S. D., A. J. Gottlieb, A. J. L. Strauss, and S. S. Spicer. 1966. Selectivity of ferritin-protein conjugates for sites on skeletal muscle. Exp. Mol. Biol. Suppl. 3: 5–20.

Duc-Nguyen, H., H. M. Rose, and C. Morgan. 1966. An electron microscopic study of changes at the surface of influenza-infected cells as revealed by ferritin-conjugated antibodies. Virology 28: 404–412.

Duc-Nguyen, H., and E. N. Rosenblum. 1967. Immuno-electron microscopy of the morphogenesis of mumps virus. J. Virol. 1: 415–429.

Duda, J. J., and J. M. Slack. 1969. Toxin production in Clostridium botulinum as demonstrated by electron microscopy. J. Bacteriol. 97: 900–904.

Easton, J. M., B. Goldberg, and H. Green. 1962a. Demonstration of surface antigens and pinocytosis in mammalian cells with ferritin-antibody conjugates. J. Cell Biol. 12: 437–443.

Easton, J. M., B. Goldberg, and H. Green. 1962b. Immune cytolysis: electron microscopic localization of cellular antigens with ferritin-antibody conjugates. J. Exp. Med. 115: 275–288.

Eckert, M., M. Gersch, and M. Wagner. 1971. Immunologische Untersuchungen des neuro-endokrinen Systems von Insekten. II. Nachweis von Gewebeantigenen des Gehirns und der Corpora cardiaca von *Periplaneta americana* mit fluorescein- und peroxydasemarkierten Antikörpern. Zool. Jahrbücher Physiol. 76: 29–35.

Eskeland, T. 1967. Hemocyanin as antibody label in electron microscopy. J. Ultrastruct. Res. 20: 305.

Franz, H. 1967a. Ferrocen-markierte Proteine. Naturwissenschaften 54: 339.

Franz, H. 1967b. Ferrocenmarkierte Proteine, Darstellung und Eigenschaften von p-Ferrocenylphenylisothiocyanat(FPITC). Z. Chemie 7: 235–236.

Franz, H. 1968. Grundlagen einer neuen Methode für die elektronenmikroskopische Immunohistochemie. Histochemie 12: 230–239.

Gitzelmann, R., T. Bächi, H. Binz, J. Lindenmann, and G. Semenza. 1970. Localization of rabbit intestinal sucrase with ferritin-antibody conjugates. Biochim. Biophys. Acta 196: 20–28.

Granick, S. 1942. Ferritin I. Physical and chemical properties of horse spleen ferritin. J. Biol. Chem. 146: 451.

Gregory, D. W. and M. A. Williams. 1967. The preparation of ferritin-labeled antibodies and other protein-protein conjugates with bis-diazotized benzidine. Biochim. Biophys. Acta 133: 319–332.

Guillien, P., S. Avrameas, and P. Burtin. 1970. Specificity of antibodies in single cells after immunization with antigens bearing several antigenic determinants: study with a new paired staining technique. Immunology, London 18: 483–491.

Guillien, P., P. Burtin, and S. Avrameas. 1968. Association de l'immunofluorescence et de l'immuno-enzymologie pour la détection d'anticorps intra-cellulaires. C.R. Acad. Sci., Ser. D, 267: 1425–1427.

Haberman, S., P. Blanton, and J. Martin. 1967. Some observations on the AB0 antigen sites of the erythrocyte membranes of adults and newborn infants. J. Immunol. 98: 150–160.

Haferkamp, O., H. Schäfer, W. Wessel, and K. C. Hsu. 1969. Studies of the antigen-antibody reaction by electron microscopy. I. On the transfer of agglutinating antibodies from sensitized sheep erythrocytes to freshly added (unsensitized) red blood cells. Int. Arch. Allergy 36: 298–316.

Hämmerling, U., T. Aoki, E. de Harven, E. A. Boyse, and L. J. Old. 1968. Use of hybrid antibody with anti-γG and anti-ferritin specificities in locating cell surface antigens by electron microscopy. J. Exp. Med. 128, 1461–1473.

Hämmerling, U., T. Aoki, H. A. Wood, L. J. Old, E. A. Boyse, and E. de Harven. 1969. New visual markers of antibody for electron microscopy. Nature, London 223: 1158–1159.

Hampar, B., P. Gerber, K. C. Hsu, L. M. Martos, J. L. Walker, R. F. Siguenza, and G. A. Wells. 1970. Immunoferritin and immunofluorescent studies with Epstein-Barr virus and Herpes simplex virus by use of human sera and hyperimmune rabbit sera. J. Nat. Cancer Inst. 45: 75–85.

Harris, G. 1964. Labelling of red cells with ferritin antibody complexes. Vox Sang. 9: 70–74.

Haust, M. D., J. C. Wyllie, and R. H. More. 1965. Electron microscopy of fibrin in human atherosclerotic lesions. Immunohistochemical and morphologic identification. Exp. Mol. Pathol. 4: 205–216.

Higashi, N., A. Matsumoto, K. Tabata, and Y. Nagamoto. 1967. Electron microscope study of development of Chikungunya virus in green monkey kidney stable (VERO) cells. Virology 33: 55–69.

Hoedemaeker, P. J., and S. Ito. 1970. Ultrastructural localization of gastric parietal cell antigen with peroxidase-coupled antibody. Lab. Invest. 22: 184–188.

Höglund, S. 1967. Electron microscopic investigations of the interaction between the T 2-phage and its IgG- and IgM-antibodies. Virology 32: 662–677.

Howe, C., C. Morgan, C. de Vaux St. Cyr, K. C. Hsu, and H. M. Rose, 1967. Morphogenesis of type 2 parainfluenza virus examined by light and electron microscopy. J. Virol. 1: 215–237.

Howe, C., C. Morgan, and K. C. Hsu. 1969. Recent virologic applications of ferritin conjugates. Progr. Med. Virol. 11: 307–353.

Howe, C., H. Spiele, F. Minio, and K. C. Hsu. 1970. Electron microscopic study of erythrocyte receptors with labeled antisera to membrane components. J. Immunol. 104: 1406–1416.

Hsu, K. C., R. A. Rifkind, and J. B. Zabriskie. 1963. Fluorescent, electron microscopic, and immunoelectrophoretic studies of labeled antibodies. Science 142: 1471–1473.

Isliker, H., B. LeMaire, and C. Morgan. 1964. The use of ferritin-conjugated antibody-fragments in electron-microscopic studies of viruses. Pathol. Microbiol. 27: 521–532.

Kalnins, V. I., H. F. Stich, and D. S. Yohn. 1966. Electron microscopic localization of virus associated antigens in human amnion cells (AV-3) infected with human adenovirus, type 12. Virology 28: 751–754.

Kalnins, V. I., H. F. Stich, C. Gregory and D. S. Yohn. 1967. Localization of tumor antigens in adenovirus-12-induced tumor cells and in adenovirus-12-infected human and hamster cells by ferritin-labeled antibodies. Cancer Res. 27: 1874–1886.

Katz, L. N., I. S. Meshcheryakova, and M. M. Ogievetskaya. 1970a. Electron microscopic study of localization of antigens in *Francisella tularensis* by means of ferritin-labelled antibodies. J. Hyg. Epidemiol. 14: 457–463.

Katz, L. N., I. S. Meshcheryakova, and M. M. Ogievetskaya. 1970b. Electron microscope studies of antigen localization in *F. tularensis* with the aid of ferritin-labelled antibodies. [In Russian.] Zh. Mikrobiol. (2) 51–55.

Kawarai, Y., and P. K. Nakane. 1970. Localization of tissue antigens on the ultrathin sections with peroxidase-labeled antibody method. J. Histochem. Cytochem. 18: 161–166.

Kendall, P. A. 1965. Labelling of thiolated antibody with mercury for electron microscopy. Biochim. Biophys. Acta 97: 174–176.

Knöll, H., and D. Tresselt. 1965. Mikrobenisolierung durch Magnetismus. Naturwissenschaften 52: 84.

Kopp, R., A. Vogt, and G. Maass. 1963. Separation of iron-containing ferritin from horse-spleen into three distinct fractions by starch-gel electrophoresis. Nature, London 198: 892–893.

Kourilsky, F. M., D. Silvestre, J. P. Levy, and A. Senik. 1970. Localisation en microscopie électronique des antigènes HL.A sur les cellules humaines. Ann. Inst. Pasteur 119: 138.

Kulberg, A. J., and N. B. Azadova. 1963. Specific contrasting in the electron microscope by use of mercury-labeled antibodies. [In Russian.] Vopros. Virusol. (1) 100–102.

Kurstak, E., S. Belloncik, and S. Garzon. 1970. Immunoperoxydase ultrastructurale: localisation d'antigènes du virus de la densonucléose (VDN) basée sur les propriétés structurales de la peroxydase. C.R. Acad. Sci., Ser. D, 271: 2426–2429.

Kurstak, E., J.-R. Côte, and S. Belloncik. 1969. Étude de la synthèse et de la localisation des antigènes du virus de la densonucléose (VDN) à l'aide d'anticorps conjugués à l'enzyme peroxydase (nouvelle méthode d'immunoperoxydase). C.R. Acad. Sci., Ser. D, 268: 2309–2312.

Lannigan, R., and S. Zaki. 1968. Location of gamma globulin in the endocardium in rheumatic heart disease by the ferritin-labelled antibody technique. Nature, London 217: 173–174.

Leduc, E. H., S. Avrameas, and M. Bouteille. 1968. Ultrastructural localization of antibody in differentiating plasma cells. J. Exp. Med. 127: 109–118.

Leduc, E. H., C. B. Scott, and S. Avrameas. 1969. Ultrastructural localization of intracellular immune globulins in plasma cells and lymphoblasts by enzyme-labelled antibodies. J. Histochem. Cytochem. 17: 211.

Leduc, E. H., R. Wicker, S. Avrameas, and W. Bernhard. 1969. Ultrastructural localization of SV 40 T antigen with enzyme-labelled antibody. J. Gen. Virol. 4: 609–614.

Lee, S. 1960. Ferritin-labelled antibody as an electron stain for phage protein. Exp. Cell Res. 21: 249–252.

Lee, R. E., and J. D. Feldman. 1964. Visualization of antigenic sites of human erythrocytes with ferritin-antibody conjugates. J. Cell Biol. 23: 396–401.

Levinthal, J. D., J. C. Cerottini, C. Ahmad-Zadeh, and R. Wicker. 1967a. The detection of intracellular adenovirus type 12 antigens by indirect immunoferritin technique. Int. J. Cancer 2: 85–102.

Levinthal, J. D., T. H. Dunnebacke, and R. C. Williams. 1969. Study of poliovirus infection of human and monkey cells by indirect immunoferritin technique. Virology 39: 211–223.

Levinthal, J. D., R. Wicker, and J. C. Cerottini. 1967b. Study of intracellular SV 40 antigens by indirect immunoferritin technique. Virology 31: 555–558.

Lindberg, L. G., and P. Biberfeld. 1967. Rous rat sarcoma studied with ferritin-conjugated antibodies. Acta Pathol. Microbiol. Scand. 69: 481–488.

Logothetopoulos, J., C. C. Yip, and M. E. Coburn. 1970. Proinsulin in B cells of bovine islets demonstrated by fluorescein or peroxidase-labeled specific antibody. Diabetes, New York 19: 539–545.

Marinis, S., A. Vogt, and G. Brandner, 1969. Isolation and characterization of immunoferritin conjugates. I. The molecular ratio. Immunology, London 17: 77–83.

Mason, T. E., R. F. Phifer, S. S. Spicer, R. A. Swallow, and R. B. Dreskin. 1969. An immunoglobulin-enzyme bridge method for localizing tissue antigens. J. Histochem. Cytochem. 17: 563–569.

Masugi, Y. 1969. Immunoelectron miscoscopic studies on local vascular changes after immunological tissue injuries—especially on the mechanism of nephrotoxic nephritis. Acta Pathol. Jap. 19: 265–281.

Matsubayashi, H., W. Stahl, and S. Akao. 1966. Immuno-electron microscopy in experimental toxoplasmosis. Proc. 1st Int. Congr. Parasitol. Rome, September, 1964, 1: 159.

McLean, J. D., and S. J. Singer. 1964. Cross-linked polyampholytes. New water-soluble embedding media for electron microscopy. J. Cell Biol. 20: 518–521.

McLean, J. D., and S. J. Singer. 1970. A general method for the specific staining of intracellular antigens with ferritin-antibody conjugates. Proc. Nat. Acad. Sci. U.S.A. 65: 122–128.

Mekler, L. B., S. M. Klimenko, G. E. Dobrezov, V. K. Naumova, J. P. Gofman, and V. M. Zhdanov. 1964. Cytochemical and immunochemical analysis at the electron microscopy level: obtaining contrasting antibodies by use of iodine. Nature, London 203: 717–719.

Mekler, L. B., N. N. Sokolov, M. I. Parfanovich, E. N. Livina, G. E. Dobrecov, and J. P. Gofman. 1967. Cytochemical and immunochemical analysis at the electron microscopic level: Obtaining of contrasted antibodies by use of iodination. [In Russian.] Vopr. Virusol. (3) 355 –361.

Mergenhagen, S. E., H. A. Bladen, and K. C. Hsu. 1966. Electron microscopic localization of endotoxin lipopolysaccharide in gram-negative organism. Ann. N.Y. Acad. Sci. 133: 279.

Meshcheryakova, I. C., L. N. Katz, I. B. Pavlova, and A. Y. Kulberg. 1967. Electron microscopy study of the localization of antigens in a virulent and an avirulent strain of *Francisella tularensis,* using mercury-labelled antibodies. J. Hyg. Epidemiol. Microbiol. 11: 147–150.

Metzger, J. F., and C. W. Smith. 1962. The application of immune electron microscopy to the demonstration of antigenic sites in biologic systems. Lab. Invest. 11: 902–911.

Micheel, B. 1970. Ferritinmarkierte Antikörper und ihre Awendung in der experimentellen Krebsforschung. Arch. Geschwulstforsch. 36: 171–184.

Micheel, B., and D. Bierwolf. 1969. Demonstration of Graffi virus-induced surface antigens of leukemia cells by indirect immunoferritin-technique. Exp. Cell Res. 54: 268–271.

Molenaar, I., J. J. Sixma, and W. H. Linssen. 1966. Immune ferritin labeling of ultrathin sections. J. Histochem. Cytochem. 14: 766.

Morgan, C., K. C. Hsu, R. A. Rifkind, A. W. Knox, and H. M. Rose. 1961a. The application of ferritin-conjugated antibody to electron microscopic studies of influenza virus in infected cells. I. The cellular surface. J. Exp. Med. 114: 825–832.

Morgan, C., K. C. Hsu, R. A. Rifkind, A. W. Knox, and H. M. Rose. 1961b. The application of ferritin-conjugated antibody to electron microscopic studies of influenza virus in infected cells. II. The interior of the cell. J. Exp. Med. 114: 833–836.

Morgan, C., K. C. Hsu, and H. M. Rose. 1962b. Structure and development of virus as observed in the electron microscope. VII. Incomplete influenza virus. J. Exp. Med. 116: 553–564.

Morgan, C., R. A. Rifkind, K. C. Hsu, M. Holden, B. C. Seegal, and H. M. Rose. 1961c. Electron microscopic localization of intracellular viral antigen by the use of ferritin-conjugated antibody. Virology 14: 292–296.

Morgan, C., R. A. Rifkind, and H. M. Rose. 1962a. The use of ferritin-conjugated antibodies in electron microscopic studies of influenza and vaccinia viruses. Cold Spring Harbor Symp. Quant. Biol. 27: 57–65.

Mott, M. R. 1963. Cytochemical localization of antigens of *Paramecium* by ferritin-conjugated antibody and by counterstaining the resultant absorbed globulin. J. Roy. Microsc. Soc. 81: 159–162.

Mott, M. R. 1965. Electron microscopy studies on the immobilization antigens of *Paramecium aurelia*. J. Gen. Microbiol. 41: 251–261.

Nakane, P. K. 1968. Simultaneous localization of multiple tissue antigens using the peroxidase-labeled antibody method: A study on pituitary glands of the rat. J. Histochem. Cytochem. 16: 557–560.

Nakane, P. K. 1970. Classifications of anterior pituitary cell types with immunoenzyme histochemistry. J. Histochem. Cytochem. 18: 9–20.

Nakane, P. K., G. E. Nichoalds, and D. L. Oxender. 1968. Cellular localization of leucine-binding protein from *Escherichia coli*. Science 161: 182–183.

Nakane, P. K., and G. B. Pierce, 1966. Enzyme-labeled antibodies: Preparation and application for the localization of antigens. J. Histochem. Cytochem. 14: 929–931.

Nakane, P. K., and G. B. Pierce. 1967. Enzyme-labeled antibodies for the light and electron microscopic localization of tissue antigens. J. Cell Biol. 33: 307–318.

Nakane, P. K., J. Sri Ram, and G. B. Pierce. 1966. Enzyme-labeled antibodies for light and electron microscopic localization of antigens. J. Histochem. Cytochem. 14: 789–791.

Néauport-Sautès, C., D. Silvestre, F. Kourilsky, J.-P. Levy, and M. Fauquet. 1970. Utilisation d'anticorps hybrides pour la localisation en microscopie électronique des antigènes d'histocompatibilité HL.A chez l'homme. C. R. Acad. Sci., Ser. D, 271: 2440–2443.

Nickerson, D. S., J. G. White, G. Kronvall, R. C. Williams, and P. G. Quie. 1970. Indirect visualization of *Staphylococcus aureus* protein A. J. Exp. Med. 131: 1031–1047.

Nii, S., C. Morgan, H. M. Rose, and K. C. Hsu. 1968. Electron microscopy of Herpes simplex virus. IV. Studies with ferritin-conjugated antibodies. J. Virol. 2: 1172–1184.

Osechinsky, I. V., L. B. Mekler, R. V. Petrov, and V. M. Mityushin. 1969. The use of iodinated antibodies for the location of antigens on the surface of *Leptospira canicola* by electron microscopy. Immunology, London 16: 427–431.

Oshiro, L. S., and R. W. Emmons. 1968. Electron microscopic observations of Colorado tick fever virus in BHK 21 and KB cells. J. Gen. Virol. 3: 279–280.

Oshiro, L. S., H. M. Rose, C. Morgan, and K. C. Hsu. 1967a. The localization of SV 40-induced neoantigen with ferritin-labeled antibody. Virology 31: 183–186.

Oshiro, L. S., H. M. Rose, C. Morgan, and K. C. Hsu. 1967b. Electron microscopic study of the development of simian virus 40 by use of ferritin-labeled antibodies. J. Virol. 1: 384–399.

Oshiro, L. S., N. J. Schmidt, and E. H. Lennette. 1969. Electron microscopic studies of rubella virus. J. Gen. Virol. 5: 205–210.

Parfanovich, M. I., N. N. Sokolov, L. B. Mekler, L. L. Fadejeva, and V. M. Zhdanov. 1965. Use of iodinized antibody for revealing viral antigens in ultra-thin sections of cells. Nature, London 206: 784–786.

Paucker, K., I. L. Shechmeister, and A. Birch-Andersen. 1970. Studies on the multiplication of vesicular stomatitis virus with fluorescein and ferritin conjugated antibodies. Acta Pathol. Microbiol. Scand. B 78: 317–329.

Paul, W. E., and A. S. Cohen. 1963. Electron microscopic studies on amyloid fibrils with ferritin-conjugated antibody. Amer. J. Pathol. 43: 721–738.

Pepe, F. A. 1961. The use of specific antibody in electron microscopy. I. Preparation of mercury-labeled antibody. J. Biophys. Biochem. Cytol. 11: 515–520.

Pepe, F. A., and H. Finck. 1961. The use of specific antibody in electron microscopy. II. The visualization of mercury-labeled antibody in the electron microscope. J. Biophys. Biochem. Cytol. 11: 521–531.

Pepe, F. A., H. Finck, and H. Holtzer. 1961. The use of specific antibody in electron microscopy. III. Localization of antigens by use of unmodified antibody. J. Biophys. Biochem. Cytol. 11: 533–547.

Pierce, G. B., A. R. Midgley, and J. Sri Ram. 1963. The histogenesis of basement membranes. J. Exp. Med. 117: 339–348.

Pierce, G. B., J. Sri Ram, and A. R. Midgley. 1964. The use of labeled antibodies in ultrastructural studies. Int. Rev. Exp. Pathol. 3: 1–34.

Reczko, E., and K. Bögel. 1963. Elektronenmikroskopische Untersuchungen über das Verhalten eines vom Kalb isolierten Parainfluenza-3-Virus in Kälbernierenzellkulturen. Arch. ges. Virusforsch. 12: 404–420.

Rifkind, R. A., K. C. Hsu, C. Morgan, B. C. Seegal, A. W. Knox, and H. M. Rose. 1960. Use of ferritin-conjugated antibody to localize antigen by electron microscopy. Nature, London 187: 1094–1095.

Rifkind, R. A., K. C. Hsu, and C. Morgan. 1964. Immunochemical staining for electron microscopy. J. Histochem. Cytochem. 12: 131–136.

Rifkind, R. A., E. F. Ossermann, K. C. Hsu, and C. Morgan. 1962. The intracellular distribution of gamma globulin in a mouse plasma cell tumor (X 5563) as revealed by fluorescence and electron microscopy. J. Exp. Med. 116: 423–432.

Ritchie, A. E., and A. L. Fernelius. 1968. Direct immuno-electron microscopy and some morphological features of hog cholera virus. Arch. ges. Virusforsch. 23: 292–298.

Samosudova, N. V., M. M. Ogievetskaya. M. B. Kalamkarova, and G. M. Frank. 1968. Use of ferritin antibodies for the electron microscopic study of myosin. III. Localization of ferritin antimyosin in the sarcomer. [In Russian.] Biofizika 13: 877.

Schäfer, H. 1970. Immunelektronenmikroskopie. Beiträge zur Methodik und Bewertung. (Veröffentlichungen aus der morphologischen Pathologie, Heft 85) Gustav Fischer Verlag, Stuttgart.

Schäfer, H., O. Haferkamp, and K. C. Hsu. 1968. Elektronenmikroskopische Untersuchungen von Antigen-Antikörper-Reaktionen. II. Über das unterschiedliche Verhalten frischer und formalinfixierter Erythrozyten unter der Einwirkung agglutinierender ferritin-markierter Antikörper. Z. Immun. Forsch. 136: 237–248.

Schiff, R., R. J. Krieg, and R. L. Hunter. 1970. Localization by peroxidase-labeled antibodies of bovine chymotrypsinogen. J. Histochem. Cytochem. 18: 195 –200.

Scott, G., S. Avrameas, and W. Bernhard. 1968. Étude au microscope électronique de la formation d'anticorps à l'aide de la phosphatase alcaline utilisée comme antigène. C.R. Acad. Sci. Ser. D, 266: 746–748.

Seegal, B. C., G. A. Andres, K. C. Hsu, and J. B. Zabriskie. 1965. Studies on the pathogenesis of acute and progressive glomerulonephritis in man by immunofluorescein and immunoferritin techniques. Fed. Proc. 24: 100.

Shalla, T. A., and A. Amici. 1967. The distribution of viral antigen in cells infected with tobacco mosaic virus as revealed by electron microscopy. Virology 31: 78–91.

Shands, J. W. 1965. Localization of somatic antigen on Gram-negative bacteria by electron microscopy. J. Bacteriol. 90: 266–270.

Singer, S. J. 1959. Preparation of an electron-dense antibody conjugate. Nature, London 183: 1523–1524.

Singer, S. J. 1964. Preparation of ferritin-antibody conjugates. Meth. Med. Res. 10: 149–151.

Singer, S. J., and J. D. McLean. 1963. Ferritin-antibody conjugates as stains for electron microscopy. Lab. Invest. 12: 1002–1008.

Singer, S. J., and A. F. Schick. 1961. The properties of specific stains for electron microscopy prepared by the conjugation of antibody molecules with ferritin. J. Biophys. Biochem. Cyt. 9: 519–537.

Siverd, N. J., and N. Sharon. 1969. Immunohistochemical method for detection of vaccinia virus. Proc. Soc. Exp. Biol. N.Y. 131: 939–941.

Smith, C. W., and J. F. Metzger. 1961. Studies of ferritin conjugates used in immune electron microscopy. Biochim. Biophys. Acta 47: 587–588.

Smith, C. W., and J. F. Metzger. 1962. Demonstration of a capsular structure on *Listeria monocytogenes*. Pathol. Microbiol. 25: 499–506.

Smith, C. W., J. F. Metzger, S. I. Zacks, and A. Kase. 1960. Immune electron microscopy. Proc. Soc. Exp. Biol. N.Y. 104: 336–338.

Sordat, B., M. Sordat, M. W. Hess, R. D. Stoner, and H. Cottier. 1970. Specific antibody within lymphoid germinal center cells of mice after primary immunization with horseradish peroxidase: a light and electron microscopic study. J. Exp. Med. 131: 77–92.

Spendlove, R. S., and S. J. Singer. 1961. On the preservation of antigenic determinants during fixation and embedding for electron microscopy. Proc. Nat. Acad. Sci. U.S.A. 47: 14–18.

Sri Ram, J., P. K. Nakane, E. G. Rawlinson, and G. B. Pierce. 1966. Enzyme-labeled antibodies for ultrastructural studies. Fed. Proc. 25: 732.

Sri Ram, J., S. S. Tawde, G. B. Pierce, and A. R. Midgley. 1963. Preparation of antibody-ferritin conjugates for immuno-electron microscopy. J. Cell Biol. 17: 673–675.

Stanislawski, M. 1970. L'emploi de la peroxydase comme marquer dans la quantification immunochimique d'antigènes et d'anticorps. C.R. Acad. Sci. Ser. D, 271: 1452–1455.

Sternberger, L. A. 1967. Electron microscopic immunochemistry: A review. J. Histochem. Cytochem. 15: 139–159.

Sternberger, L. A. 1969. Some new developments in immunocytochemistry. Mikroskopie 25: 346–361.

Sternberger, L. A., and J. J. Cuculis. 1969. Method for enzymatic intensification of the immunocytochemical reaction without use of labeled antibodies. J. Histochem. Cytochem. 17: 190.

Sternberger, L. A., E. J. Donati, and C. E. Wilson. 1963. Electron microscopic study on specific protection of isolated *Bordetella bronchiseptica* antibody during exhaustive labelling with uranium. J. Histochem. Cytochem. 11: 48–58.

Sternberger, L. A., E. J. Donati, J. J. Cuculis, and J. P. Petrali. 1965. Indirect immunouranium technique for staining of embedded antigen in electron microscopy. Exp. Mol. Pathol. 4: 112–125.

Sternberger, L. A., E. A. Donati, J. S. Hanker, and A. M. Seligman. 1966a. Immuno-diazothioether-osmium tetroxide (immuno-DTO) technique for staining embedded antigen in electron microscopy. Exp. Mol. Pathol., Suppl. 3: 36–43.

Sternberger, L. A., J. S. Hanker, E. J. Donati, J. P. Petrali, and A. M. Seligman. 1966b. Method for enhancement of electron microscopic visualization of embedded antigen by bridging osmium to uranium antibody with thiocarbohydrazide. J. Histochem. Cytochem. 14: 711–718.

Sternberger, L. A., P. H. Hardy, J. J. Cuculis, and H. G. Meyer. 1970. The unlabeled antibody enzyme method of immunohistochemistry. Preparation and properties of soluble antigen-antibody complex (horseradish peroxidase – antihorseradish peroxidase) and its use in identification of spirochetes. J. Histochem. Cytochem. 18: 315–333.

Stich, H. F., V. I. Kalnins, E. MacKinnon, and D. S. Yohn. 1967. Electron microscopic localization of adenovirus type 12 antigens. J. Ultrastruct. Res. 19: 556–562.

Straus, W. 1968. Cytochemical detection of sites of antibody to horseradish peroxidase in spleen and lymph nodes. J. Histochem. Cytochem. 16: 237–248.

Straus, W. 1970a. Location of antibody to horseradish peroxidase in popliteal lymph nodes of rabbits during the primary and early secondary response. J. Histochem. Cytochem. 18: 120–130.

Straus, W. 1970b. Localization of the antigen in popliteal lymph nodes of rabbits during the formation of antibodies to horseradish peroxidase. J. Histochem. Cytochem. 18: 131–142.

Striker, G. E., E. J. Donati, J. P. Petrali, and L. A. Sternberger. 1966. Post-embedding staining for electron microscopy with ferritin-antibody conjugates. Exp. Mol. Pathol., Suppl. 3: 52–58.

Suzuki, I., and M. Takahashi. 1969. Ultrastructure of human myeloma cells studied by peroxidase conjugated antibodies directed to human immunoglobulin component chains. Experientia 25: 1307–1309.

Suzuki, I., M. Takahashi, and H. Kamel. 1969. Ultrastructural localization of heavy- and light-polypeptide chains in human long-term culture cells detected by peroxidase-conjugated antibodies. Experientia 25: 1309–1311.

Suzuki, T. 1970. Blood grouping of blood-stains by immuno-electron microscopy. Tohoku J. Exp. Med. 101: 1–7.

Swanson, J., K. C. Hsu, and E. C. Gotschlich. 1969. Electron microscopic studies on streptococci. I. M antigen. J. Exp. Med. 130: 1063–1091.

Swope, A. E., R. H. Kahn, and J. L. Conklin. 1970. A comparison of alcian blue-aldehyde fuchsin and peroxidase-labeled antibody staining techniques in the rat adenohypophysis. J. Histochem. Cytochem. 18: 450–454.

Tajima, M., T. Ushijima, S. Kishi, and J. Nakamura. 1967. Electron microscopy of cytoplasmic inclusion bodies in cells infected with Rinderpest virus. Virology 31: 92–100.

Tanaka, H., and D. H. Moore. 1967. Electron microscopic localization of viral antigens in mouse mammary tumors by ferritin-labelled antibody. I. Homologous systems. Virology 33: 197–214.

Tawde, S. S., and J. Sri Ram. 1962. Conjugation of antibody to ferritin by means of p,p'-difluoro-m,m'-dinitrodiphenylsulphone. Arch. Biochem. 97: 429–430.

Thomson, R. O., P. D. Walker, and R. D. Hardy. 1966. Location of spore and vegetative antigens of *Bacillus cereus* by means of ferritin-labelled antibodies. Nature, London 210: 760–761.

Tonietti, G., G. A. Andres, L. Accinni, M. Purpura, and K. C. Hsu. 1969. Immuno-electronmicroscopic studies of surface antigens of blood elements. I. Autoantibody on erythrocytes in acute hemolytic anemia. Blood 33: 179–185.

Vickerman, K., and A. G. Luckins. 1969. Localization of variable antigens in the surface coat of *Trypanosoma brucei* using ferritin-conjugated antibody. Nature, London 224: 1125–1126.

Vogt, A., H. Bockhorn, K. Kozima, and M. Sasaki. 1968. Electron microscopic localization of the nephrotoxic antibody in the glomeruli of the rat after intravenous application of purified nephritogenic antibody-ferritin conjugates. J. Exp. Med. 127: 867–878.

Vogt, A., R. Caesar, and J. Müller. 1966. In vivo localization of ferritin-labeled anti-kidney antibodies in rats. J. Histochem. Cytochem. 14: 767.

Vogt, A., and R. Kopp. 1964. Loss of specific agglutinating activity of purified ferritin-conjugated antibodies. Nature, London 202: 1350–1351.

Vogt, A., and R. Kopp. 1965. Über die spezifische Aktivität ferritin-markierter Antikörper. Zbl. Bakt. I. Orig. 198: 270–274.

Vogt, A., R. Kopp, K. Nakanoin, and K. Kozima. 1967. Ferritinmarkierte Antikörper. Acta histochem., Suppl. 7: 237–247.

Wagner, M. 1967a. Reinigung ferritin-markierter Antikörper durch Gelfiltration an Agarose. Naturwissenschaften 54: 444.

Wagner, M. 1967b. Fluoreszierende Antikörper und ihre Anwendung in der Mikrobiologie. VEB Gustav Fischer Verlag, Jena.

Wagner, M., and A. Veckenstedt. 1970. Elektronenmikroskopischer Nachweis des Mengovirus in L-Zellen mit ferritinmarkierten Antikörpern. Arch ges. Virusforsch. 32: 147–156.

Wagner, M., and B. Wagner. 1972. Glutaraldehyd als Kupplungsagens für die Herstellung ferritin-markierter Antikörper. Zbl. Bakt. Hyg., I. Abt. Orig. A, 221: 100–105.

Wagner, B., and M. Wagner, 1973. Immunelektronenmikroskopischer Nachweis von Zellwandantigenen bei Streptokokken. I. Vergleichende Darstellung des M-Proteins von *Streptococcus pyogenes* mit ferritin-, peroxydase- und ferrocenmarkierten Antikörpern. Zbl. Bakt. Hyg., I. Abt. Orig. A (in press).

Wagner, M., and M. Wunderwald. 1964. Unpublished results.

Walker, P. D., A. Baillie, R. O. Thomson, and I. Batty. 1966. The use of ferritin labelled antibodies in the location of spore and vegetative antigens of *Bacillus cereus*. J. Appl. Bacteriol. 29: 512–518.

Walker, P. D., R. O. Thomson, and A. Baillie. 1967a. Fine structure of Clostridia with special reference to the location of antigens and enzymes. J. Appl. Bacteriol. 30: 444–449.

Walker, P. D., R. O. Thomson, and A. Baillie. 1967b. Use of ferritin labelled antibodies in the location of spore and vegetative antigens of *Bacillus subtilis*. J. Appl. Bact. 30: 317–320.

Wicker, R., and S. Avrameas. 1969. Localization of virus antigens by enzyme-labelled antibodies. J. Gen. Virol. 4: 465–471.

Wicker, R., and S. Avrameas. 1970. Application de l'autoradiographie associée aux technique immuno-enzymatiques à l'étude des antigènes et des anticorps. C.R. Acad. Sci., Ser. D, 270: 431–433.

Wilson, C. E., E. J. Donati, J. P. Petrali, J. V. Vuicich, and L. A. Sternberger. 1966. Cytochemical timing of ultrastructural events: formation of bacterial flagella studied by immunouranium technique. Exp. Mol. Pathol., Suppl. 3: 44–51.

Wyllie, J. C. 1964. Identification of fibrin with ferritin-conjugated antifibrinogen. Exp. Mol. Pathol. 3: 468–474.

Zacks, S. I., J. Metzger, C. W. Smith, and J. M. Blumberg. 1962. Localization of ferritin-labelled botulinus toxin in the neuromuscular junction of the mouse. J. Neuropathol. Exp. Neurol. 21: 610–633.

Zacks, S. I., and M. F. Sheff. 1967. Tetanus toxin: Fine structure localization of binding sites in striated muscle. Science 158: 643–644.

Zeromski, J. 1970. Immunological findings in sensory carcinomatous neuropathy. Application of peroxidase labelled antibody. Clin. Experim. Immunol. 6: 633–637.

Zhdanov, V. M., N. B. Azadova, and A. J. Kulberg. 1962. Labelling of antibodies with an organic mercury compound. [In Russian.] Vopr. Virusol. (4) 110–111.

Zhdanov, V. M., N. B. Azadova, and A. J. Kulberg. 1965. Transport of S-antigen of Sendai virus as revealed by means of antibody labelled with an organic mercury compound. Nature, London 207: 554–555.

Supplementary References

Since the completion of this review the following publications have appeared.

An, T., K. Miyai, and S. Sell. 1972. Electron microscopic localization of rabbit immunoglobulin allotype b 4 on blood lymphocytes by an indirect ferritin immune complex labeling technique. J. Immunol. 108: 1271.

Aoki, T., and T. Takahashi. 1972. Viral and cellular surface antigens of murine leukemias and myelomas. Serological analysis by immunolectron microscopy. J. Exp. Med. 135: 443.

Atanasiu, P., P. Dragonas, H. Tsiang, and A. Harbi. 1971. Immunopéroxydase. Nouvelle technique spécifique de mise en évidence de l'antigène rabique intra- et extra-cellulaire en microscopie optique. Ann. Inst. Pasteur 121: 247.

Avrameas, S., B. Taudou, T. Ternynck. 1971. Specificity of antibodies synthesized by immunocytes as detected by immunoenzyme techniques. Int. Arch. Allergy 40: 161.

Avrameas, S., and T. Ternynck. 1971. Peroxidase labelled antibody and Fab conjugates with enhanced intracellular penetration. Immunochemistry 8: 1175.

Billard, R., B. Breton, and M. P. Dubois. 1971. Immunocytologie et histochimie des cellules gonadotropes et thyréotropes hypophysaires chez la carpe *Cyprinus carpio*. C.R. Acad. Sci., Ser. D, 272: 981.

Booyse, F. M., L. A. Sternberger, D. Zschocke, and M. E. Rafelson. 1971. Ultrastructural localization of contractile protein (thrombosthenin) in human platelets using an unlabeled antibody-peroxidase staining technique. J. Histochem. Cytochem. 19: 540.

Breese, S. S., and W. H. McCollum. 1971. Equine arteritis virus: Ferritin tagging and determination of ribonucleic acid core. Arch. ges. Virusforsch. 35: 290.

Bretton, R., T. Ternynck, and S. Avrameas. 1972. Comparison of peroxidase and ferritin labeling of cell surface antigens. Exp. Cell Res. 71: 145.

Burns, J., and A. G. MacIver. 1971. Immuno-electron microscopy of the glomerular basement membrane in Goodpasture's syndrome. Europ. J. Clin. Biol. 16: 48.

Coulter, J. R., and T. M. Mukherjee. 1971. Electron microscopic localization of alpha toxin within the staphylococcal cell by ferritin-labeled antibody. Infect. Immunity 4: 650.

Coward, J. E., D. H. Harter, K. C. Hsu, and C. Morgan. 1971. Electron microscopic study of development of vesicular stomatitis virus using ferritin-labelled antibodies. J. Gen. Virol. 13: 27.

Cox, J. C., E. Pihl, R. S. D. Read, and R. C. Nairn. 1972. Rapid localization of bacterial surface antigens by whole-mount immunoperoxidase technique. J. Gen. Microbiol. 70: 385.

Davis, W. C. 1972. H-2 antigen on cell membranes: An explanation for the alteration of distribution by indirect labeling techniques. Science 175: 1006.

Davis, W. C., M. A. Alspaugh, J. H. Stimpfling, and R. L. Walford. 1971. Cellular surface distribution of transplantation antigens: discrepancy between direct and indirect labelling technique. Tissue Antigens 1: 89.

DeGrandi, P. B., J. P. Kraehenbuhl, and M. A. Campiche. 1971. Ultrastructural localization of calcitonin in the parafollicular cells of pig thyroid gland with cytochrome c-labeled antibody fragments. J. Cell Biol. 50: 446.

Dimmock, E., D. Franks, and A. M. Glauert. 1972. The location of blood group antigen A on cultured rabbit kidney cells as revealed by ferritin labelled antibody. J. Cell Sci. 10: 525.

Eng, J., and L. O. Frøholm. 1971. Immune electron microscopy of not cell-bound antigen of Mycoplasma pneumoniae. Acta Path. Microbiol. Scand. 79 b: 759.

Faulk, W. P., and G. M. Taylor. 1971. An immunocolloid method for the electron microscope. Immunochemistry 8: 1081.

Francois, D., R. Oriol, and R. A. Binaghi. 1972. Immunoperoxidase localization of antihapten antibodies in rats responding unequally to antigenic stimulation. J. Histochem. Cytochem. 20: 527.

Francois, D., V. Van Tuyen, H. Febvre, and F. Haguenau. 1972. Étude au microscope électronique de la fixation de lectines marquées à la peroxydase de raifort sur des cellules embryonnaires humaines transformées in vitro par le virus du sarcome de Rous(RSV), souche Bryan. C.R. Acad. Sci., Ser. D, 274: 1981.

Franz, H., and W. Wildführ. 1971. Chemische und immunologische Aspekte der Ferrocenmarkierung von Antikörpern. Z. Immun.-Forsch. 142: 334.

Fresen, K. O., and A. Vogt. 1971. Die hämolytische Aktivität von ferritinmarkierten Antikörpern gegen Schafserythrocyten (Ambozeptor). Med. Microbiol. Immunol. 157: 24.

Gelderblom, H., H. Bauer, and T. Graf. 1972. Cell-surface antigens induced by avian RNA tumor viruses: Detection by immunoferritin technique. Virology 47: 416.

Gonatas, N. K., J. C. Antoine, A. Stieber, and S. Avrameas. 1972. Surface immunoglobulins of thymus and lymph node cells demonstrated by the peroxidase coupling technique. Lab. Invest. 26: 253.

Hamanaka, N., O. Tanizawa, T. Hashimoto, S. Yoshinari, and Y. Okudaira. 1971. Electron microscopic study on the localization of human chorionic gonadotropin (HCG) in the chorionic tissue by enzyme-labeled antibody technique. J. Electr. Microsc. 20: 128.

Horisberger, M., H. Bauer, and K. A. Bush. 1971. Mercury-labelled concanavalin A as a marker in electron microscopy-localization of mannan in yeast cell walls. FEBS Letters 18: 311.

Hoshino, M., and K. Maeno. 1971. The usefullness of enzyme-labeled antibody method for ultrastructural localization of Newcastle disease virus antigens in infected HeLa cells. J. Electr. Microsc. 20: 49.

Hoshino, M., K. Maeno, and M. Inuma. 1972. Ultrastructural localization of Newcastle disease virus surface antigen in infected HeLa cells as revealed by an enzyme-labelled antibody method. Experientia 28: 611.

Huang, S. N., I. Millman, A. O'Connell, A. Aronoff, H. Gault, and B. S. Blumberg. 1972. Virus-like particles in Australia antigen-associated hepatitis: An immunoelectron microscopic study of human liver. Am. J. Pathol. 67: 453.

Ikonikoff, L. K. de, C. Hubert, and L. Cedard. 1972. Études histochimique du plazenta humain. Localisation de l'hormone gonadotrope chorionique par la technique immunohistoenzymologique à la peroxydase. C. R. Acad. Sci., Ser. D, 274: 3431.

Kapikian, A. Z., J. D. Almeida, and E. J. Stott. 1972. Immune electron microscopy of rhinoviruses. J. Virology 10: 142.

Kelen, A. S., A. E. Hathaway, and D. A. McLeod. 1971. Rapid detection of Australia/SH antigen and antibody by a simple and sensitive technique of immunoelectronmicroscopy. Canad. J. Microbiol. 17: 993.

Kelley, V. E., and R. S. Cotran. 1972. Mesangial and subepithelial localization of ferritin immune complexes in mouse glomerulus. Lab. Invest. 27: 144.

Kendall, P. A. 1972. Antibody labelling for electron microscopy: Immunochemical properties of immunoglobulin G heavily labelled with methylmercury after thiolation by homocystein thiolactone. Biochim. Biophys. Acta 257: 101.

Killby, V. A. A., and P. H. Silverman. 1971. Preliminary studies on the use of ferritin-conjugated antibodies to *Plasmodium berghei*. J. Protozool. 18: 73.

Kind, J., and J. Krieg. 1972. Glutaraldehyd als Kopplungsreagenz von Ferritin an Antikörper. Ein Beitrag zur Herstellung und Reinigung Ferritin-markierter Antikörper. Cytobiologie 6: 22.

Knüsel, A. 1971. Hybridization of guinea pig anti-ferritin and anti-rabbit intestinal sucrase. Path. Microbiol. 37: 337.

Knüsel, A., T. Bächi, R. Gitzelmann, and J. Lindenmann. 1971. Electron microscopic recognition of surface antigen by direct reaction and ferritin capture with guinea pig hybrid antibody. J. Immunol. 106: 583.

Kourilsky, F. M., D. Silvestre, J. P. Levy, J. Dausset, M. G. Nicolai, and A. Senik. 1971. Immunoferritin study of the distribution of HL.A antigens on human blood cells. J. Immunol. 106: 454.

Kraehenbuhl, J. P., P. B. DeGrandi, and M. A. Campiche. 1971. Ultrastructural localization of intracellular antigen using enzyme-labelled antibody fragments. J. Cell Biol. 50: 432.

Kraehenbuhl, J. P., and J. D. Jamieson. 1972. Solid-phase conjugation of ferritin to Fab-fragments of immunoglobulin G for use in antigen localization on thin sections. Proc. Nat. Acad. Sci. USA 69: 1771.

Kuhlmann, W. D., and S. Avrameas. 1971. Glucose oxidase as an antigen marker for light and electron microscopic studies. J. Histochem. Cytochem. 19: 361.

Kuhlmann, W. D., and S. Avrameas. 1971. Reliability of glucose oxidase staining at the ultrastructural level for immunohistochemical studies. J. Histochem. Cytochem. 19: 810.

Kurstak, E. 1971. The immunoperoxidase technique: Localization of viral antigens in cells. Methods in Virology 5: 423.

Kurstak, E., S. Belloncik, P. A. Onji, S. Montplaisir, and B. Martineau. 1972. Localisation par l'immunoperoxydase des antigènes du virus cytomégalique en culture cellulaire de fibroblastes humains: Microscopie photonique et électronique. Arch. ges. Virusforsch. 38: 67.

Kurstak, E., M. Lanzon, C. Kurstak, and R. Morrisset. 1972. Nouvelle possibilité de diagnostic rapide par l'immunoperoxydase photonique de l'infection de cellules humaines par le virus Herpes simplex hominis. C.R. Acad. Sci., Ser. D, 274: 3145.

Machida, M., and M. Hoshino. 1971. The ultrastructural localization of antigens in Ehrlich ascites tumor cells against antinuclear factors in lupus erythematosus sera by peroxidase-labelled antibody method. Experientia 27: 201.

Matsakura, Y. 1972. Demonstration of ferritine-labelled antibodies bound to human erythrocytes fixed with glutaraldehyde. Vox sanguinis 22: 549.

McLean, J. D., and S. J. Singer. 1971. A technique for the specific staining of macromolecules and viruses with ferritin-antibody conjugates. J. Mol. Biol. 56: 633.

Micheel, B. 1972. Die Verwendung von Glutaraldehyd als Kopplungsreagens für die Präparation ferritinmarkierter Antikörper. Acta biol. med. germ. 28: 391.

Micheel, B., D. Bierwolf, A. Randt, H. Franz, J. Mohr, and G. Pasternak. 1971. Nachweis GRAFFI-Virus-induzierter und Spezies-specifischer Oberflächenantigene in Ratten-GRAFFI-Leukämiezellen mit immunoelektronenmikroskopischen Techniken. Acta biol. med. germ. 27: 639.

Miyamoto, K., C. Morgan, K. C. Hsu, and B. Hampar. 1971. Differentiation by immunoferritin of Herpes simplex virion antigen with the use of rabbit 7S and 19S antibodies from early (7-day) and late (7-week) immune sera. J. Nat. Cancer Inst. 46: 629.

Morgan, C. 1972. The use of ferritin-conjugated antibodies in electron-microscopy. Intern. Rev. Cytol. 32: 291.

Moriarty, G. C., and N. S. Halmi. 1972. Electron microscopic study of the adrenocorticotropin-producing cell with the use of unlabeled antibody and the soluble peroxidase-antiperoxidase-complex. J. Histochem. Cytochem. 20: 590.

Neauport-Sautes, C., and D. Silvestre. 1972. Ferritin-antibody coupling with glutaraldehyde. Transplant. 13: 536.

Neauport-Sautes, C., D. Silvestre, M. G. Niccolai, F. M. Kourilsky, and J. P. Levy. 1972. Ultrastructural localization of human HL-A membrane antigens by use of hybrid antibodies. Immunology 22: 833.

Nicolson, G. L. 1971. Different distribution of ferritin-conjugated concanavalin A on surfaces of normal and tumor cell membranes. Nature (New Biology) 233: 244.

Nicolson, G. L., R. Hyman, and S. J. Singer. 1971. The two-dimensional topographic distribution of H-2 histocompatibility alloantigens on mouse red blood cell membranes. J. Cell Biol. 50: 905.

Nicolson, G. L., V. T. Marchesi, and S. J. Singer. 1971. The localization of spectrin on the inner surface of human red blood cell membranes by ferritin-conjugated antibodies. J. Cell Biol. 51: 265.

Nicolson, G. L., and S. J. Singer. 1971. Ferritin-conjugated plant agglutinins as specific saccharide stains for electron microscopy: Application to saccharides bound to cell membranes. Proc. Nat. Acad. Sci. USA, 68: 942.

Nöthiger, R., D. S. McDevitt, and T. Yamada. 1971. Detection of γ-crystallins in the developing amphibian lens by peroxidase-labelled antibodies. Experientia 27: 423.

Rigby, C., and C. M. Johnson. 1972. Immuno-electron microscopy of Herpes simplex virus. Canad. J. Microbiol. 18: 1337.

Shabo, A. L., J. C. Petricciani, and R. L. Kirschstein. 1972. Immunoperoxidase localization of Herpes zoster virus and simian virus 40 in cell culture. Appl. Microbiol. 23: 1001.

Shahrabadi, M. S., and T. Yamamoto. 1971. A method for staining intracellular antigens in thin sections with ferritin-labeled antibody. J. Cell Biol. 50: 246.

Shahrabadi, M. S., and T. Yamamoto. 1972. Localization of canine adenovirus capsid antigens in a MDCK cell line by immunoferritin and immunofluorescence techniques. Canad. J. Microbiol. 18: 1299.

Shigematsu, T., L. Dmochowski, and W. C. Williams. 1971. Studies on mouse mammary tumor virus (MTV) and mouse leukemia virus (MuLV) by immunoelectron microscopy. Cancer Res. 31: 2085.

Shigematsu, T., E. S. Priori, L. Dmochowski, and J. R. Wilbur. 1971. Immunoelectron microscopic studies of type C virus particles in ESP-1 and HEK-1-HRLV cell lines. Nature, London 234: 412.

Shirasawa, K., B. P. Barton, and A. B. Chandler. 1972. Localization of ferritin-conjugated anti-fibrin/fibrinogen in platelet aggregates produced in vitro. Am. J. Pathol. 66: 379.

Siess, E., O. Wieland, and F. Miller. 1971. A simple method for the preparation of pure and active gamma-globulin-ferritin conjugates using glutaraldehyde. Immunology 20: 659.

Silvestre, D., F. M. Kourilsky, J. P. Levy, and A. Senik. 1969. Localisation des antigènes HL-A à la surface des lymphocytes humains à l'aide d'anticorps conjugués à la ferritine. C.R. Acad. Sci., Ser. D, 268: 1145.

Sinden, R. E. 1971. The synthesis of the immobilization antigens in Paramecium aurelia: in situ localization of immobilization antigen using fluorescein- or ferritin-conjugated antibodies. J. Microscopy 93: 129.

Straus, W. 1971. Inhibition of peroxidase by methanol and by methanol-nitroferricyanide for use in immunoperoxidase procedures. J. Histochem. Cytochem. 19: 682.

Straus, W. 1972. Improved staining for peroxidase with benzidine and improved double staining immunoperoxidase procedures. J. Histochem. Cytochem. 20: 272.

Strobel, P. L., and S. J. Kraus. 1972. An electron microscopic study of the FTA-ABS "beading" phenomenon with lupus erythematosus sera, using ferritin-conjugated anti-human IgG. J. Immunol. 108: 1152.

Sugawara, K., and T. Osato. 1970. An immunoferritin study of a Burkitt lymphoma cell line harboring EB virus particles. Gann 61: 279.

Ubertini, T., B. N. Wilkie, and F. Noronha. 1971. Use of horseradish peroxidase-labelled antibody for light and electron microscope localization of a reovirus antigen. Appl. Microbiol. 21: 534.

Wagner, R. R., J. W. Heine, G. Goldstein, and C. A. Schnaitman. 1971. Use of antiviral-antiferritin-hybrid antibody for localization of viral antigen in plasma membrane. J. Virol. 7: 274.

Ward, H. A., S. Yamana, E. Pihl, and R. C. Nairn. 1972. Ultrastructural localization of antilymphocyte globulin on viable lymphocytes by immunoperoxidase tracing. Immunology 23: 61.

Wildführ, W., and H. Franz. 1971. Immunelektronenmikroskopische Untersuchungen mit 3-Carboxy-4-ferrocenylisothiocyanat-markierten Antikörpern an Toxoplasma gondii. Zbl. Bakt. I Orig. 216: 532.

Author's address: Dr. rer. nat. habil. Manfred Wagner, Zentralinstitut für Mikrobiologie und experimentelle Therapie, DDR-69 Jena, Beuthenbergstrasse 11 (German Democratic Republic).

Immunochemistry of Fusobacteria

TORE KRISTOFFERSEN AND TOR HOFSTAD

University of Bergen, School of Dentistry, Bergen, Norway

Contents

I.	Introduction. The Genus *Fusobacterium*.	253
II.	Early Immunological Studies	255
III.	Cell Wall Composition and Structure	256
	A. Preparation	256
	B. Composition	256
	1. Quantitative Data	256
	2. Amino Acids	257
	3. Sugar Components	259
	C. Ultrastructure	259
IV.	Cell Wall Antigens	260
	A. Antigens Extracted from Crushed Cells	260
	B. Immunochemistry of Lipopolysaccharide from Fusobacteria	261
	1. Preparation	261
	2. Chemical Composition	262
	3. Ultrastructure	263
	4. Immunological Properties	265
	C. The Group Reactive "Precipitinogen 2"	270
	1. Preparation	270
	2. Chemical Composition	271
	3. Biological Activities	271
V.	Other, Less Thoroughly Characterized, Antigens	277
VI.	Summary and Comment	278
	Literature Cited	280

I. Introduction. The Genus Fusobacterium

While the immunochemistry of gram-negative aerobic bacteria has been of great interest to immunochemists for many years, the study of gram-negative anaerobes has attracted much less attention. There may be several reasons for this. The pathogenic potential of many of these organisms and their possible role in disease have been largely unknown or uncertain. Their nomenclature and taxonomy, particularly with regard to gram-negative anaerobic bacilli, have been confusing, and the organisms are frequently somewhat difficult to cultivate and cumbersome to work with. All of these problems are encountered in the study of bacteria of the genus *Fusobacterium*.

The genus *Fusobacterium* was proposed by Knorr (1922) for anaerobic, nonsporulating, gram-negative bacilli having pointed ends, and found in the oral cavity of man. In the past these organisms have attracted interest as ever-present members of the mixed anaerobic flora of Plaut-Vincent's angina, or fusospirochetal disease. More recently, *Fusobacterium* has received attention among oral microbiologists as a prominent member of the anaerobic part of the bacterial flora of dental plaque and gingival debris (Socransky et al., 1963; Gibbons et al., 1963). In particular, the renewed interest in the immunochemistry and serology of these and other gram-negative anaerobes found in dental plaque can be ascribed to their intimate and possibly causative association with periodontitis, the chronic inflammatory disease of the supporting structures of the teeth, which is a predominant cause of tooth loss after the age of forty (Schultz-Haudt, Bruce, and Bibby, 1954; Löe, Theilade, and Jensen, 1965; Theilade et al., 1966).

Fusobacterium is also part of the indigenous microflora of the intestine and the upper respiratory tract of man and presumably of animals (Rosebury, 1962). It has been isolated under pathological conditions from these and contiguous areas, including the blood, and from abscesses elsewhere in the human body (Böe, 1941; Lahelle, 1945).

There is some confusion in the taxonomy and nomenclature of *Fusobacterium,* mainly because other spindle-shaped bacteria have often been designated as fusobacteria (Rosebury, 1962). In the seventh edition of *Bergey's Manual of Determinative Bacteriology* (Breed et al., 1957), *Fusobacterium* is included in the family Bacteroidaceae and separated from the other genera of this family, *Bacteroides, Sphaerophorus,* and *Dialister,* on the basis of morphological characteristics. Fusobacteria are described as "straight or curved rods, usually with tapering ends, occurring singly, in pairs and sometimes in chains; filaments are common."

The biochemical properties of fusobacteria were extensively

studied by Böe (1941) and have been investigated by Jackins and Barker (1951), Berger (1956, 1957), Omata and Braunberg (1960), Baird-Parker (1960), Beerens and Tahon-Castel (1965), and others. According to these investigators, *Fusobacterium* is nutritionally exacting and weakly saccharolytic, produces indole and hydrogen sulfide, and gives a fetid odor. *Leptotrichia buccalis,* which has frequently been mistaken for *Fusobacterium,* is a strong sugar fermenter, and produces neither indole nor hydrogen sulfide. The main characteristic used to differentiate fusobacteria from *Bacteroides* is the production of butyric acid by all strains of *Fusobacterium* (Beerens, 1970).

In this chapter we present principally data derived from investigations carried out on oral fusobacteria isolated in our laboratory. Our strains correspond morphologically and biochemically to *F. polymorphum* Knorr or *F. nucleatum* Knorr as described by Omata and Braunberg (1960), and to the descriptions of *F. fusiforme* by Rosebury (1962) and of *F. fusiformis* by Smith and Holdeman (1968).

II. Early Immunological Studies

Most early immunological studies of microorganisms designated as fusobacteria (Pratt, 1927; Varney, 1927; Slanetz and Rettger, 1933; Spaulding and Rettger, 1937; Brocard, 1939) were of limited value. The organisms frequently reacted spontaneously in the conventional agglutination tests used, and did not readily lend themselves to serological analysis based on complement fixation tests. Observations related to the chemistry of antigens involved in serological reactions were not reported in these early studies. Spaulding and Rettger (1937) made unsuccessful attempts to isolate type-specific carbohydrates from fusobacteria. Weiss and Mercado (1938), on the basis of precipitin tests with extracts from four different strains, reported the presence of type-specific proteins and group-specific carbohydrates. Even the outstanding studies of Böe (1941) contributed relatively little to our knowledge of the immunochemistry of the genus *Fusobacterium*. Böe was, however, able to demonstrate that *Fusobacterium* differs immunologically from *L. buccalis* Trevisan, and concluded that the antigenic composition of *Fusobacterium* is very complex. In retrospect, probably his most significant contribution with regard to the immunochemistry of these organisms was the demonstration of factors which he found to be similar to endotoxins and which were capable of eliciting the local Shwartzman reaction.

III. Cell Wall Composition and Structure

Studies of the composition and structure of cell walls of fusobacteria have furnished at least some information with regard to the immunochemistry of these bacteria.

A. Preparation

Cell walls from fusobacteria were first stuided by Davis and Baird-Parker (1959). Baird-Parker (1960) later studied the composition of walls prepared from whole cells by the method of Cummins and Harris (1956). Criteria of purity were not reported by these authors. More recently, cell walls prepared from five strains of fusobacteria by a method which included rupturing of the cells, differential centrifugation, and digestion with trypsin were included in a study by Baboolal (1969). Some of his preparations were checked for purity by electron microscopy. Kristoffersen (1969b) reported on some properties of "undigested" cell walls, also from five strains, prepared from ruptured cells by differential and gradient centrifugation by the method of Yoshida et al. (1961). His cell walls were checked for purity by electron microscopy and for absence of nucleic acid components by paper chromatographic and colorimetric methods.

B. Composition

1. Quantitative Data

Quantitative data have been reported only by Baboolal (1969) and Kristoffersen (1969b). Selected data from their investigations are given in Table 1.

Baboolal (1969) found his trypsin-digested walls to contain 20%

Table 1. Selected data from quantitative analyses of *Fusobacterium* cell walls

Constituent	Percentage of dry weight	Constituent	Percentage of dry weight
Nitrogen	10.7[a]	Methyl pentose	0.9[a]
Phosphorus	0.5[a]	Fatty acid esters	10.5[a]
Neutral sugar		Lipid (gravimetric)	20[b]
(orcinol)	5.1[a]	Peptidoglycan	6[b]
Hexosamine	9.2[a]		

[a] Mean values for "undigested" walls of five strains (Kristoffersen, 1969b).

[b] Data from trypsin-digested cell walls from the five strains of Baboolal (1969).

lipids, based on the gravimetric method of Salton (1953). Only 6% of his wall preparations were recovered as peptidoglycan after repeated extraction with hot formamide. With cell walls from gram-positive, filamentous organisms, the yield of mucopeptide was 46–58%. Kristoffersen (1969b) found his cell walls to contain 9–12% fatty acid esters, as measured by the hydroxamic acid method (Snyder and Stephens, 1959), with tripalmitin as the arbitrarily chosen standard. Different preparation methods, as well as different methods for estimating lipid content, probably account for the variance of results in these two studies. A high content of protein, as calculated from Kjeldahl nitrogen values, was reported (Kristoffersen, 1969b).

The high percentage of lipid and protein and the low recovery of peptidoglycan are the outstanding features in these studies. The overall composition of the cell walls of fusobacteria therefore is similar to that of other gram-negative bacteria (Salton, 1964).

2. Amino Acids

Both trypsin-digested (Baboolal, 1969; Baird-Parker, 1960) and "undigested" (Kristoffersen, 1969b) cell walls of fusobacteria contain a wide range of amino acids. Kristoffersen (1969b) detected 17 amino acids in his preparations (Table 2). The results of his quantitative amino acid analysis are in good agreement with the visual estimates of Baboolal (1969), who found alanine, glutamic acid, glycine, and lysine to be major components, and also reported relatively high quantities of aspartic acid and leucine. According to Cummins and Harris (1956) and Baboolal (1969), the amino acid pattern of *Fusobacterium* cell

Table 2. Quantitative amino acid analysis of "undigested" cell
wall preparation from *Fusobacterium* strain F1

Amino acid	Moles per 100 moles total amino acids
Lysine	11.24
Histidine	1.16
Arginine	3.58
Aspartic acid	11.57
Threonine	4.68
Serine	4.62
Glutamic acid	12.99
Proline	5.01
Glycine	8.36
Alanine	10.00
Diaminopimelic acid	0.26
Valine	6.17
Methionine	1.84
Isoleucine	6.30
Leucine	8.14
Tyrosine	3.00
Phenylalanine	1.00

Data from Kristoffersen (1969b).

walls as observed in paper chromatograms can be considered typical of
gram-negative bacteria, a conclusion which is in agreement with the
results of quantitative analyses. The mucopeptide fraction of *Fusobacterium* cell walls was, however, found to contain lysine and not, as one
might expect, diaminopimelic acid (Baboolal, 1969). The status of
diaminopimelic acid in *Fusobacterium* cell walls appears unsettled or
perhaps variable. Baird-Parker (1960) reported that diaminopimelic
acid was present in cell walls from some of his strains but not from
others. Kristoffersen (1969b) found small amounts of diaminopimelic
acid in whole undigested cell walls (Table 2). The amino acid composition of peptidoglycan prepared from our *Fusobacterium* strain F1
by a modification of the method of Mandelstam (1962) has recently
been studied in our laboratory (Kristoffersen and Endresen, unpublished). The preparations contained diaminopimelic acid, as indicated

by gas chromatography and paper and thin-layer chromatography using various solvents. In addition, glutamic acid and alanine were present. The molar ratio between the two was approximately 1 : 2. Trace amounts of a few other amino acids, including small amounts of lysine, were detected.

3. Sugar Components

Glucosamine and muramic acid have been detected in cell walls (Baird-Parker, 1960; Baboolal, 1969; Kristoffersen 1969b) and in peptidoglycan preparations (Baboolal, 1969) from fusobacteria. Small amounts of galactosamine were found in whole preparations by Baboolal (1969), while Baird-Parker (1960) and Kristoffersen (1969b) did not report the presence of this amino sugar.

Glucose and galactose appear to be major neutral sugar components (Baird-Parker, 1960; Baboolal, 1969; Kristoffersen, 1969b). Trace amounts of xylose as well as rhamnose have also been reported (Kristoffersen, 1969b). Kristoffersen (1969b) found evidence of the presence of an unidentified aldoheptose in *Fusobacterium* cell walls. He also demonstrated the presence of a component which was different from sialic acid but which did react in the thiobarbituric acid assay for 2-keto-3-deoxy-sugar acids of Weissbach and Hurwitz (1959). These observations, together with the presence of heptose, suggested the presence in *Fusobacterium* of a lipopolysaccharide endotoxin with a composition similar to those of gram-negative aerobic bacilli.

C. Ultrastructure

The ultrastructure of whole cells and cell walls of fusobacteria have been studied by several authors (Hampp, Scott, and Wyckoff, 1960; Takagi and Nuyama, 1963; Ueda and Takagi, 1965). In carbon replicas and ultrathin sections, three distinct layers were recognized (Takagi and Nuyama, 1963). The outer trilaminar layer is wavy and consists of two electron-dense and one intermediate electron-lucent layer. Between this and the cytoplasmic membrane is a slightly granular layer. The wavy appearance of the outer layer is probably responsible for the corrugated, brain-like appearance of the surface of negatively stained whole cells (Ueda and Takagi, 1965). Cells of *Veillonella* were shown by Bladen and Mergenhagen (1964) to have a similar surface pattern. These authors further showed that the cell wall of *Veillonella* also has an outer, wavy trilaminar layer which could be removed by extraction of cells with 45% phenol. From the aqueous phase of this extract they extracted an endotoxic lipopolysaccharide with a characteristic ultrastructural appearance. An endotoxic lipopolysaccharide from *Fusobacterium* has recently been shown to have similar electron microscopic features.

IV. Cell Wall Antigens

A. Antigens Extracted from Crushed Cells

Kristoffersen (1969a) extracted crushed cells of 20 strains of fusobacteria at neutral pH in the cold, and studied the precipitinogens present in these extracts. Cross-reactivity was found between all strains. One of the strains, strain F1, was selected for closer study. With homologous antiserum, the extract from this strain formed three major precipitation lines in agar double diffusion and immunoelectrophoretic experiments (Figure 1). Two of these (lines 1 and 3) fused

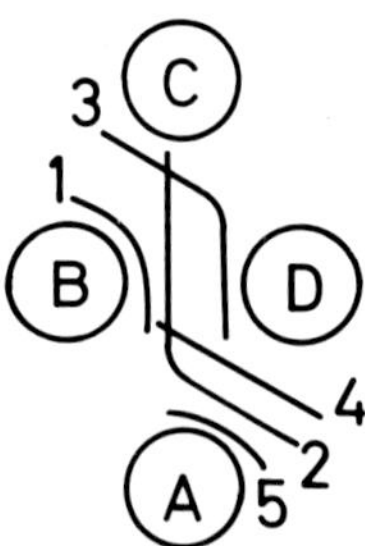

Fig. 1. Schematic drawing of principal lines formed on agar double diffusion with extracts from *Fusobacterium* strain F1. Antiserum to strain F1 was in well B. Antiserum to strain Fev1 was in well A. Wells C and D contained phenol-water extract (water phase) and crude buffer extract from strain F1, respectively. Figure indicates principal lines as described in the text. (From Kristoffersen, 1969a.)

with lines formed with the dialyzed water phase after phenol-water extraction of crushed cells according to Westphal, Lüderitz, and Bister (1952). The pellet obtained after ultracentrifugation of the dialyzed water phase gave positive epinephrine skin tests when 50 γg quantities were tested in rabbits. It contained both the precipitating antigens found in the aqueous phase after phenol-water extraction. It was later demonstrated that these two precipitinogens correspond to the endotoxic lipopolysaccharide and the related polysaccharide hapten.

The third precipitinogen demonstrated with homologous antiserum was provisionally termed "precipitinogen 2" (Figure 1, line 2). This precipitating antigen and two additional precipitinogens, which were demonstrable with buffer extract from strain F1 and antiserum to other strains (Figure 1, lines 4 and 5), were found most likely to be dependent upon protein constituents for their serological activity. None of them appeared to be identical to the group-reactive antigen—probably also of protein nature—which was demonstrated in supernatants of heat-killed whole bacteria by de Araujo, Varah, and Mergenhagen (1963) and considered by them to be responsible for the broad group-reactivity found in their bacterial extracts in indirect hemagglutination experiments.

All of the five precipitinogens found in this one strain of *Fusobacterium* could be shown either directly by precipitin reactions or through absorption experiments to be present in "undigested" cell wall preparations of these bacteria (Kristoffersen, 1969a,b).

B. Immunochemistry of Lipopolysaccharide from Fusobacteria

1. Preparation

In 1941 Böe produced the local Shwartzman reaction in rabbits with cell-free filtrates of cultures of fusobacteria. Twenty years later Mergenhagen, Hampp, and Scherp (1961) used the phenol-water extraction procedure of Westphal et al. (1952) to isolate endotoxic lipopolysaccharide (LPS) from acetone-dried cells of a strain of *F. nucleatum*. Extractions were performed at room temperature under constant stirring for 10–15 min. By precipitation of the water phase with cold acetone, they obtained a protein-lipid-carbohydrate complex which produced the Shwartzman phenomenon and was highly pyrogenic in rabbits. In later experiments the crude LPS was purified by precipitation in the ultracentrifuge (de Araujo et al., 1963; Jensen and Mergenhagen, 1964a,b).

Extractions with 45% aqueous phenol at room temperature and further purification by ultracentrifugation were also used by Kristoffersen and Hofstad (1970a) for preparation of LPS from whole cells of oral fusobacteria, or from bacteria that had been crushed in a bacterial press (the "X-press"), defatted with acetone and by ethanol-ether at $-25°C$, and extracted with 0.05 phosphate buffer, pH, 7.4, at 4°C overnight (Kristoffersen, 1969c).

2. Chemical Composition

The crude LPS prepared by Mergenhagen et al. (1961) was contaminated with protein and nucleic acids. By purification in the ultracentrifuge, the protein content decreased to 2–7% (de Araujo et al., 1963). Purified LPS from oral strains listed as *F. nucleatum* showed percentage compositions of lipid and carbohydrate of 19.7–37.3% and from 18.6–62.4%, respectively.

LPS prepared by Kristoffersen and Hofstad (1970a) from acetone-dried whole cells of three oral strains of *Fusobacterium* contained relatively large amounts of protein (Table 3, preparation 1) and were contaminated with nucleic acids. By extraction of crushed, defatted, and washed bacteria, these workers obtained LPS preparations containing small amounts of protein and no demonstrable nucleic acid components. The chemical composition of a representative batch of LPS prepared in this manner from strain F1 is listed in Table 3 (preparation 2). 2-Keto-3-deoxy-octonate (KDO) was measured by the thiobarbituric acid method as modified by Weissbach and Hurwitz (1959), using a KDO standard prepared from 2,4,5,7,8-penta-O-acetyl-KDO-methyl ester (Ghalambor, Levine, and Heath, 1966). Compared with LPS isolated from strains within Enterobacteriaceae (Lüderitz, Staub, and Westphal, 1966) and from the anaerobic *Veillonella* (Hofstad and Kristoffersen, 1970), the KDO content was low. Very small amounts of KDO have also been found in LPS purified from phenol-water extracts of a strain of *Sphaerophorus necrophorus* (Hofstad and Kristoffersen, 1971). The relatively low content of lipid in these preparations (Table 3), as compared with the values found by

Table 3. Chemical composition of LPS prepared from acetone-dried whole cells (preparation 1) and from crushed, defatted, and buffer-extracted bacteria (preparation 2) of *Fusobacterium* strain F1

Constituent	Preparation 1 (%)	Preparation 2 (%)
Protein (folin)	29.1	2.5
Fatty acid ester	12.9	15.2
Neutral sugar (orcinol)	18.7	50.1
Nitrogen		2.0
Phosphorus		2.1
Hexosamine		15.7
Methyl pentose		2.3
KDO		1.4

Data from Kristoffersen and Hofstad (1970a).

de Araujo et al. (1963) in their purified LPS preparations, may be at least partially explained by the different methods used to estimate lipid. de Araujo et al. (1963) measured the amounts of lipid in LPS by weighing choloroform-extractable material (Mergenhagen, Martin, and Schiffman, 1963).

The sugar components of the LPS preparations of Kristoffersen and Hofstad (1970) were identified by paper chromatography of acid hydrolysates (Table 4). LPS from the three strains examined all contained glucosamine, heptose, and KDO, but varied with respect to other sugars. The heptose was tentatively identified to be D-glycero-D-manno-, D-glycero-L-manno-, or D-glycero-D-gulo-heptose.

The qualitative composition of the lipid and protein moieties of LPS from fusobacteria has not been investigated.

3. Ultrastructure

The morphology of LPS isolated from *Fusobacterium* has been examined by Hofstad, Kristoffersen, and Selvig (1972). Lyophilized, positively stained preparations of LPS appeared in the electron microscope as straight or curved rod-like particles with diameters of 90 Å (Figure 2). Large numbers of disc-like bodies, 250– 1250 Å in diameter,

Table 4. Sugar components in LPS from three strains of fusobacteria

Component	Strain		
	F1	Fev1	ATCC 10953
Glucosamine	+	+	+
KDO	+	+	+
Heptose	+	+	+
Glucose	+	+	− [a]
Galactose	−	−	+
Mannose	−	+	+
Rhamnose	+	−	−

Data from Kristoffersen and Hofstad (1970).

[a] − , Sugar not detected.

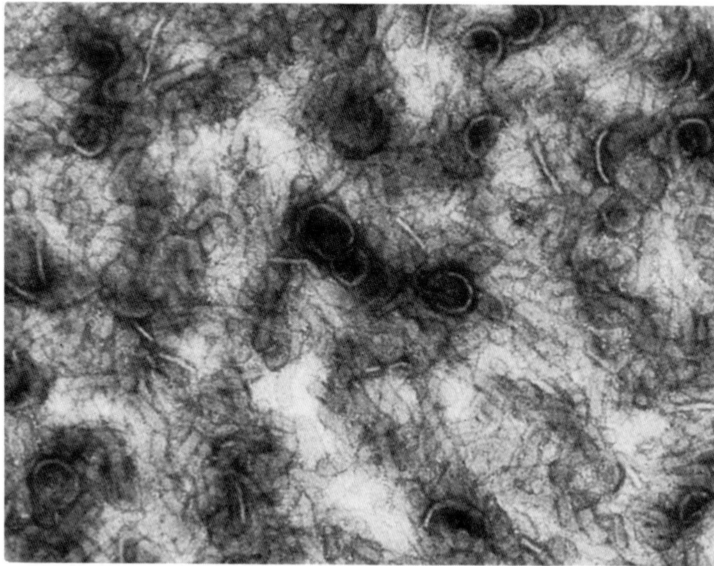

Fig. 2. Lyophilized lipopolysaccharide endotoxin (LPS) extracted from *Fusobacterium* strain F1 with phenol-water and purified by ultracentrifugation. Suspension stained with uranyl acetate. × 100,000. (Courtesy Dr. K. A. Selvig.)

were also seen. Most of these appeared to be circumscribed by a triple-layered surface structure. Structures with a striking similarity to the particles described in LPS preparations have been seen in sections of dental plaque in association with bacterial cells with a gram-negative cell wall profile (Selvig, Hofstad, and Kristoffersen, 1971). The three-dimensional structure of the particles remains uncertain.

4. Immunological Properties

The serological activity of *Fusobacterium* LPS has been examined by hemagglutination and precipitation techniques.

de Araujo et al. (1963), employing hemagglutination inhibition, found that phenol-water–extracted LPS purified by ultracentrifugation exhibited a high degree of serological specificity. Within 21 oral strains of *Fusobacterium,* several serological types appeared to exist. However, none of the LPS preparations from these strains cross-reacted with LPS extracted from the *Fusobacterium* type strain ATCC 10953. The findings of de Araujo et al. were corroborated and extended by Kristoffersen, Maeland, and Hofstad (1971), who worked with purified LPS from the strains F1, F4, Fev1, and ATCC 10953. These workers found that antisera to strains F1 and F4 agglutinated sheep erythrocytes sensitized with LPS prepared from either of the two strains, but not erythrocytes sensitized with LPS from strains Fev1 or ATCC 10953 (Table 5). Sheep cells sensitized by LPS F1 or LPS F4 were also agglutinated by antiserum to strain Fev1. Antiserum ATCC 10953 did not agglutinate sheep erythrocytes sensitized with heterologous LPS preparations. This indicates that in the LPS preparations exam-

Table 5. Titers in indirect hemagglutination tests of antibody to LPS in rabbit antisera to *Fusobacterium* strains F1, F4, Fev1, and ATCC 10953

Source of LPS	Anti-F1	Anti-F4	Anti-Fev1	Anti-10953
Strain F1	2048	1024	128	< 16
Strain F4	2048	1024	128	< 16
Strain Fev1	< 16	< 16	2048	< 16
Strain ATCC 10953	< 16	< 16	< 16	2048

Data from Kristoffersen, Maeland, and Hofstad (1971).

ined there were at least four determinant groups with different immunological specificity, that is, one determinant group common to LPS F1 and LPS F4, a second shared by LPS F1, LPS F4, and LPS Fev1, a third in LPS Fev1, and a fourth in LPS ATCC 10953. The findings were confirmed in hemagglutination inhibition and cross-absorption experiments. The effect on titers in indirect hemagglutination tests of absorption and cross-absorptions of antisera to strains F1, F4, and Fev1 are shown in Table 6. Adsorption with LPS ATCC 10953 did not affect the titers of antibodies in antisera-F1, -F4, or -Fev1, and the titers of antibodies in antiserum ATCC 10953 did not decrease following absorption of this antiserum with LPS from any of the three other heterologous *Fusobacterium* strains. Ring test precipitations with undiluted antisera and serial dilutions of the LPS preparation corroborated the observations made by the indirect hemagglutination experiments.

All serological activity of the LPS preparations of Kristoffersen,

Table 6. Effects of absorption with various LPS preparations on titers in the indirect hemagglutination of rabbit antisera to *Fusobacterium* strains F1, F4, and Fev1

Antiserum	Source of LPS	Titers in hemagglutination tests with erythrocytes sensitized with LPS from strain		
		F1	F4	Fev1
Anti-F1 unabsorbed		2048	2048	< 16
Anti-F1	F1	< 16	< 16	< 16
	F4	< 16	< 16	< 16
	Fev1	2048	2048	< 16
Anti-F4 unabsorbed		1024	1024	< 16
Anti-F4	F1	< 16	< 16	< 16
	F4	< 16	< 16	< 16
	Fev1	1024	1024	< 16
Anti-Fev1 unabsorbed		128	128	2048
Anti-Fev1	F1	< 16	< 16	2048
	F4	< 16	< 16	2048
	Fev1	< 16	< 16	< 16

Data from Kristoffersen, Maeland, and Hofstad (1971).

Maeland, and Hofstad (1971) was destroyed by oxidation with periodate, but remained unchanged following treatment with pronase. By examination of immunoprecipitates, it was found that the two determinant groups of LPS from strain F1 or from strain Fev1 could not be separated by precipitation with antibodies to one of the two groups. This clearly indicates that, like the O-factors of enterobacterial LPS (Lüderitz, Staub, and Westphal, 1966), the determinant groups of any one LPS preparation from *Fusobacterium* are carried by one and the same molecular complex, which was assumed to be the carbohydrate moiety of the LPS. Hemagglutination inhibition studies with monosaccharides and disaccharides supported this concept, and also yielded information on the chemical composition of at least one of the determinant groups detected in LPS from the four strains studied. Table 7 shows that maltose exhibited a strong inhibitory effect on the agglutination of sheep erythrocytes sensitized with LPS F1 in antiserum Fev1. Some inhibition was also observed when glucose and cellobiose were used as inhibitors in the same test system. It is therefore probable that terminal glucose is linked to another glucose residue in the structure responsible for the cross-reactivity between LPS isolated from strains F1, F4, and Fev1. Other results obtained by the inhibition studies suggest that glucose and mannose are present in the antigenic determinant found in LPS Fev1 only. Similarly, galactose may be the terminal sugar in one or more of the immunologically active groups in LPS from strain ATCC 10953 (Table 7).

By double diffusion in agar it has been shown that the aqueous phase from phenol-water extraction, as well as purified LPS from *Fusobacterium,* contains two precipitinogens, one a rapidly diffusing component and a second which moves more slowly (de Araujo et al., 1963; Kristoffersen, 1969a,b) (Figure 3; see also Figure 1, lines 1 and 3). de Araujo et al. (1963) separated the two immunologically distinct components by centrifugation at $50,000 \times g$ for 4 hr, and found that both of them sensitized sheep erythrocytes to agglutination in antiserum made against the parent strain. Kristoffersen (1969a) showed that brief hydrolysis of a crude LPS preparation from strain F1 in 0.1 N acetic acid at 100°C resulted in the disappearance of the slowest moving agar precipitation line. At the same time, the concentration of the rapidly diffusing component increased approximately 128-fold, as

Table 7. Inhibition of indirect hemagglutination in various test systems with monosaccharides and disaccharides

Test system[a]	Sugar present in LPS[b]	Sugar giving inhibition				
		Glucose	Mannose	Galactose	Maltose	Cellobiose
Anti-Fev1/LPS from Fev1	Glucose, mannose	+[d]	+	−[c]	−	−
Anti-Fev1/LPS from F1	Glucose, rhamnose	+	−	−	++[e]	+
Anti-10953/LPS from ATCC 10953	Galactose, mannose	−	−	+	−	−

Data from Kristoffersen, Maeland, and Hofstad (1971).

[a] Antiserum used/erythrocytes sensitized with LPS from strain designated.

[b] In addition, all LPS preparations contained glucosamine, heptose, and 2-keto-3-deoxyoctonate.

[c] −, No inhibition.

[d] +, Titer reduced 4- to 8-fold.

[e] ++, Titer reduced more than 8-fold.

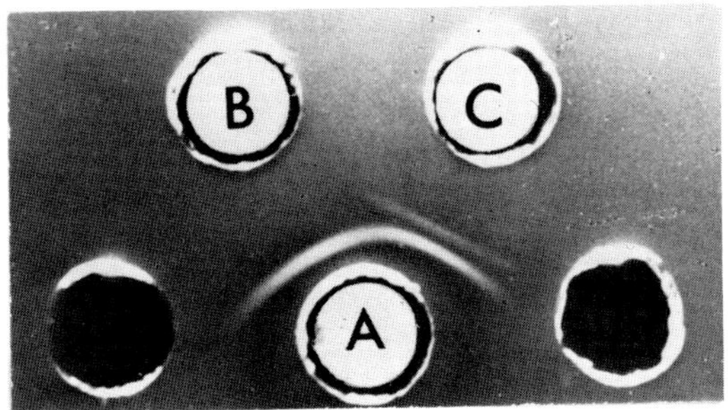

Fig. 3. Precipitation lines in agar with cell fractions from *Fusobacterium* strain F1. Well A contained antiserum to microorganisms strain F1. Well B contained unconcentrated protoplasmic fraction, and well C contained phenol-water extract (water phase) from cell walls of the same strain. (From Kristoffersen, 1969b.)

judged by titer (Table 8). These observations are analogous to the findings made by Ribi et al. (1962) with LPS prepared in different ways from various Enterobacteriaceae. The rapidly diffusing component is a polysaccharide hapten similar to the acid hapten that Freeman (1942) found in this group of bacteria (Staub, 1954; Landy et al., 1955).

Evidence has also been found for the presence in *Fusobacterium* of a "native protoplasmic hapten" analogous to that found in the protoplasm of *Escherichia coli* cells (Anacker et al., 1964). By immunological examination of a protoplasmic fraction of strain F1, Kristoffersen (1969b) was able to demonstrate an agar precipitation line which showed deviation and complete fusion with the line pro-

Table 8. Effect on agar precipitation titer of brief acid hydrolysis of the dialyzed aqueous phase from phenol-water extracts of *Fusobacterium*, strain F1

Precipitation line	Highest dilution of antigen giving precipitation with homologous antiserum		
	Unhydrolyzed	Hydrolyzed, 2 min	Hydrolyzed, 7 min
3	4096	256	1
1	8	256	1024

Data from Kristoffersen (1969a).

duced by the rapidly diffusing component in the crude LPS preparation (Figure 3).

C. The group-reactive "Precipitinogen 2"

One of the five precipitinogens demonstrated by Kristoffersen (1969a) in buffer extracts was found in preliminary studies to be present in all of his 20 strains of fusobacteria. In subsequent experiments attempts were made to purify this material, provisionally called "precipitinogen 2," and to characterize it chemically and serologically (Kristoffersen, 1969c,d,e,f).

1. Preparation

The isolation of this antigen was complicated by its instability, especially after a certain degree of purification had been achieved (Kristoffersen, 1969c). Flocculent precipitates appeared in solutions of the antigen with concomitant loss of immunological activity. The purification procedure finally adopted included the following steps:

1. Preparation of an acetone powder from crushed bacteria and further removal of lipids with ethanol : ether (2 : 1) at $-25°C$;
2. extraction of dried, defatted microorganisms with 0.05 M phosphate buffer, pH 7.4, at 4°C;
3. fractional precipitation with ammonium sulphate (all buffers used after this step contained 0.005 M 2-mercaptoethanol and 0.001 M ethylenediaminetetra-acetate);
4. ultracentrifugation for 1 hr at $100,000 \times g$;
5. gel filtration of the supernatant fluid on Sephadex G-200;
6. ion exchange chromatography on DEAE-cellulose at pH 6.3.

Concentration and desalting were achieved by the use of Sephadex G-25 (Flodin, 1962). The loss of active material through these procedures was considerable, but other methods proved even less suitable. The overall purification was about 75-fold. The purity of the isolated material was studied by paper- and immunoelectrophoresis, agar double diffusion, and by gel filtration (Kristoffersen, 1969c).

2. Chemical Composition

The chemical composition of different preparations varied somewhat (Kristoffersen, 1969d), although the same chemical components were present in the various preparations. One preparation contained approximately 85% protein, including 15 amino acids, a carbohydrate component consisting of 9.1% glucose and 0.7% xylose, and a small amount of fatty acid esters (Table 9). Although no amino sugars were detected, several indications were found that the carbohydrate and the protein components were linked together.

3. Biological Activities

The isolated material was active in interfacial ring test precipitation experiments in concentrations of 6 μg/ml (Kristoffersen, 1969e). It fixed complement, concentrations of 6.25–50 μg giving the highest serum titers with rabbit immune sera. The antigen could be adsorbed to tanned sheep erythrocytes, and indirect hemagglutination was found to be the most sensitive method for demonstration of antibody. The purified antigen also was immunogenic in rabbits (Figure 4, wells 5, 6, and 7). Rabbit immune sera to whole bacteria were found to contain both high and low molecular weight specific antibodies to the antigen.

Table 9. Chemical composition of "precipitinogen 2" from *Fusobacterium* strain F1

Constituent	Percentage
Nitrogen	13.8
Phosphorus	0.17
Neutral sugar (orcinol) as glucose	9.1
Pentose (cysteine-H_2SO_4) as xylose	0.7
Fatty acid esters (hydroxamic acid assay) as tripalmitin	0.3

Data from Kristoffersen (1969d).

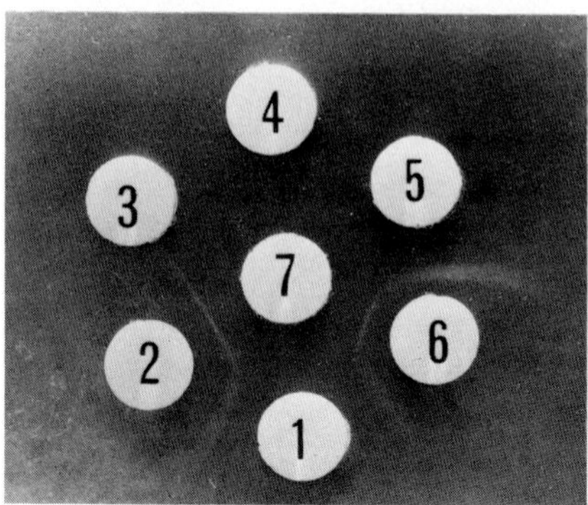

Fig. 4. Agar double diffusion plate showing lines formed with purified "precipitinogen 2" and different homologous antisera. Well contents were as follows: *1,* Rabbit antiserum to autologous erythrocytes sensitized with purified antigen. *3,* Normal rabbit serum. *5,* Rabbit antiserum to purified antigen. *7,* Rabbit antiserum to whole microorganisms strain F1. Wells 2 and 6 contained purified antigen, 0.1 mg/ml. (From Kristoffersen, 1969e.)

Further studies revealed that the antibody-neutralizing capacity as measured by inhibition of hemagglutination and the precipitating ability both were retained after heating solutions of the antigen to 70°C for 15 min, whereas the ability to sensitize tanned sheep erythrocytes was destroyed by such treatment. Heating to 100°C for 15 min completely destroyed all these activities.

A number of other experiments were carried out in attempts to elucidate the nature of the antigenic determinant or determinants present. Apparently, both the polysaccharide and the peptide or protein component are important for the serological reactivity of the antigen, as indicated by the effect of various enzymes on the different immunological activities. Furthermore, there were indications that the antigenic determinant or determinants responsible for the precipitating and the hemagglutinating activities of the antigen were parts of the same molecule, and that they may be identical. Thus, serum from rabbits immunized with autologous erythrocytes sensitized with purified "precipitinogen 2" produced a line on agar precipitation which gave a "reaction of identity" with the line formed with antiserum to whole microorganisms (Figure 4, wells 1, 2, and 7).

The antigen reacted in precipitation and indirect hemagglutination experiments with all of 11 rabbit immune sera to different strains of *Fusobacterium* (Kristoffersen, 1969f). Similarly, all of 29 strains of fusobacteria reacted in precipitin tests with specific antisera to the antigen, and cells of these strains absorbed specific antibodies to the antigen. None of ten other species of oral and enteric bacteria, including *L. buccalis, Bacteroides melaninogenicus, Veillonella, E. coli, Salmonella typhi,* and *S. paratyphi,* reacted in precipitation or absorption experiments. The strain of *Sphaerophorus necrophorus* used in these experiments, strain ATCC 12290, has since been shown to belong to the genus *Bacteroides* (Barnes and Goldberg, 1969; Werner, 1970; Hofstad and Kristoffersen, 1971). This strain showed no evidence of cross-reaction with "precipitinogen 2." The *S. necrophorus* strain N167 (Hofstad and Kristoffersen, 1971) has recently been tested in precipitin reactions. Extracts from this organism reacted in interfacial ring test experiments and produced a line in agar with specific antisera to "precipitinogen 2." The line gave a "reaction of partial identity" with the line produced with the same antiserum and an extract from *Fusobacterium* strain F1 (Kristoffersen and Hofstad, unpublished).

In one series of experiments antibodies to the antigen were found in 86% of sera from "healthy" adult humans tested in indirect hemagglutination experiments (Table 10) (Kristoffersen, 1969f). Antibodies were also present in 75% of umbilical cord sera. The titers in mothers' and infants' sera paralleled each other very well. Gel filtration experiments and reductional cleavage with 2-mercaptoethanol indicated that antibodies in most human sera were primarily of the IgG and not of the IgM class of antibodies, as might have been expected (LoSpalluto et al., 1962; Bauer, Mathies, and Stavitsky, 1963; Evans, Spaeth, and Mergenhagen, 1966; Pike, 1967). Commercial preparations of human gamma globulin also agglutinated tanned sheep erythrocytes sensitized with the purified antigen and, in addition, produced a precipitation line in agar with the antigen. This line fused with the line produced with rabbit immune serum, although with a strong "spur" formation (Figure 5A and B). A faint line of precipitation was also produced with a few human sera which gave high titers in indirect hemagglutination tests. No antibodies were found by indirect hemagglutination in sera from five children 3–11 months of age (Table 10). Sera from three out of eight children in the 1–3-year-old group reacted with the antigen, and the incidence of positive reactions, as well as titer levels, increased with age in childhood and adolesence.

The observation that antibodies were present in sera of

Table 10. Antibody to "precipitinogen 2" in various human sera; distribution of sera according to titers in indirect hemagglutination tests

Source of serum	Reciprocal of titers in indirect hemagglutination						Number of sera with titer > 8	Total in age group
	< 8	8 + 16	32 + 64	128 + 256	512 + 1.024	2.048 + 4.096		
Umbilical cord	6	1	7	3	2	2	15	21
Children								
3–11 months	5	0	0	0	0	0	0	5
1–3 years	5	1	0	1	1	0	3	8
4–6 years	5	0	1	1	0	0	2	7
7–10 years	2	0	1	2	1	1	5	7
13–15 years	2	0	1	4	4	2	11	13
Blood donors								
18–68 years	13	6	36	24	13	7	86	99

Data from Kristoffersen (1969f).

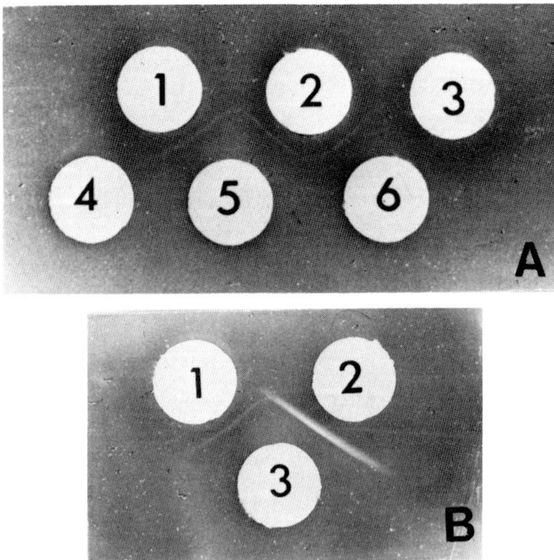

Fig. 5. Agar doubled diffusion plates showing lines formed with purified "precipitinogen 2" and human gamma globulin. *A,* Wells 1 and 2: human gamma globulin 16% (Kabi); well 3: the same, but absorbed with "precipitinogen 2"; well 4: buffered saline; wells 5 and 6: "precipitinogen 2," 0.1 mg/ml in buffered saline. *B,* Well 1: human gamma globulin 16% (Kabi); well 2: antiserum to purified "precipitinogen 2"; well 3: "precipitinogen 2," 0.1 mg/ml in buffered saline. (From Kristoffersen, 1969f.)

one-year-old children is in accordance with the findings of Berger, Kapovits, and Pfeifer (1959), who found that at this age fusobacteria are regularly present in the oral cavity.

It is not known how the antigen gains access for antigenic stimulation. However, *Fusobacterium* is one of several gram-negative, anaerobic bacterial genera which are both relatively and absolutely increased in inflammatory periodontal disease (Schultz-Haudt et al., 1954; Socransky et al., 1963; Löe, Theilade, and Jensen, 1965; Theilade et al., 1966). The antigen may gain access to the interior of the body through other parts of the gastrointestinal or nasopharyngeal tracts or possibly through other ports of entry (Rosebury, 1962; Lahelle, 1945). However, Evans et al. (1966) found significantly elevated titers of bactericidal antibody to fusobacteria in sera from six individuals with periodontal disease as compared to five "normal" sera. The sera of 31 otherwise healthy patients in whom the severity of

　　　　　　　　　　　　　　　TORE KRISTOFFERSEN AND TOR HOFSTAD

inflammatory periodontal disease had been scored on a numerical scale (Russell, 1956) were therefore examined for antibodies to "precipitinogen 2" in indirect hemagglutination tests (Kristoffersen and Hofstad, 1970b). No clear-cut correlation between titer levels and severity of periodontal disease was observed in these patients, although there appeared to be a tendency for patients with more severe periodontal disease to have slightly higher titers.

Intradermal injections of 0.1–0.4 mg of "precipitinogen 2" in 0.2 ml of sterile, buffered saline into rabbits which had received intravenous injections of 160 mg of human gamma globulin 20–45 min earlier produced rapidly developing skin reactions which reached a maximum in 4–6 hrs in five out of eight animals (Kristoffersen and Hofstad, 1970b). The lesions were characterized by hemorrhage, redness, and swelling, and, when maximal, covered an area with a maximum diameter of 2 cm (Figure 6). After 8 hr the centers of these

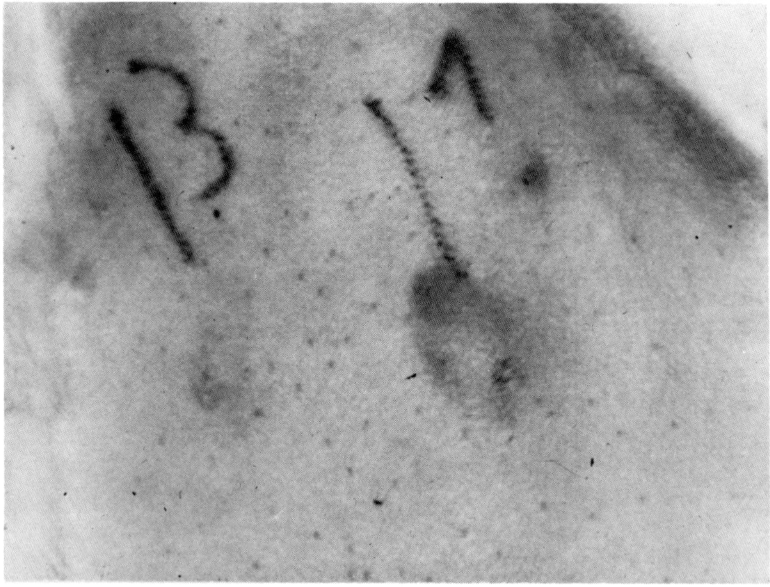

Fig. 6. Arthus-like reaction (marked "1") produced in rabbit by intradermal injection of 0.4 mg of "precipitinogen 2," 20 min after intravenous injection of 160 mg of human gamma globulin (Kabi). Photograph was taken eight hours after intradermal injection. The "3" indicates the site of injection of 0.1 mg of the antigen. (From Kristoffersen and Hofstad, 1970b.)

lesions frequently paled, and after 20 hr they were often markedly pale and slightly elevated. When no preparatory injection was given, no hemorrhagic lesions were produced, although a mild inflammatory reaction, usually developing slowly, was seen. Intravenous injection of 250 μg of lipopolysaccharide endotoxin 24 hr after intradermal injection of "precipitinogen 2" did not influence the appearance of the lesions, regardless of whether gamma globulin had been given.

Although histological and preferably immunohistochemical studies will be necessary for a definite classification, the experimental procedure, the rapidity of development, and the appearance of the hemorrhagic lesions are consistent with an immediate, Arthus-type hypersensitivity reaction. The experiments of Gustafson, Sjöquist, and Stålenheim (1967) indicate that the reactions observed can hardly be caused by the accumulation of preformed aggregates of gamma globulin in the commercial preparations used, at a preexisting local site of inflammation.

Whether, and to what extent, the mechanisms behind the reactions observed in rabbits also function in humans is, of course, not known. However, our investigations demonstrate that circulating antibodies to "precipitinogen 2" from *Fusobacterium* are frequently found in humans, that such antibodies and corresponding human immunoglobulins may give rise to immune precipitates, and that the reaction of the antibodies with the corresponding antigen *in vivo* may contribute to tissue injury, as, for example, in inflammatory periodontal disease, through immediate type, Arthus-like reactions.

V. Other, Less Thoroughly Characterized, Antigens

In experiments with supernatants of heat-killed cells of *Fusobacterium* ("crude antigen"), de Araujo et al. (1963) reported the presence of one or more antigens responsible for a broad cross-reactivity among strains of this genus (see also de Araujo, 1963). No cross-reactions with strains of *L. buccalis* were observed. The cross-reactivity was destroyed by treatment of extracts with phenol or trypsin, possibly indicating that the antigen or antigens involved were protein in nature. The residual immunological activity corresponded to that of phenol-water–extracted endotoxic lipopolysaccharide. The "crude antigen" of these workers gave three precipitation lines on agar double diffusion with homologous antiserum. Two of these lines corresponded to the slow- and the fast-moving components of endotoxic lipopolysaccharide as shown by absorption experiments. The third line observed was considered to correspond to the protein antigen or antigens responsible for the broad cross-reactivity observed in indirect hemagglutination. The chemical nature and other characteristics of this antigen apparently have not been studied further. The difference in heat stability and resistance to enzymatic digestion indicate, however, that this antigen is not identical to the "precipitinogen 2" studied by Kristoffersen (1969c,d,e).

Mashimo and Ellison (1968, 1969) have reported briefly on soluble antigens released by strains of fusobacteria into protein-free culture media and detectable by agar double diffusion and immunoelectrophoresis. Typical strains were reported to produce four or more "major" antigens and several "minor" ones. The bacterial strains apparently could be divided into groups according to these antigens. The nature of the antigens has not been reported, although it is implied (Mashimo and Ellison, 1968) that they are soluble proteins. It should be noted, however, that secretion of endotoxic lipopolysaccharide into the culture fluid during the growth of gram-negative bacteria has also been observed (Crutchley, Marsh, and Cameron, 1967).

VI. Summary and Comment

Our knowledge of the immunochemistry of the genus *Fusobacterium* has expanded considerably in recent years. Indeed, it appears that, with respect to immunochemistry at the present time, we know more about these microorganisms than about any other gram-negative anaerobic bacterium. The most important information gathered during the past years' studies on the immunochemistry of fusobacteria are briefly summarized below.

The structure and the overall chemical composition of the cell wall of the *Fusobacterium* are similar to those of other gram-negative bacteria. The cell wall lipopolysaccharide is analogous to lipopolysaccharides of most other gram-negative bacteria, with respect to both ultrastructure and overall qualitative and quantitative chemical composition. An exception is the relatively low content of 2-keto-3-deoxyoctonate. The LPS acts as a powerful endotoxin, and the carbohydrate moiety of the macromolecular LPS complex exhibits serological type-specificity similar to that of the somatic O-antigens of the Enterobacteriaceae and the antigenic determinants of LPS of *Neisseria gonorrhoea* (Maeland, 1969; Maeland, Kristoffersen, and Hofstad, 1971). An "acid hapten" and a "native protoplasmic hapten" have also been demonstrated.

In the group-reactive antigen "precipitinogen 2," carbohydrate and protein appear to be bound together without involvement in the linkage of amino sugars. Antibodies in most human sera against this antigen appear to be predominantly immunoglobulins with low molecular weights.

Immunochemical studies also have yielded information of interest with regard to taxonomy. They have, for instance, corroborated Böe's conclusion (1941) that the lack of serological cross-reactivity between *Fusobacterium* and *L. buccalis* suggests that these bacteria belong to separate genera. The presence within *Fusobacterium* LPS of KDO and heptose distinguishes fusobacteria from *Bacteroides,* since the LPS of the latter does not contain these sugar constituents. The cross-reactivity of *S. necrophorus* with the group-reactive "precipitinogen 2" from *Fusobacterium,* as well as the similarity in chemical composition of LPS from *S. necrophorus* strain N167 with LPS from fusobacteria (Kristoffersen and Hofstad, 1970a; Hofstad and Kristoffersen 1971), support the suggested close relationship between these bacteria (Werner, 1968).

The demonstration of type-specificity of LPS from *Fusobacterium* shows that tools are available for a classification of fusobacteria into serotypes. Thus, LPS provides us with an immunological marker which may reveal that some serotypes are more significant than others in the host-parasite relationship of some endogenous bacterial infections, as, for instance, in periodontal disease (Mergenhagen, 1967).

Antigens from *Fusobacterium* may well be implicated in hypersensitivity mechanisms in certain bacterial infections. The occurrence *in vivo* of an interaction of endotoxin from certain other bacterial species and the complement system, causing the generation of products that are biologically active in inflammation (Mergenhagen et al., 1969), most likely also holds true for *Fusobacterium* LPS. If immune injury through Arthus-like reactions contributes to tissue damage—for example, in human periodontal disease—the group-reactive "precipitinogen 2" fulfills the requisites for antigens capable of eliciting such reactions. Precipitating antibodies to this antigen are present in human serum, and when given together with pooled human gamma globulin, the antigen produces hemorrhagic lesions in rabbit skin.

Although a great deal is known about the immunochemistry of *Fusobacterium,* we are still at the beginning of our chemical and immunological investigations of this organism. The fine structure of the various macromolecular cell-wall components, including the peptidoglycan and the LPS, for instance, largely remains obscure. The status of diaminopimelic acid and lysine in the peptidoglycan is still unsettled. Antigens other than the somatic O-antigen and the group-reactive "precipitinogen 2" have not been isolated and characterized. It is hoped that many of these aspects of the immunochemistry of this pathogenic microorganism will be elucidated in the near future.

Literature Cited

Anacker, R. L., R. A. Finkelstein, W. T. Haskins, M. Landy, K. C. Milner, E. Ribi, and P. W. Stashak. 1964. Origin and properties of a naturally occurring hapten from *Escherichia coli.* J. Bacteriol. 88: 1705–1720.

Araujo, W. C. de. 1963. The specific status of *Fusiformis fusiformis* (Prevot). An. Microbiol. (Rio de F.) 11: 99–104.

Araujo, W. C. de, E. Varah, and S. E. Mergenhagen. 1963. Immunochemical analysis of human oral strains of *Fusobacterium* and *Leptotrichia.* J. Bacteriol. 86: 837–844.

Baboolal, R. 1969. Cell wall analysis of oral filamentous bacteria. J. Gen. Microbiol. 58: 217–226.

Baird-Parker, A. C. 1960. The classification of fusobacteria from the human mouth. J. Gen. Microbiol. 22: 458–469.

Barnes, E. M., and H. S. Goldberg. 1968. The relationship of bacteria within the family *Bacteroidaceae* as shown by numerical taxonomy. J. Gen. Microbiol. 51: 313–324.

Bauer, D. C., M. J. Mathies, and A. B. Stavitsky. 1963. Sequences of synthesis of γ-1 macroglobulin and γ-2 globulin antibodies during primary and secondary responses to proteins, salmonella antigens and phage. J. Exp. Med. 117: 889–907.

Beerens, H. 1970. Report of the International Committee on Nomenclature of Bacteria, Taxonomic Subcommittee for Gram-negative anaerobic rods. Int. J. System. Bact. 20: 297–300.

Beerens, H., and M. Tahon-Castel. 1965. Infections humaines à bactéries anaérobies non toxigènes. Presses Académiques Européennes. Bruxelles.

Berger, U. 1956. Untersuchungen an Fusobakterien. I. Mitteilung. Systematik, Züchtung und Morphologie. Zbl. Bakt. I. Abt. Orig. 166: 484–497.

Berger, U. 1957. Untersuchungen an Fusobakterien. II. Mitteilung. Zur Toxinbildung *in vitro*. Zbl. Bakt. I. Abt. Orig. 167: 372–383.

Berger, U., M. Kapovits, and G. Pfeifer. 1959. Zur Besiedlung der kindlichen Mundhöhle mit anaeroben Mikroorganismen. Z. Hyg. Infekt. -Kr. 145: 564–573.

Bladen, H. A., and S. E. Mergenhagen. 1964. Ultrastructure of *Veillonella* and morphological correlation of an outer membrane with particles associated with endotoxic activity. J. Bacteriol. 88: 1482–1492.

Böe, J. 1941. *Fusobacterium:* Studies on its bacteriology, serology and pathogenicity. Skr. Norske Vitensk.-akad. I. Mat.-Nat. Kl. no. 9 Oslo.

Breed, R. S., E. G. D. Murray, and N. R. Smith. 1957. Bergey's manual of determinative bacteriology, 7th ed. Williams and Wilkins, Baltimore.

Brocard, H. 1939. Le pouvoir agglutinogène du *Bacille fusiforme*. Application de la reaction d'agglutination au diagnostic de l'infection humaine. Compt. Rend. Soc. Biol. 130: 435–437.

Crutchley, M. J., D. G. Marsh, and J. Cameron. 1967. Free endotoxin. Nature, London 214: 1052.

Cummins, C. S., and H. Harris. 1956. The chemical composition of the cell wall in some gram-positive bacteria and its possible value as a taxonomic character. J. Gen. Microbiol. 14: 583–600.

Davis, G. H. G., and A. C. Baird-Parker. 1959. Cell wall composition of *Leptotrichia* spp. Nature, London 183: 1206–1207.

Evans, R. T., S. Spaeth, and S. E. Mergenhagen. 1966. Bactericidal antibody in mammalian serum to obligatorily anaerobic gram-negative bacteria. J. Immunol. 97: 112–119.

Flodin, P. 1962. Dextran gels and their applications in gel filtration. Pharmacia, Uppsala.

Freeman, G. G. 1942. The preparation and properties of a specific polysaccharide from *Bact. typhosum* Ty_2. Biochem. J. 36: 340–355.

Ghalambor, M. A., E. M. Levine and E. C. Heath. 1966. The biosynthesis of cell wall lipopolysaccharide in *Escherichia coli*. III. The isolation and characterization of 3-deoxyoctulosonic acid. J. Biol. Chem. 241: 3207–3215.

Gibbons, R. J., S. S. Socransky, S. Sawyer, B. Kapsimalis, and J. B. Macdonald. 1963. The microbiota of the gingival crevice area of man. II. The predominant cultivable organisms. Arch. Oral Biol. 8: 281–289.

Gustafson, G. T., J. Sjöquist, and G. Stålenheim. 1967. "Protein A" from *Staphylococcus aureus*. II. Arthus-like reaction produced in rabbits by interaction of Protein A and human γ-globulin. J. Immunol. 98: 1178–1181.

Hampp, E. G., D. B. Scott, and R. W. G. Wyckoff. 1960. Morphological characteristics of oral fusobacteria as revealed by the electron microscope. J. Bacteriol. 79: 716–728.

Hofstad, T. and T. Kristoffersen. 1970. Chemical composition of endotoxin from oral *Veillonella*. Acta Pathol. Microbiol. Scand., Section B.78: 760–764.

Hofstad, T., and T. Kristoffersen. 1971. Preparation and chemical characteristics of endotoxic lipopolysaccharide from three strains of *Sphaerophorus necrophorus*. Acta Pathol. Microbiol. Scand., Section B, 79: 385–390.

Hofstad, T., T. Kristoffersen, and K. A. Selvig. 1972. Electron microscopy of endotoxic lipopolysaccharide from *Bacteroides, Fusobacterium* and *Sphaerophorus*. Acta Pathol. Microbiol. Scand. Section B. 80: 413–419.

Jackins, H. C., and H. A. Barker. 1951. Fermentative processes of the fusiform bacteria. J. Bacteriol. 61: 101–114.

Jensen, S. B., and S. E. Mergenhagen. 1964a. Influence of endotoxin on resistance of mice to intraperitoneal infection with human oral bacteria. Arch. Oral Biol. 9: 229–239.

Jensen, S. B., and S. E. Mergenhagen. 1964b. Influence of endotoxin on the dermal response of rabbits to human oral bacteria. Arch. Oral. Biol. 9: 241–254.

Knorr, M. 1922. Über die fusospirilläre Symbiose, die Gattung *Fusobacterium* (K. B. Lehmann) und *Spirillum sputigenum*. II. Mitteilung. Die Gattung *Fusobacterium*. Zbl. Bakt. I. Abt. Orig. 89: 4–22.

Kristoffersen, T., 1969a. Immunochemical studies of oral fusobacteria. 1. Major precipitinogens. Acta Pathol. Microbiol. Scand. 77: 235–246.

Kristoffersen, T. 1969b. Immunochemical studies of oral fusobacteria. 2. Some properties of undigested cell wall preparations. Acta Pathol. Microbiol. Scand. 77: 247–257.

Kristoffersen, T. 1969c. Immunochemical studies of oral fusobacteria. 3. Purification of a group reactive precipitinogen. Acta Pathol. Microbiol. Scand. 77: 447–456.

Kristoffersen, T. 1969d. Immunochemical studies of oral fusobacteria. 4. Some chemical properties of a group reactive precipitinogen. Acta Pathol. Microbiol. Scand. 77: 457–464.

Kristoffersen, T. 1969e. Immunochemical studies of oral fusobacteria. 5. Serological characterization of a group reactive antigen. Acta Pathol. Microbiol. Scand. 77: 707–716.

Kristoffersen, T. 1969f. Immunochemical studies of oral fusobacteria. 6. Distribution of a group reactive antigen among some bacteria and occurrence of antibodies in human sera to this antigen. Acta Pathol. Microbiol. Scand. 77: 717–726.

Kristoffersen, T., and T. Hofstad. 1970a. Chemical composition of lipopolysaccharide endotoxins from human oral fusobacteria. Arch. Oral. Biol. 15: 909–916.

Kristoffersen, T., and T. Hofstad. 1970b. Antibodies in humans to an isolated antigen from oral fusobacteria. J. Periodont. Res. 5: 110–115.

Kristoffersen, T., J. A. Maeland, and T. Hofstad. 1971. Serological properties of lipopolysaccharide endotoxins from oral fusobacteria. Scand. J. Dent. Res. 79: 105–112.

Lahelle, O. 1945. Finger infection caused by *Fusobacterium* and spirochetes with a discussion of fusospirochetal infection of the fingers. Acta Derm. Venereol. 25: 266–274.

Landy, M., A. G. Johnson, M. E. Webster, and J. F. Sagin. 1955. Studies on the O antigen of *Salmonella typhosa*. II. Immunological properties of the purified antigen. J. Immunol. 74: 466–478.

Löe, H., E. Theilade, and S. B. Jensen. 1965. Experimental gingivitis in man. J. Periodont. 36: 177–187.

LoSpalluto, J., W. E. Miller, B. Dorward, and C. W. Fink. 1962. The formation of macroglobulin antibodies. I. Studies on adult humans. J. Clin. Invest. 41: 1415–1421.

Lüderitz, O., A. M. Staub, and O. Westphal. 1966. Immunochemistry of O and R antigens of Salmonella and related Enterobacteriaceae. Bacteriol. Rev. 30: 192–255.

Maeland, J. A. 1969. Serological cross-reactions of aqueous ether extracted endotoxin from *Neisseria gonorrhoeae*. Acta Pathol. Microbiol. Scand. 77: 515–517.

Maeland, J. A., T. Kristoffersen, and T. Hofstad. 1971. Immunochemical investigations on *Neisseria gonorrhoeae* endotoxin. 2. Serological Multispecificity and Other Properties of Phenol-Water Preparations. Acta Pathol. Microbiol. Scand., B, 79: 233–236.

Mandelstam, J. 1962. Preparation and properties of the mucopeptides of cell walls of gram-negative bacteria. Biochem. 84: 294–299.

Mashimo, P. A., and S. A. Ellison. 1968. Soluble antigens of oral anaerobic bacteria. I.A.D.R. 46th Gen. Meeting. (Abstr.).

Mashimo, P. A., and S. A. Ellison. 1969. Antigenic structure of fusiform bacteria. I.A.D.R. 47th Gen. Meeting. (Abstr.).

Mergenhagen, S. E. 1967. Nature and significance of somatic antigens of oral bacteria. J. Dent. Res. 46 (Suppl.): 46–52.

Mergenhagen, S. E. 1960. Endotoxic properties of oral bacteria as revealed by the local Shwartzman reaction. J. Dent. Res. 39: 267–272.

Mergenhagen, S. E., E. G. Hampp, and H. W. Scherp. 1961. Preparation and biological properties of endotoxins from oral bacteria. J. Infect. Dis. 108: 304–310.

Mergenhagen, S. E., G. R. Martin, and E. Schiffman. 1963. Studies on an endotoxin of a group C *Neisseria meningitidis*. J. Immunol. 90: 312–317.

Mergenhagen, S. E., R. Snyderman, H. Gewurz, and H. S. Shin. 1969. Significance of complement to the mechanism of action of endotoxin. Curr. Top. Microbiol. Immunol. 50: 37–77.

Omata, R. R. and R. C. Braunberg. 1960. Oral fusobacteria. J. Bacteriol. 80: 737–740.

Pike, R. M. 1967. Antibody heterogenicity and serological reactions. Bacteriol. Rev. 31: 157–174.

Pratt, J. S. 1927. On the biology of *B. fusiformis*. J. Infect. Dis. 41: 461–466.

Ribi, E., W. T. Haskins, K. C. Milner, R. L. Anacker, O. B. Ritter, G. Goode, R.-J. Trapani, and M. Landy. 1962. Physiochemical changes in endotoxin associated with loss of biological potency. J. Bacteriol. 84: 803–814.

Rosebury, T. 1962. Microorganisms Indigenous to Man. McGraw-Hill, New York.

Russell, A. L. 1956. A system of classification and scoring for prevalence surveys of periodontal disease. J. Dent. Res. 35: 350–359.

Salton, M. R. J. 1953. Studies on the bacterial cell wall. IV. The composition of the cell walls of some gram-positive and gram-negative bacteria. Biochim. Biophys. Acta 10: 512–523.

Salton, M. R. J. 1964. The Bacterial Cell Wall. Elsevier, Amsterdam.

Schultz-Haudt, S. D., M. A. Bruce, and B. G. Bibby. 1954. Bacterial factors in nonspecific gingivitis. J. Dent. Res. 33: 454–458.

Selvig, K. A., T. Hofstad, and T. Kristoffersen. 1971. Electron microscopic demonstration of bacterial lipopolysaccharides in dental plaque matrix. Scand. J. Dent. Res. 79: 409–421.

Slanetz, L. W., and L. F. Rettger. 1933. A systematic study of the fusiform bacteria. J. Bacteriol. 26: 599–622.

Smith, L. D. S., and L. V. Holdeman. 1968. The pathogenic anaerobic bacteria. Charles C Thomas, Springfield Ill.

Snyder, F., and N. Stephens. 1959. A simplified spectrophometric determination of ester groups in lipids. Biochim. Biophys. Acta 34: 244–245.

Socransky, S. S., R. J. Gibbons, A. C. Dale, L. Bortnick, E. Rosenthal, and J. B. Macdonald. 1963. The microbiota of the gingival crevice area of man. I. Total microscopic and viable counts, and counts of specific organisms. Arch. Oral Biol. 8: 275–280.

Spaulding, E. H., and L. F. Rettger. 1937. The *Fusobacterium* genus. I. Biochemical and serological classification. J. Bacteriol. 34: 535–548.

Staub, A.-M. 1954. Role des anticorps antipolyosidiques dans l'agglutination des bacilles typhiques. Ann. Inst. Pasteur 86: 618–635.

Takagi, A., and K. Nuyama, 1963. Characteristic cell wall structure of a *Fusobacterium*. Jap. J. Microbiol. 7: 43.

Theilade, E., W. H. Wright, S. B. Jensen, and H. Löe. 1966. Experimental gingivitis in man. II. A longitudinal clinical and bacteriological investigation. J. Periodont. Res. 1: 1–13.

Ueda, M., and A. Takagi. 1965. Surface pattern of *Fusobacterium polymorphum*. Jap. J. Microbiol. 9: 145–148.

Varney, P. L. 1927. The serological classification of fusiform bacilli. J. Bacteriol. 13: 275–314.

Weiss, C., and D. G. Mercado. 1938. Demonstration of type specific proteins in extracts of fusobacteria. J. Exp. Med. 67: 49–59.

Weissbach, A. and J. Hurwitz. 1959. The formation of 2-keto-3-deoxyheptonic acid in extracts of *Escherichia coli B*. I. Identification. J. Biol. Chem. 234: 705–709.

Werner, H. 1968. Die Gramnegativen anaeroben sporenlosen Stäbchen des Menschen. Infektionskrankheiten und ihre Erreger, 9: Gustav Fischer, Jena.

Werner, H. 1970. Glutaminsaüredecarboxylaseaktivität bei *Bacteroides*-arten. Zbl. Bakt. I. Abt. Orig. 215: 321–326.

Westphal, O., O. Lüderitz, and F. Bister. 1952. Über die Extraktion von Bakterien mit Phenol/Wasser. Z. Naturforsch. 7, B: 148–155.

Yoshida, A., C.-G. Heden, B. Cedergren, and L. Edebo. 1961. A method for the preparation of undigested bacterial cell walls. J. Biochem. Microbiol. Technol. Eng. 3: 151–159.

Author's address: Dr. T. Kristoffersen, University of Bergen, School of Dentistry, Aistadvei 17, 5000 Bergen (Norway).

Index

Adsorption, nonselective, 75
Analysis, immunological distribution,
    41–90
    multicompartment, 55
    nonselective, 76
    sequential adsorption, 72–83
Antibody
    antitumor, 51
    enzyme labeled, 217
    ferritin labeled, 201
    iodination, 228
    labeling, 186–233
Antigen
    localization, 186–233
    microbial, 204–226
    parasitic, 204
    tagging with antibodies, 218
Antitumor antibodies, 51
Enzyme-labeled antibodies, 217–226
Ferritin, 187
    labeled antibodies, 195, 201–208
    labeling with, 189
    staining with, 197
Ferrocene, 229
Fusobacteria, immunochemistry,
    253–284
    antigens, 260–278
    cell wall antigens, 260
    cell wall composition, 256
    lipopolysaccharides, 261
    ultrastructure, 259
Immunoenzyme technique, 208–233
    applications, 222
    coupling reagents, 209
    enzymes, 209
    principle, 208
    procedures, 209
    staining methods, 218
Immunoferritin technique, 187–208
    applications, 201
    assays, 195
    conjugation procedures, 191

coupling agents, 189
hybrid-antibody method, 200
specificity control, 201
Immunoglobulin A, immunochemis-
    try, 93–106
affinity, 158
α-chains, 120
biological properties, 141–160
carbohydrate composition, 118
chemical properties, 116–141
constitutive polypeptide chains,
    116–139
determinants, 128
electron microscopy, 113
electrophoretic mobility, 109–111
half life, 150
identification, 94
immunological assays, 157
immunological cross reactions,
    108
J-chains, 134
light chains, 117
in man, 141
model, 117
molecular size, 112, 114
molecular weight, 126
in nonhuman vertebrates, 94–106
physiology, 107–116
proteolytic fragmentation, 139
reduction, 131, 139
in rodents, 134
in ruminants, 130, 153
secretary component, 109, 125
serum concentration, 141
synthesis, 150
units, 113
valence, 158
Immuno-osmium technique, 232
Immuno-uranium technique, 230,
    232
Immunozoning *in vitro*, 66
Immunozoning *in vivo*, 70

Iodine-conjugated antibodies, 228
Lipopolysaccharides
    in bacteria, 23–28
    side chains, 18–20
Mercury-conjugated antibodies, 229
Osmium-conjugated antibodies, 230
Polysaccharides, 1–40
    capsular, 3
    constituents, 6
    C-polysaccharide, 3
    of *Enterobacteriaceae,* 19
    immunodominant groups, 12
    of *Klebsiella,* 22
    meningococcal, 18
    mycobacterial, 27

periodate-oxidized, 2
pneumococcal, 2–11
of *Salmonella,* 17
Radioantibody
    adsorption, 56
    distribution analysis, 48–88
    kinetics, 82
    localization *in vivo,* 82
    negative localization, 87
    stability, 85
Radioglobulin compartmentalization,
    51
Specificity parameters, 44
Uranium-conjugated antibodies, 230